FASD Relationships

What I have learned about Fetal Alcohol Spectrum Disorder

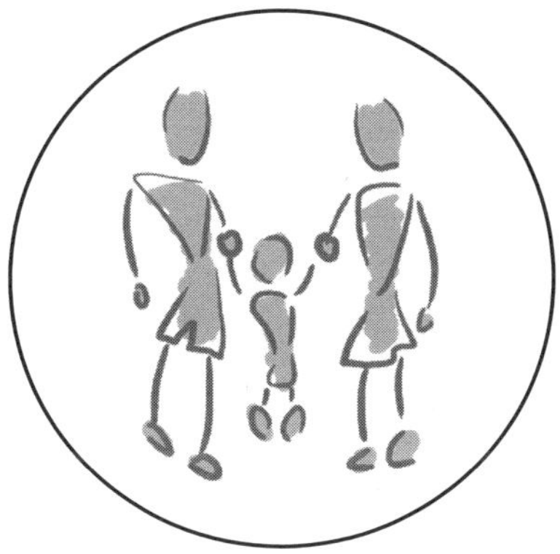

Rod Densmore, M.D., Father of a young adult who has FAS

Cover and graphic design by Julia Densmore

Production Services: Mareike Klem, The Urban Think Tank
Printer: Friesens Corporation, Altona, MB, Canada.

Published by Dory Spirit Books Ltd.
P.O. Box 10006
Salmon Arm, British Columbia, Canada V1E 3B9

Printed in Canada

Densmore, Roderick J.
FASD Relationships: What I have learned about Fetal Alcohol Spectrum Disorder
Illustrations by Julia G. Densmore
Includes bibliographical references and index.

ISBN 978-0-9813818-0-0

1. Fetal Alcohol Spectrum Disorder 2. Developmental Disabilities. 3. Human Attachment

With sincere thanks, the author acknowledges these permissions:

The images of the Lip-Philtrum guides reproduced on page 214 and in the DVD lecture, "Neurobiology of FASD for Health Professionals" appeared on page 30 in the 2004 Diagnostic Guide for Fetal Alcohol Spectrum Disorders: The 4-Digit Diagnostic Code, Third Edition published by Center on Human Development and Disability and are included with permission from Dr. Susan Astley, Director, Washington State FAS Diagnostic and Prevention Network, Center on Human Development and Disability School of Public Health and Community Medicine, University of Washington, Seattle, Washington, USA, 98195

The diffusion tensor MRI image reproduced on the cover and several DVD lectures was generated by the diffusion tensor MRI group at the University of Alberta and provided to me for this book by Catherine Lebel and Dr. Christian Beaulieu, Department of Biomedical Engineering, Faculty of Medicine and Dentistry, University of Alberta, Research Transition Facility, Room 1098, Edmonton, Alberta, Canada, T6G 2V2

The lyrics for the song "Lay Your Hands" by Cary Landry, reproduced on page 283, appeared in the album, "Abba Father" and are included with permission from NALR, 5536 NE Hassalo, Portland, Oregon, USA, 97213

The song "This is Worth Fighting For" by Greg Sczebel, reproduced on the DVD Interview with Myles Himmelreich, appears in Greg's 2009 album, "Love and The Lack Thereof" produced by Soultone Records and is included with permission of Jerry Sczebel, Manager of Greg Sczebel Music

The text and graphics around the Getty Image of three friends, reproduced on pages 122 and 201 and in the DVD Genetics and FASD lectures appears on the National Institute on Alcohol Abuse and Alcoholism website and is included with permission of Maureen B. Gardiner, Technical Writer/ Editor

The image "sb100613275-001 (RF) Three friends having meal in restaurant, smiling," reproduced on pages 122 and 201 and in the DVD Genetics and FASD lectures, photographed by Dream Pictures is available through Getty Images Website Collection: Digital Vision and is included with permission of Getty Images

Quotes and content from Dr. Gordon Neufeld's "Vital Connection" (attachment-parenting) DVD series, reproduced on pages 225-282, appear in Dr. Neufeld's 2010 release of Power to Parent, Part One, The Vital Connection, Second Edition DVD Series, produced by The Neufeld Institute, 2155 West 36th Avenue, Vancouver, BC, Canada, V6M 1L and are included with permission of Dr. Neufeld who generously stated to me, "Just be sure to make it clear what's yours and what's mine."

Dedication

I don't know what condition affected Gene, my grade two classmate. In 2011, I can imagine Gene might be diagnosed with asperger disorder but in 1964 I doubt he was diagnosed with anything other than being a bit slow. He took longer to learn new things; he struggled. What I remember was his lunch. He always had the most interesting sandwich and nicest cookies. We were all jealous. Gene got as dirty as the rest of us, mucking around in puddles, dusty baseball diamonds and muddy soccer fields—but every morning he would show up to class immaculate with a nice fresh shirt and clean *pressed* jeans. Even to me, his eight year-old classmate, Gene made an impression—wow! His mum sure loved him and looked after him. Some classmates teased or even bullied him but Gene didn't seem to be bothered much by his learning difficulties or taunting. Now, I can see Gene's mum's love and care might well have helped him overcome ostracism.

I was fortunate to grow up surrounded by thoughtful, nurturing adults. These folks share Gene's Mum's vision:

My (adoptive) mum and dad, Chris and Jim Densmore—both, the epitome of supportive, unconditional love

My parents' wonderful child-care network including Roger and Joan Williams, "Gramma" Lindsay, Margaret and Hugh Clarke

My courageous birth mum, Margaret

Lillis Bremnes, my child's superb youth group leader who figured out how to be validating but not a "pushover"

My wife, Shannon, who has an enormous heart and passion for kids

And Shannon's amazing Aunt Shirley and Uncle Garth Waines

This book is dedicated to Gene's mum and the individuals listed above that, like her, get up each morning dedicating themselves to improving the lives of children in their care. Their selflessness and heart for kids makes our world a much better place.

Contents

Introduction

The brain has many different cell types and they mediate a huge number of functions. The brain allows us to love, laugh, walk, talk, sleep, wake-up, hate and interact with each other in productive relationships. At its core, the brain allows us to sense our environment, process these sensations, share perspectives, perceive others' perspectives and act. Even with all this complexity, there is actually, in some ways, a very simple list of three tasks that the brain allows us to do:

1) Promote survival of our groups.

2) Procreate.

3) Protect dependants.

Even these basic functions—survival, procreation and protection of dependants—are subsets of a bigger "domain." All require the capacity to form and maintain relationships. All depend on our ability to interact with and respond to other people. [1]

FASD Relationships: What I have learned about Fetal Alcohol Spectrum Disorders is about how caring adults, siblings and professionals can help people with FASD transcend their disabilities. Love is not enough. Burnout and emotional exhaustion are unwelcome but frequent companions on the journey of parenting those with FASD.

The book explains:

» What brain differences—both strengths and difficulties—affect kids who have FASD

» Do not take (disability-caused) behavioural problems personally

» Dream big and maintain hope about your child. Yes, they need accommodations for their disabilities—but neuroplasticity (new nerve growth) allows everyone's brain to change and grow (yours too!)

» The value of maintaining and strengthening relationships with your children

» Ways to stay attached when kids resist connection

» That caregivers and the professionals who work with our children have finite energy and resources…which strategies are most likely to be effective and where anticipatable pitfalls are.

A core message of this book—understand body and brain differences caused by prenatal alcohol exposure so you can respond more effectively—is the same for parents, persons with FASD or professionals caring for patients, clients or students with FASD. Each group, however, uses different language. Thus, some parts of the book are designed for professionals familiar with medical/psychological language and some are for a general audience.

More difficult interactions such as discipline or redirection might have a chance of success if they occur in the setting of a caring relationship. On the other hand, even constructive criticism, when delivered outside the context of a nurturing attachment is likely to meet with resistance. Caring relationships are the conduit through which any lessons, interventions, strategies, or corrections are delivered. Viable relationships are the key for children's success and caregivers' effectiveness and satisfaction. Regrettably, in FASD, fractured, strained relationships are everywhere.

Understanding where behaviour comes from can heal estrangement so this book probes recent brain science for answers to why children misbehave or act in strange or even alienating ways. Optimal ways to respond follow when caregivers and counselors know why certain behaviours happen. Sometimes a serious problem cannot be completely corrected, but if parents know they have done whatever is possible in the situation, they can at least hang on to some sense of effectiveness. Knowing they can be a positive force for their kids and that their efforts make a difference, gives caregivers a sense of self-efficacy. Self-efficacy, though often battered, is a life-blood for parents, counselors and other professionals who work with children; self-efficacy allows hope and makes it possible to persist despite setbacks.

This book is about real people—maybe your son, or nephew, or granddaughter. Maybe it describes you or your patient. Last week I saw a fellow in the clinic for a long term drinking problem. I started to review the Power Point: *Genetics and FASD for a General Audience* with him—he found the material to be relevant to his family's situation. A foster mother came in with her daughter—who is strongly attached to her birthfather. Dr. Neufeld's concepts of *Polarized attachment* broke an isolating impass for this family. A man molested as a child in Indian Residential School disclosed his abuse and PTSD symptoms—he found the PTSD module near the end of the *Our Brain* DVD lecture to be empowering.

A lady with FASD, let's call her Eva, recently released from jail, told me she missed playing her guitar while she was in custody. "That guitar keeps me sane," she explained. Eva was in jail because she fought with a policeman in the hospital emergency room. That was two weeks after she got evicted, tried living on the streets, had her guitar, music and backpack (with her organizer in it) ripped off, quit taking her meds, couldn't sleep because of danger (on the street) and nightmares (from her PTSD), ran out of money, got assaulted and would not wait patiently in Emergency when she needed stitches. Eva yelled a lot in jail. They put her in solitary confinement. That punishment *did not* settle her down. *Quelle surprise*! The music chapter and the sensory processing discussions in the book describe this lady—and offers ideas to help her. Authorities interacting with Eva violated just about every principle for constructive engagement of clients that Grace Gerry, Social Worker, describes in Chapter Six (*Stakeholders*).

Chapter One: *FASD 101: Fetal Alcohol Spectrum Disorder for a General Audience* is a book within a book. It is designed to provide everyone with a succinct update on common pitfalls concerning how children with FASD are approached, the nature of brain changes and ideas for how to work around difficulties. It discusses areas of strength, sensory processing difficulties and ideas to help, and problems with how FASD is diagnosed and classified. The chapter also explains how these issues might cause delays in diagnosis and effective management ideas from professionals. Chapter one concludes with information about what a child has inherited from his/her birth parents and strategies to help genetic traits not express themselves as what we now call Secondary disabilities.

FASD discussions often abound in gloom and doom. Negativity impairs our ability to make good choices and sabotages success. However, superficially pretending hard times don't exist is also unproductive. An admirable role model and inspiring young man who has lived through difficulties caused by FASD is Myles Himmelreich. Open to constructive advice from caring adults he works alongside, focusing efforts within his (many) areas of strength, Myles has been able to transcend turmoil, drugs and alcohol. Chapter Two: *Interview with Myles Himmelreich* consists of a detailed interview with Myles (on DVD) along with a study guide so viewers can note his strengths, difficulties and responses to my questions.

People learn best in various ways. Some prefer to read about a topic; for others, a lecture or viewing a DVD works best. Experiential learning is best of all. I have included a DVD with narrated Power Point presentations with the book. Copies of the lecture slides are provided in Chapter Three: *DVD Power Point Slides*. This entire book, and chapter three in particular, is about learners moving past knowing to understanding and using information. Many FASD conferences include fast-paced discussions with numerous slides; this hurried format seldom results in deep understanding. I encourage readers to use these narrated Power Point DVD lectures differently. Grab a coffee, stop and start the DVD as often as you like, and be unhurried but thorough about making notes on aspects of a topic that are directly relevant for you and the kids you care for. Lectures presented on the DVD for a general audience include:

1. Genetics and FASD for a General Audience
2. Sensory Processing and FASD
3. Neurobiology of FASD for a General Audience
4. Neurobiology of Attachment
5. Our Brain: a review of brain processes important for depression, posttraumatic stress disorder, addictions, and dementia

Health care professionals will find more detailed DVD lectures on:

6. Genetics and FASD for Health Professionals
7. Neurobiology of FASD for Health Professionals

Practical ideas on maintaining and even rebuilding vibrant relationships with children are well described by developmental psychologist, Gordon Neufeld, in his widely available DVD series, *The Vital Connection*. I have been trained in facilitation of Dr. Neufeld's video course and have found his material to be especially helpful for caregivers of children who have FASD. I developed Chapter Four of the book to describe *Relevant FASD brain biology differences to consider when viewing Dr. Gordon Neufeld's "Vital connection" attachment-parenting DVD series*. Dr. Neufeld's topics in this series are almost a "short list" of key concerns of caregivers:

» Becoming and staying attached

» Harnessing the power of attachment

» Competing attachments (such as to peers or the computer!)

» Preserving and restoring the ties that empower

» Handling aggression

» Handling counterwill

» Guidelines for discipline

Chapter Four will also include copies of material from a poster entitled *Restoring Hope: An Adapted Attachment-parenting DVD Series Empowers Caregivers of Children who have FASD* that I presented at the 2010 Fetal Alcohol Canadian Expertise (FACE) meeting.

Chapter Five is *Music and FASD*. Music can be fun, engaging and very helpful for children and adults with FASD. Though not a musicologist or music therapist, I have been an active musician for over forty years and have taken musical training through to the third year level of a Bachelor of Fine Arts in Music. So, from the perspective of an educated layperson, this short chapter offers a look at how music can help FASD. I have been absolutely fascinated by the power of music to:

» allow access to and allow expression of emotions

» help resolve turmoil, and

» access the feelings encountered in intense situations such as yearning or grief that can sometimes be very difficult to describe using words.

Very diverse groups of people from the wider community have keen interest in people affected by FASD. A foster and adoptive parent, sibling, developmental paediatrician, primary care physician, medical office receptionist, music therapist, occupational therapist, educator, residential care coordinator for developmentally disabled adults, social worker/assessment clinic coordinator, parent educator, and family respite coordinators all share their perspectives about FASD in Chapter Six: *Insights from FASD Stakeholders*.

At the root of relationships are human affiliative systems such as the mirror neuron system and the oxytocin receptor system. Chapter Seven: *Interpersonal Affiliation Systems and FASD* reviews how such systems might be changed in FASD and how caregivers can respond. I know that this pioneering science, advancing daily, so insights of today, 2011, might seem backward in a few years. Despite this, I hope readers might be "infected" with a little of the enthusiasm I have for the work described in this chapter—and Chapter Eight. I suspect within ten years affiliative system science and genetics/epigenetics will transform mental health care and the FASD field.

Chapter Eight: *Genetics and FASD: Heritability information gives us a deeper perspective on "Secondary Disabilities"* offers health care professionals a review of relevant genetics that expands on ideas presented in their Genetics and FASD Power Point. Chapter eight aims to offer a 2011 answer to the question, "What did this child I am caring for inherit from his/her birthparents and what ought I to do about it?" Genetics and epigenetics are fast moving sciences and I know this material is—to some degree—dated before it is even published. Nevertheless, I hope the genetics material in this book can serve as a helpful introduction to the field.

The book concludes with Chapter Nine: *Terminology, diagnosis, epidemiology and pathogenesis of Fetal Alcohol Spectrum Disorder (FASD) for health professionals*. This material is designed to be a resource for health professionals to consult when they need a concise well-referenced summary of FASD.

Rod Densmore, January 25, 2011

[1] Perry B. 2010. Understanding the impact of trauma and neglect in the developing child; clinical implications and applications of neurodevelopmentally-informed treatment strategies. (Conference presentation) New Westminister, BC, Canada. Justice Institute of BC. June 2nd and 3rd, 2010.

How to use this book

Chapters can be considered a series of modules about FASD. Although they build on one another, for the most part, each chapter can stand alone. This means readers can start anywhere they'd like. Some chapters display a small amount of redundancy and overlap, for example, results of the attachment-parenting educational initiative are described in both chapters one and four, and power point slides describing subtypes of sensory processing disorder are shown in several of the power point lectures.

Chapters one, two, (most of) three, four, five, and six are written in language accessible to a general audience. Chapters seven, eight, nine and two of the lectures from chapter three are designed as references and possible curriculae for health professional training.

My main aim with this book is to add a practical, well referenced, accessible, engaging, and inexpensive teaching tool to existing resources. If parents and professionals that work with our kids can glean a few new ideas and feel equipped and empowered by this book, my goal will be met.

Request for feedback

This is the book's first printing. My editor suggested references be provided in the (Densmore, 2011) format—so I did this in Chapter One: *FASD 101: Fetal Alcohol Spectrum Disorder for a General Audience*. However, I think this format can get intrusive, especially when there are numerous references such as in Chapter Nine: *Terminology, diagnosis, epidemiology and pathogenesis of Fetal Alcohol Spectrum Disorder (FASD) for health professionals.* Thus, I decided to use numbers such as [2] to mark references in chapters two through nine. I am hoping readers will let me know which method they find easiest to use so I can adjust future printings accordingly.

Every effort possible has been taken to ensure accuracy. Nevertheless, human and mechanical errors occur. I appreciate suggestions from readers about any corrections they think ought to be made.

Feedback could be sent to:

FASD Relationships,

PO Box 10006

Salmon Arm, BC, Canada V1E 3B9

Chapter One

FASD 101: Fetal Alcohol Spectrum Disorder For A General Audience

1) Introduction

I am Dr. Rod Densmore, a primary care physician. Welcome to my world! Thank you for your interest in FASD. Our family adopted a child who has Fetal Alcohol Syndrome fifteen years ago and we've been students of this condition ever since. I have a passion for understanding the underlying brain mechanisms of behaviour - but always with a view to how this knowledge can be applied in practical ways for my family members and patients. *FASD Relationships: What I Have Learned About Fetal Alcohol Spectrum Disorder* summarizes my experiences thus far.

Fetal Alcohol Spectrum Disorder (FASD) is an umbrella term describing the various patterns of how prenatal alcohol can affect people. FASD is caused by consumption of alcohol during pregnancy. Physical, learning, social and behavioural effects of prenatal exposure to alcohol last a lifetime. People affected by FASD can be helped. The brain, although permanently changed by prenatal exposure to alcohol and adverse early life events, can regenerate. I am more optimistic about my child's future now than at any point in the last fifteen years. This book puts forward suggestions and strategies that have worked for families, other caregivers and professionals. There is hope.

The disorders covered by the term FASD are Fetal Alcohol Syndrome (FAS), which includes facial changes, growth deficiency, brain changes affecting thought, social and adaptive functions and a history of maternal intake of alcohol; Partial Fetal Alcohol Syndrome (PFAS), which includes brain changes, proven maternal alcohol intake and lesser degrees of facial and growth changes; Alcohol-related Neurodevelopmental Disorder (ARND), which includes brain changes and confirmed maternal alcohol intake, but even lesser degrees of growth or facial abnormalities; and Alcohol-related Birth Defects (ARBD), which describes body changes due to prenatal alcohol exposure, often including kidney problems, heart murmurs or heart septum problems, bone issues including small 5th fingers and toes, visual focus and eye movement problems, dental problems, and hearing impairment.

FASD is common - although many estimates suggest a prevalence of about one per cent, some recent school studies suggest that three or four percent of the students *whose parents consented* to testing have FASD. Conjecture? - Yes - but isn't it likely that the *fifty percent* of kids whose parent chose *not* to allow testing have an even higher likelihood of FASD? Furthermore, in specific populations - special education classes, homeless individuals, those in prison, children in foster care - the rate is even higher. To make progress tackling drug abuse, alcoholism, repeat criminal offences, homelessness, learning disorders, foster or adoptive parent burnout, child abuse and neglect - some of society's most costly and heart wrenching issues - caregivers and policy makers must understand FASD.

But most people with FASD look "normal". Sadly, people with F A S D are Frequently Abused and Seldom Diagnosed. This book's primary aim is to help inform and equip caregivers, policy makers and the professionals who work with our kids. Better prepared, with a few handy tools and strategies at our disposal, maybe we can help F A S D stand for Myles Himmelreich's guiding values and aspirations: "Faith, Ability, Strength and Determination." These values have helped Myles, whose interview with me is streamed on the fasdrelationships.ca website and included in the DVD enclosed with this book, transcend some of FASD's limitations - and these values are something we can all aspire to.

Please do not use the term "FASD kid." I ask this, in part, to spare you the wrath of my friend and colleague, Jan Lutke, who has correctly pointed out that the suitable title is "a child who has FASD," and in part because the latter is more accurate and respectful.

Unlike Hollywood movies, the illustrations I use *are* real stories from my kids, my patients, and myself. They are not "adaptations of" or "based on" real stories. I have changed only irrelevant details in order to respect patient confidentiality.

Chemistry of FASD Relationships

Dan Dubovsky is a social worker and FASD expert for the Substance Abuse and Mental Health Services Administration (SAMHSA) in Maryland, USA. Dan is also an adoptive parent of Bill, a young man with FASD who was tragically killed in a car accident several years ago. Dan has created the acronym NURMU (noncompliant, uncooperative, resistant, manipulative, unmotivated) to describe *how our kids are often viewed* by adults that work with them (including, I am ashamed to say, parents and physicians like me!)

I will add a rather cheeky acronym, PTHD (PMS, tired, hungry, depleted), which describes the *internal state of caregivers*, again including me! Before hissing at me for talking about premenstrual syndrome (PMS) in the first part of this book please be aware I have four daughters and a wife and have lived with them through a total of one hundred ten "girl-years" so, in-so-far as a guy can talk about PMS, I consider myself at least "experienced". Besides, I think men can fulfill diagnostic criteria for PMS too; my symptoms usually appear after being "on call" for a weekend (Post too Much work Syndrome) and after meetings with particularly odious colleagues (Post Meeting Syndrome.)

If the catalyst of righteous indignation (e.g. "I've told him a hundred times not to sneak money from my wallet! - and he is 15! I should not have to keep a lock on the bedroom door at his age!") is added to the toxic duo (of seeing kids as NURMU and being in a state of PTHD) then the inevitable result is what our kids will view as an attack. This attack could be as innocent as a sigh of frustration or a look of exasperation. Caregivers are often certain that they are not angry. (But subjective self-assessment of how angry you are is spectacularly inaccurate!) Kids who have FASD, despite being less responsive in many areas, often have hyper-responsive "criticism detectors" (not unlike their parents - again I am guilty!), so productive social exchanges and civility can be quickly lost in an interpersonal cycle of perceived rejection, negativity and detachment following what caregivers view as legitimate correction, redirection or discipline. If parents' or teachers' corrective efforts are not received, then their goal (to help kids not repeat similar mistakes) *cannot* be accomplished. Getting angrier will *certainly not* help kids see the light. Curiosity can re-direct this angry response - "*why ever* did that kid snitch the i-Pod?"

Dr. Ron Minon, a psychiatrist from Denver who has spent years developing therapeutic listening systems for kids who have handicaps, suggested we call this dynamic the "replacement of righteous indignation with insatiable curiosity." In the melodramatic tradition of psychologist, John Gottman, who calls his four most important "relationship busters" (criticism of character, contempt, defensiveness and stonewalling) "The Four Horsemen of the Apocalypse," I propose we take Dr. Minon's ideas a step further: *Parents and all who work with children who have FASD must replace righteous indignation with insatiable curiosity - or perish!*

I do not know of a more potent force than insatiable curiosity to maintain attachments and preserve relationships with those affected by FASD. Yet this curiosity, this life-blood of maintaining relationships, can seem a distant mirage to depleted mums and dads who are weary from lack of sleep, emotionally exhausted and feeling that they have absolutely nothing more to give. I've been there. However, because of their disability, many people with FASD depend *even more than the rest of us* on supportive, secure relationships with caring adults to help their development and maintain optimal functioning in the world. Creating and maintaining these relationships must be a main priority of all those who work with people (of all ages) who have FASD. *Only* through the communication channel that comes from a vital, caring relationship can a caregiver have any hope of being able to influence and help a child with FASD.

Simulation - one way non-affected people can understand FASD

Myles Himmelreich's vivid descriptions of personal struggles and problems as a child and teen can give the rest of us a glimpse of what it feels like to have FASD. I suggest readers start their foray into FASD by watching the interview with Myles which is found in this book's accompanying DVD or on the fasdrelationships.ca website. Myles and I have found simulations help others to get a clearer picture of what FASD is. What follows is a description of how I present a simulation. You, the reader, might find it more realistic if I phrase it in the first person. In your imagination, be a student in grade 6 again!

Chemistry of FASD Relationships: Figure 1.

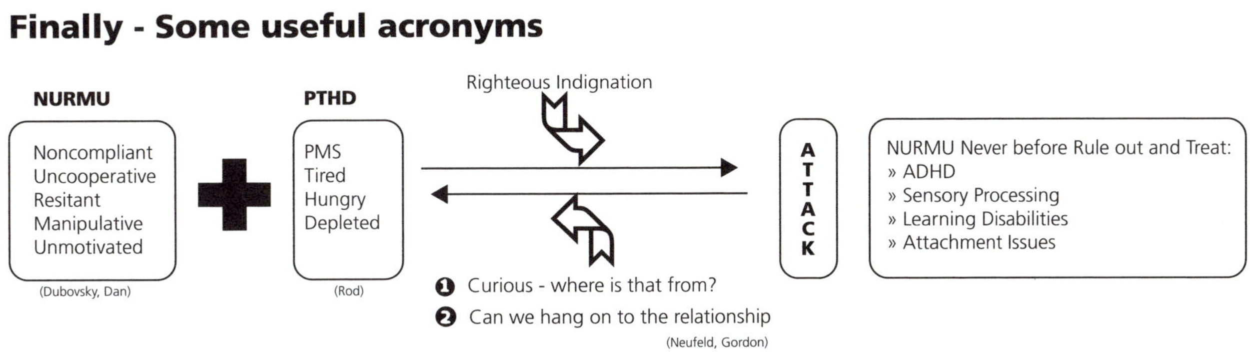

Figure 1. notes: If we view kids as NURMU, especially if we are a bit PTHD ourselves, and work ourselves up with righteous indignation, an all-too-common result is the child perceiving an attack and withdrawing from the relationship. Caregivers able to question, "where in heck did that behaviour come from?" or take the position "I have no idea what to do but I'll try to at least keep the connection open with my kid" can possibly avoid the destructive attack/withdrawal situation. Vibrant, effective relationships between caregivers and their children are the most important factor in optimal development for all children, according to psychologist Gordon Neufeld. Kids with undiagnosed and/or untreated ADHD, FASD, sensory processing difficulties, learning disorders, attachment issues, abuse, or posttraumatic stress disorder (PTSD) might look like they are NURMU, but NURMU will disappear with correct diagnosis and appropriate interventions.

Barry Fawcett, my daughter's Grade 6 teacher, initially suggested I develop this simulation for FASD. I usually do a lecture right out of my daughter's Grade 6 Social Studies textbook, describing early missionaries to Canada. The lecture lasts 3 minutes and is followed by a test on content. I attempt to simulate FASD for all students in the class.

Children with FASD often are easily distracted. Imagine that the little boy behind you whispering to his neighbour was as loud to your ears as the teacher's voice. (I ask two or three people to talk loudly to the "classmates" next to them.) Imagine that the irritation from the label in your shirt or your itchy new socks was so distracting that you could not concentrate on the lecture. (I ask "students" to sit on their car keys or a tennis ball...something to make them feel *really* uncomfortable and distracted.) Imagine that the ventilation fan was a loud, obnoxious buzz. (I have an awful, old, rattly fan that I turn on.) Imagine that your processing speed could not possibly keep up to the speed of the lecture. (I deliver the lecture *very* quickly and leave out a few random words.) Seizures, sometimes quite subtle but troublesome enough to cause students to miss parts of a lecture, are common. (I intentionally leave out parts of the lecture.) Learning of facts (via circuits involving the hippocampus) and learning of procedures (via circuits involving the cerebellum) can often be impaired. Most academic skills (such as how to print an "s" or how to spell the word "cat") are actually learned in the muscle-memory procedural circuits. (To simulate impaired automatic functioning in procedural circuits I ask students to write their exam using their wrong hand.)

Before the pandemonium begins I usually ask some pleasant earnest-looking person if she or he would not mind participating in a bit of theatre after the lecture and test - just to help illustrate a point. Almost everyone agrees - let's call that person you, the reader, in this simulation. The lecture is then delivered at break-neck speed amidst all the distractions. Then class members attempt to answer a brief quiz on the contents of the lecture. Few get more than two or three correct answers out of a possible ten "What did you get?" "Two out of ten teacher," you'd likely say. Then comes the key point: *"Did you even try?"* I ask. "I just looked at your test results from the psychologist...you are a smart boy...I don't understand why you only got two correct answers!" Then I list off some rather unhelpful things that kids who have FASD have told me were said to them: "I think you are a daydreamer. I wish your brain was here as well as your body; when it is time to come to class *all* of you needs to show up. I wish you'd put more effort into this. Why did you not study? You are going to need to pull your socks up or you will fail. If you would sit up and pay more attention instead of choosing to watch the cars out the window and squirm around you might achieve more."

Despite knowing that the simulation is theatre, most actors who play the humiliated child feel dreadful - some have cried. How about you? Everyone comes to understand the distressing reality: students with FASD often fail *even though they try very hard - and often they are labeled or criticized as not trying or not performing up their potential, or NURMU* as Dan Dubovsky suggests.

Functional MRI (fMRI) neuroimaging studies (Malisza, 2005) have compared patterns of brain activation required to do simple tasks in kids who are affected by FASD to brain activation in control subjects. "N minus one" tasks ask a study participant to look at a panel of four lights and indicate which was lit up *the previous time* they were flashed. Minimal levels of brain activation were required for most control subjects to do the N minus one task, but children who had been exposed to alcohol prenatally showed *significant* activation of *many* brain areas - in other words, they had to work much harder to accomplish this simple task. "N minus two" tasks ask that participants identify the pattern of lights that were lit up not the last time but the second last time they flashed. Most control study participants were successful at completing N minus two and showed more brain activation while completing this more complex task, but those with prenatal alcohol exposure showed *less* brain activation and very few succeeded in this more challenging task. They were overwhelmed and gave up. I don't blame them! Trying harder won't "fix" brain damage.

If we keep these fMRI findings in mind when considering the end of a very taxing day at school we could understand that "I don't want to do homework" might mean "my brain is maxed out - it has been all day - and I need to do some non-brain stuff now to recoup some mental energy." Bouncing on a trampoline, strumming a guitar, or playing a game of foosball with Dad 'til the angst and tension of being on edge all day abates are all winning strategies. If the child was older, had been developing normally and then became disabled by a head injury, she or he might be able to tell us, "I used to be able to sit down and concentrate for an hour after school to do homework but now, since the injury, even if you bribed me with a million dollars to sit still for ten minutes *I can't*. Let me run around for a while and listen to my music and then I will try homework in half an hour." This kind of self-awareness that can lead to self-advocacy is difficult for kids born with disabilities, including FASD, because they cannot compare how they feel and act now to something different previously; they have *always been the way they are*.

Questions, Answers and Comments regarding the simulation

Question: How did it feel to be singled out/ shamed in front of your classmates?

Usual Answer: Alienating, distressing, vulnerable and alone.

Comment: Have a heart. Kids' struggles are profound. See the dignity in their struggle.

Question: What is the result of dealing with this degree of put-down and *invalidation* over and over?

Usual Answer: Destroys motivation, willingness to learn and willingness to be vulnerable and open.

Comment: *Don't corner, don't give up on the kids; encourage them.* When you are tired (or PTHD), get someone else to take over or you might "attack," which you will regret later. When stressed, we all become very thin-skinned, easily wounded by even subtle put-downs such as a sigh, frown or exasperated look. Try to create a no-lose situation in which the kids know they will not be embarrassed in front of classmates because they know they will be respectfully coached into giving the right answer. (e.g. figure 2, page 10.)

The "cost" of judgmental disapproval

According to psychologist Daniel Goleman in his 2006 book, *Social Intelligence*, criticism, especially if delivered in a shaming and shunning manner pushes the buttons of our stress response system more strongly than any other toxic stressor. Our very self-worth, sense of social value and status are threatened; rejection shakes our core. Bullies that engage in publically humiliating others can turn their victims into "frozen" speechless "bundles of nerves" by nasty hostile criticism. (Goleman, 2006) The quaking, mortified victim probably finds it impossible to intelligently respond or rebut the attack because they are literally immobilized by stress chemicals such as cortisol and adrenaline. Stress chemicals even highjack victim's abilities to process and understand the meaning of words; more primal needs for safety become paramount so their brain's resources shift from verbal processing and problem solving to worried, tense surveillance of the environment in an attempt to circumvent further attack. (Perry, 2010) Those with FASD have an over-reactive stress response system so move to this immobilized, guarded, defensive state quicker than their peers. (Weinberg, 2007) Clearly, shaming, hostile criticism and rejection sabotage learning or constructive exchange and must be completely removed from the classroom, the family home and the workplace. Those using their strength or power to ostracize, insisting that weaker people "need to be taught a lesson" spurn recent science of the stress response system and must be reigned in. Readers that believe I am overstating the destruction caused by harsh judgment should review the references cited above.

Rant Number One: Diagnostic Discrimination

One of the primary purposes of this book is to teach, and nothing helps me sit up and take notice *and remember* better than a good rant. Here in Canada we are blessed with Rex Murphy and Rick Mercer, ranters extraordinaire. I do not possess the razor-sharp wit of either of my rant heroes, but I am full of passion about what I see as some injustices within the FASD system that have hurt my kid - after all, I am a dad. So, with apologies to Rex and Rick I offer these fledgling attempts by a "ranter-in-training:"

I am irritated by lack of widespread acceptance of FASD in standard medical diagnostic manuals - this situation is inconsistent with both good science and basic principles of fairness. Because not all children with FASD present *identical* symptoms, it has been hard to convince bodies such as the committee overseeing the DSM (the psychiatric Diagnostic and Statistical Manual) to include FASD in their list of "legitimate" diagnoses. "Too many different clinical presentations, too much variability of the symptom patterns, too many genes, too complex to be a workable diagnosis" are the tired old mantras that have excluded FASD from mainstream statistical manuals in the past. All I can say is, "Yeah, yeah - why is there one set of rules for Major Depression and Autism Spectrum Disorder and a much-harder-to-satisfy set of rules for FASD?" Patients with either depression or autism *seldom present identical patterns of symptoms. Many genes* contribute to the risk of developing depression or autism, yet both conditions are included in diagnostic manuals. Insurance companies and even some government support programmes insist that patients meet diagnostic criteria for certain DSM diagnostic categories before they can receive benefits or be granted access to certain therapy programmes.

One might think, with legal considerations, and eligibility for insurance and government services dependent on a DSM diagnosis, that there is *a great deal of scientific validity* justifying DSM diagnostic categories. However, I don't think psychiatry is that sophisticated yet - I wish it were. Let's look at Dr. Bruce Perry's (Perry, 2010) perspective:

The problem with the DSM diagnostic system is that these lists of symptoms (that fit criteria for Oppositional Defiant Disorder [ODD], Attention Deficit Hyperactivity Disorder [ADHD] and so on) aren't really clearly connected to a (cont'd pg 12)

Non-Shaming Solutions

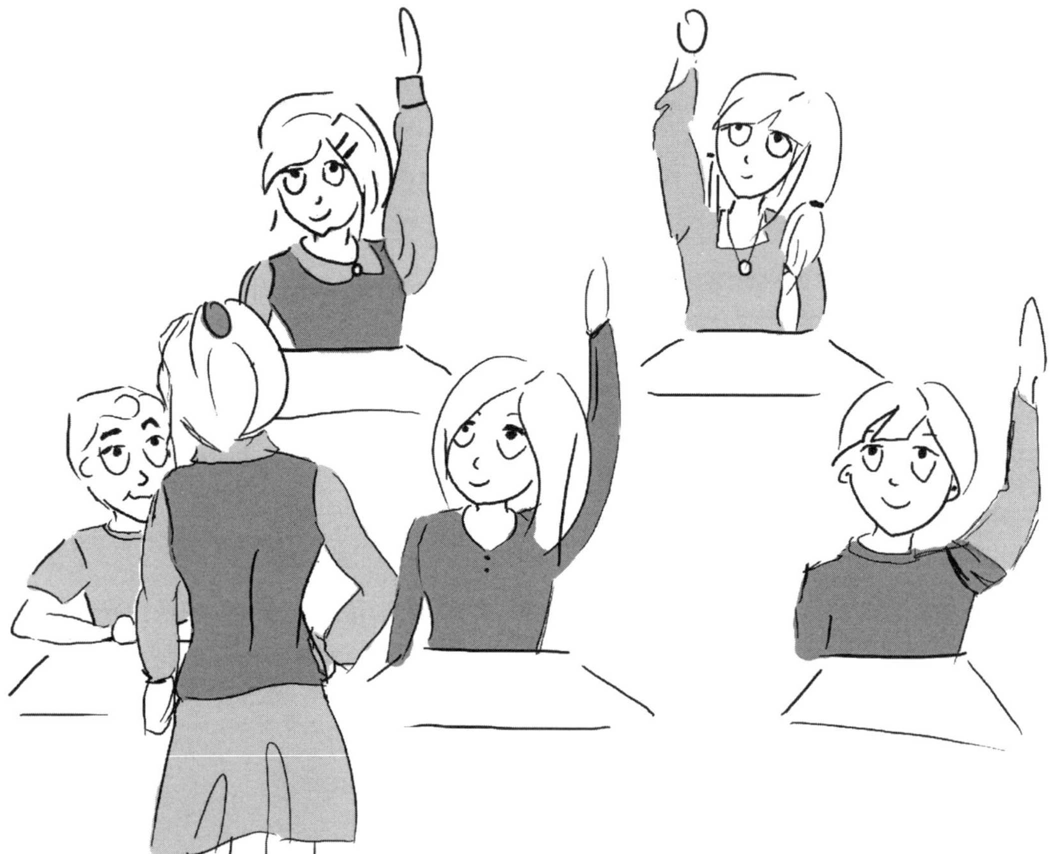

Non-Shaming Solutions: Figure 2.

Figure 2. Notes: The boy on the left now has his turn to answer teacher's question. He is a slow language processor. He was processing question one while classmates were already on question four. This very astute teacher has made some strategic secret deals with her student:

1. *I will only ask you the next question if I am standing right in front of your desk - so you'll need to try really hard to stay focused on the question I am asking you, but don't drive yourself silly trying to keep up with all the other (too-fast-for-you-to-be-able-to-process) questions.*
2. *If you need a bit of help to get the right answer that's okay - whatever it takes, I will coach you so you can get the answer if you try to participate.*

In other words: You can't lose; it is safe to put yourself out there and try to answer questions; you'll never be embarrassed in front of your class. This grade seven student (who had wanted to quit school) actually enjoyed his classes for the first time thanks to these strategies. Don't you wish your child could be in this teacher's class?

Question: *When the student becomes upset, what happens to his ability to answer questions?*

Answer: *Memory and learning, already impaired for kids who have FASD, are profoundly affected by stress. (To be precise, memory and learning are sabotaged and derailed by stress.)*

Comment: *Don't corner or put down because these approaches just lead to negativity, withdrawal, resistance, and reluctance to participate.*

physiologic or pathological cause. In a way, psychiatry is at the "diagnosis-based-on-symptoms" point in its evolution. A hundred years ago, doctors might have diagnosed a patient as having "fever." That is a symptom the patient had. Now, we wouldn't use "fever" as a diagnosis. We would say the fever was caused by a urinary tract infection or pneumonia or some other specific diagnosis; knowing this diagnosis would lead to a more accurate treatment. Part of the problem with this situation is that the brain is so complex. It consists of maybe a hundred billion neurons, many of which are very different cell types, and many many times that number of supportive glial cells and yet 90% of child psychiatry is four or five diagnoses such as ADHD, Bipolar Disorder, Anxiety Disorder, etc. Almost by definition, these diagnoses are in a similar category to the diagnosis of fever one hundred years ago. They are not precise enough to have an accurate pathophysiologic cause which can lead to a precise diagnosis and treatment plan.

In 2011, shamefully, there is still racial discrimination - but at least it has a bad name and is repugnant to most thinking people. Diagnostic discrimination (for example, against those affected by FASD) is disgusting too. In B.C. if your children are diagnosed with autism they might qualify for early childhood interventions - this is real money, enough to hopefully improve the trajectory of your child's development, maybe ten thousand dollars a year. Enough to do more than an assessment, of sensory needs for example; it is also enough to purchase equipment and pay for therapy. Scientific knowledge underpins this work: damaged nerve circuits can be reprogrammed by *an adequate "dose"* of therapy.

Let's be clear - the goal is not "covering up" damaged parts of the brain. The goal to grow new circuits and new connections between nerve cells to improve brain function is not a pipe dream. If skeptics visited Bruce D. Perry's Child Trauma Academy in Houston or Lucy Jane Miller's Sensory Processing Disorder (SPD) Foundation in Denver or read Norman Doige's book, *The Brain That Changes Itself* they would find their dubious position (that we cannot remodel circuits in damaged brains) simply untenable. If skeptics *chose not* to make themselves aware of the potential for the brain to grow new circuits that will help self-regulation, attention and function such people fit my definition of a menace: *Someone that does not know what they don't know - and wants to stay that way!* I used to be more tolerant of menaces - after all, how long can it be 'til that guy retires - but bad decisions can lead to the hopelessness that wrecks lives. Knowing the brain can remodel itself restores hope. We all need hope. A diagnosis that leads to effective treatments restores hope.

The day of harnessing the power of neuroplastic change (how nerves and brain circuits grow in response to a rich environment) is here *now*. Lasting improvements in function and objective testing are seen *if therapy is frequent enough*. For example, in Denver, lasting functional and Evoked Response Potential (ERP) improvements were seen in kids given thirty to forty 45-minute sessions of Multisensory Integration Treatment, usually at a frequency of three to five per week. (Brett-Green, 2008) "That much therapy might cost $4000!" bean counters shriek. Okay, bean counters - count *all* the beans - be sure to include money saved if the treatment helps kids stay in school, stay out of prison, avoid mental health problems and avoid the need to take Ritalin because their ability to self-regulate was improved.

Diagnoses not in the DSM are a bit off the radar of many practicing primary care doctors, psychiatrists, psychologists and their training institutions. At this point, new brain imaging tests like MRI and brain *function* tests like Evoked Response Potentials (ERP) are helping us link abnormal behaviours, thoughts, and emotions to their biological causes - specific areas of nerve cells that function abnormally. Can we diagnose, plan interventions and assess progress based on brain imaging (e.g. functional MRI) results? "Not yet," says PhD candidate Catherine Lebel in her presentation *Brain Imaging and Neurocognitive Functioning in Children and Twins with FASD.* (Lebel, 2010) Lebel explains that today, these advanced techniques are research tools - what is learned will guide future interventions but *very few clinics* use neuroimaging to diagnose and plan treatments at this point. (An exception is The Amen Clinic - unusual in that it dispenses medical advice based on current neuroimaging technology. See Clinical use of Neuroimaging Today, below.)

Perhaps DSM Advisory Groups would like to be able to have the neurobiology worked out for each diagnosis, but that will not happen before the DSM-5 comes out in May 2013. Current medical literature (Norman, et al., 2009), supports *neurobiological mechanisms underlying specific symptoms* at least as well for FASD as for depression or autism. Unrecognized and untreated, FASD can cause *severe impairments*; useful *preventive and therapeutic approaches* exist for treatment. FASD is *distinct* from related diagnoses and affects a large number of people. To be considered for inclusion in DSM a condition must be distinct from others, diagnosable, treatable and, ideally, linked to clear genetic and biological causes. I believe FASD meets these criteria as satisfactorily as other spectrum disorders such as Autism Spectrum Disorder. However, it is a complex condition, not easily recognized even by pediatricians. (Gahagan, et al., 2006) In September, 2010, I questioned residents from numerous psychiatric training programmes across Canada. All knew what the acronym FASD stood for; none knew details of how to diagnose or treat it and none had participated in thorough, didactic teaching sessions about the condition.

As of 2011, I know FASD will *not* be considered for the DSM-5, which is a shame because some jurisdictions will continue the unscientific practice of denying support due to lack of a DSM diagnosis. Maybe diagnostic systems from the Institute of Medicine, or the World Health Organization can do better. Fetal Alcohol Syndrome (FAS) (not FASD) *is being considered* for inclusion in DSM-5 as a "Condition Proposed by Outside Sources."

Being considered for inclusion in DSM-5 is a useful *first* step - if FAS is accepted - but I have two big concerns:

1. 85%+ of those affected with significant brain injury due to prenatal exposure to alcohol *do not* have the growth impairment and facial abnormalities that would fulfill criteria for an FAS diagnosis - to exclude this larger group from diagnosis is wrong because we have evidence that they have *a higher likelihood* of school failure, trouble with the law and other secondary disabilities than people who are diagnosed with FAS. (Streissguth AP, et al., 1996) Society recognizes small stature and facial anomalies and thus makes allowances for those with FAS. Those who look normal are expected to perceive, think and act normally; these are barriers that 85% of those with FASD share. Furthermore, the facial anomalies in FAS are often subtle and can be easily overlooked even by physicians so many patients, even those with all the symptoms of FAS, are not recognized.

2. Revisions of DSM are not frequent. Although it was revised in 2000, the

DSM-4 was published in 1994. The next revision (DSM-6) may not be published for another generation - in that case, thousands of people will miss out on a diagnosis that could grant them access them to services that may significantly improve their lives. If I knew society would fund FASD diagnosis and treatment strategies effectively without the badge of "legitimacy" that inclusion in the DSM affords, I would not care so much about this issue. Even if FAS were included in DSM-5, exclusion of other FASD disorders would be analogous to inclusion of Asperger's disorder *but exclusion of the other 75% of autism spectrum disorders* (ASD). Quite rightly, advocates for those with autism spectrum disorders would never let this happen. Children born with FASD have as many learning and health issues to contend with as those born with ASD, and deserve the same level of support for diagnosis and therapy.

Interested readers can add their perspectives to the DSM database on FAS by accessing the DSM website listed in the appendix.

Clinical use of Neuroimaging *Today*

The Amen Clinic plans treatment approaches based on currently available neuroimaging technology. Daniel Amen is an American psychiatrist and brain-imaging specialist; he serves as the Amen Clinic's medical director. The usual technique he uses to examine the brain is the Single Photon Emission Computed Tomography (SPECT) scan. He looks for SPECT findings that fit with clinical symptoms. For example: does already reduced function in the middle of the frontal lobes *get even worse* when a patient tries to concentrate? This pattern (on the SPECT scan) fits with the type of ADHD that often responds to stimulants such as methylphenidate (Ritalin) in Dr. Amen's experience.

Jay, an energetic young man I met 3 years ago, exemplifies another pattern Dr. Amen often sees on SPECT scans. Jay does not have FASD, but his experience is instructive. Despite using two alarm clocks, carrying a diary and really trying hard, Jay kept arriving late for work. Eventually his boss had to fire him from his minimum-wage job. Jay's self-described "ADHD from hell" resisted all types of treatment. Dexedrine and Ritalin made him feel "wired" and lose his creativity, Wellbutrin made him feel "wingy" and even more inattentive, and Strattera made him jittery and did not help to focus his attention. He became depressed. He tried Paxil, Celexa and

Prozac with no success. At about this time I took a plane to Toronto and learned that the pleasant East Indian lady sitting next to me was a pediatric psychiatrist. Her idea re Jay: "rule out temporal lobe epilepsy, maybe try a mood stabilizer medicine like Epival whether an electroencephalogram (EEG) shows seizure activity or not, and suspect an *undiagnosed Traumatic Brain Injury* (TBI)." Jay got a SPECT scan at the Amen Clinic which showed temporal lobe damage (from a head injury - "Oh yeah, I did fall off a log and bang my head. I 'lost' a day and I was dizzy for two weeks," he recalled. "Ever tell your mum?" "No, I wasn't supposed to be down on the beach!") Dr. Amen suggested the mood stabilizer Lamotrigine. Jay now takes 100mg per day. Last year he won an entrance scholarship to a university. Jay's situation illustrates a useful way of approaching SPECT scanning. If counseling and meds are working really well, there is no need to consider alternatives; if therapies are not working, consider testing such as a SPECT scan to hopefully lead to more effective treatments.

Dream: I see lots of folks like Jay in my clinical work but often they've had 10-15 severe blows to the head. They might be homeless or recently released from jail. If standard treatments were not working well I would like to be able to order a scan, diagnose traumatic brain injuries like Jay's and treat them with mood stabilizers like lamotrigine or valproic acid. As taxpayers, think of the money saved for society in Jay's case: this fellow, who could not manage to function in a minimum wage job, became a scholarship student.

A few of my patients who have FASD have attended the Amen Clinic in Tacoma, Washington and found the experience helpful and worthwhile. The cost for an assessment and treatment plan including rest and concentration scans is approximately $3000. The Amen Clinic website is listed in the appendix.

Bruce Perry's Rant for Functional, not DSM, Diagnoses

Bruce Perry, Author of *The Boy Who Was Raised as a Dog* (Basic Books, 2006) and *Born for Love* (Harper Collins, 2010) is the Senior Fellow of Houston's ChildTrauma Academy. Dr. Perry presented "Introduction to the Neurosequential Model of Therapeutics: Application in Children Impacted by FASD" at the Feb 2010 Alberta FASD Conference. Assessment of *functional domains* determines skills and deficits in important areas such as the ability to focus attention, memorize, detect and process sensations, perform calculations, successfully problem solve and effectively use language. Dr. Perry says that *functional* diagnoses, not DSM diagnoses, are a much more effective foundation for planning interventions to improve kids' development. "We figured there might be something wrong with our diagnostic process - five percent of the (traumatized) kids I ever worked with fit nicely into the DSM," he explained. "Nobody got much better in our clinical work, we were just slugging along (diagnosing and treating the way we were taught using DSM). The patients and their families knew it too - they'd show up an average of only four visits before stopping coming to see us, and that was 'good' compared to the (even more pathetic) two and a half visit average in other clinics. So we decided to do something different. Everyone thought that FASD, ADHD, Major Depression were very different (they might require similar treatments, however) - our approach first figures out how the brain functions and then plans sequential interventions based on this information. (- Not the DSM diagnosis).

2) How The Brain Works in FASD

Part One: Primary Disabilities – What Brain Differences (Problems/Issues and Strengths/Assets) are kids who have FASD born with?

"Invisible" disability

If you are diagnosed with FAS, your *growth restriction and facial appearance* may make your disability more recognizable. This often leads to the provision of support services (such as family and school support), which are associated with better outcomes. As "Rant Number One" suggests, only fifteen percent of those with brain damage from prenatal exposure to alcohol have the facial changes and growth restriction that would allow them to be recognized physically and diagnosed with Fetal Alcohol Syndrome. Eighty-five percent of those with brain damage look normal, and there are only a few well-trained physicians who are able to recognize the subtle facial changes in the fifteen percent that do have these physical signs. *FASD, for the most part, is an "invisible" disability.*

Alcohol can affect brain and nerve development at any stage of fetal development. Two things are true: 1) No two kids will show *identical* patterns of brain damage because each individual carries different genes, each was affected by prenatal alcohol at different times in the pregnancy, and each had different patterns of prenatal exposure to other environmental factors such as stress, cigarettes, other drugs, physical injury or poor nutrition. However, 2) a number of specific areas of the brain are *more likely to sustain damage* when prenatally exposed to alcohol.

Think First of Gifts, Relative Strengths

Keep gifts and strengths uppermost in your mind. By working within these areas of success children will be able to tackle (and maybe work around or even transcend) whatever is problematic.

Furthermore, being good at something helps *anyone's* self-confidence. Pursuing passions, interests and gifts leads to forming an *identity.* Not knowing who you are, not having a sense of your own identity, adds to turmoil, impulsiveness and emotional distress. Conversely, having a clear sense of identity can be your refuge in life's storms, and a key part of resisting peer pressure, such as when friends are trying to get you into drugs or alcohol. ("I *can't* smoke pot because *I am a dancer and a singer* and I don't want to be coughing!")

Common Gifts/Strengths of those who have FASD (adapted from Kapp, 2001):

1. *High energy, exuberant.* Activity ideas: Using the climbing wall, bowling, hiking, cross-country skiing, camping, canoeing.
2. *Making up stories and improvising.* Activity ideas: theatre, acting, class comedian who tells the joke of the day.
3. *Artistic in drama, visual art, dance, music.* Activity ideas: music or art therapy, music classes, dance classes, playing instruments or singing, amateur theatre.

For example: The Chicken Shed Theatre in North London, UK engages handicapped and college-level actors working together to produce magic on the stage. Pete LaFlamme in Prince Albert, Saskatchewan shows juvenile delinquents from the jail how to make (some darned gorgeous) copies of Fender Stratocaster guitars in his shop, and he then teaches them how to play. How cool is that? I could get sidetracked by talking about how music is good for *all parts of our brains* but will limit comments here to a few key thoughts. A core issue in FASD is *alexithymia* (which means "no words for emotions"). If we cannot *name* emotions, how can we *process* emotions? How could we ever *explain* or *control* emotions? How could we ever avoid acting impulsively, in simple reaction to raw urges? (Sullivan, 2007) When deficiencies in language processing fail to allow expression of emotions, music can help because the brain circuits that process music, also involved in processing of emotions, are *not* identical to language processing circuits. Music allows an individual to partially work around the language-based circuits of emotional processing that are often harmed by prenatal exposure to alcohol.

4. *A heart for animals or people who are younger, older or ill.* Activity ideas: supervised help in an old folks home, therapeutic riding, having a dog.

For example: An after-school and weekend sled dog training/ handling programme for high schoolers affected by prenatal exposure alcohol in Comox, B.C. Kids in this programme learn how to care for the dogs and work with them in "mushing" races. This programme helps kids stay on track, show up even if they don't feel like it, commit to each other and follow through.

Diane Malbin, a talented social worker, educator, and long-time advocate of kids who have FASD (including her own), adds to the above list some strengths that she has seen in those she works with: skills/ relative strengths in *spelling, reading, writing, poetry, mechanics, woodworking and skilled vocations such as welding.* (Malbin, 2002) I have seen children compose some really touching poetry despite having significant language limitations.

Perceptions of sensory signals can be increased, decreased, or scrambled enough to confuse children.

1. **Hearing.** "Normal" sounds can be perceived as overwhelmingly loud; nuisance noise can be impossible to tune out. Some kids complain they feel swamped by "too many words." Others can't focus on the teacher's voice when there is background noise.

2. **Vision.** Some kids are very sensitive to lights; fluorescent lights, especially if they flicker, can be very distracting. Direct eye contact can be "over the top", i.e. far too invasive of personal comfort boundaries to be tolerable - this could lead to aggression or bolting. People prenatally exposed to alcohol may have difficulty moving their eyes across a page in a well-coordinated way, a skill that is essential for efficient reading. Depth perception issues, and problems in anticipation of movement of objects in space - "is that car coming too fast for

me to be able to get across the road?" - contribute to safety concerns.

3. **Touch.** Some kids are insensitive to hot or cold. Others may be oversensitive to pain, or not sensitive enough to pain (and thus at risk of burns or other injuries). If shirt collar labels, wool or other scratchy materials, or unexpected touch bothers a person, he or she could be "tactile defensive."

4. **Taste/oral.** Certain food textures and tastes may be unbearable. Some people affected this way cannot brush their teeth because this activity is too irritating.

5. **Smell.** Sometimes children find it hard to function because they are distracted by certain smells. Strong perfume or cooking smells can be almost impossible to tune out.

6. **Vestibular** (balance and movement). Knowing where your body is with respect to gravity - are you upright or leaning - is critical to planning accurate muscle movements. Some kids *have* to spin or rock in order to feel relaxed or be able to concentrate - they may be "vestibular input seekers" - whereas some kids *have* to be still (movement bugs them - they may be "vestibular hyper-responsive").

7. **Proprioception.** This refers to the sense of where muscles and joints are with respect to other joints and muscles. This information is vital for coordination of muscle movement. If proprioception is not well developed, clumsiness results, which often leads to teasing from peers, poor self-esteem and feelings of anxiety.

8. **Body signals (from gut, etc.)** Accurate perception of these sensory messages allow people to know, for example, if they need to stop the car and pee in the bush, or if they can wait ten minutes for the next rest stop. This sense also tells people if their abdominal pain is just cramping or if it might be a ruptured the appendix and need assessment by a surgeon.

Sensory issues are *very* common in FASD. Understanding an individual's pattern of sensory processing can lead to helpful intervention strategies that *have the potential to permanently improve* brain circuitry, which, in turn, allays anxiety and permanently improves self-regulation, performance of tasks, and ability to sustain attention. If this information excites you, learn more at the SPD Foundation website listed in the appendix. I am very enthusiastic about sensory interventions. I have seen sensory processing treatments help my own kids' attention, sleep, and self-esteem, so I have taken some extra training in this emerging field. Although many of these ideas may seem new they are anything *but* "fringy". I invite skeptics to view Brett-Green's 2008 ERP (Evoked Response Potential) study (see references). Whenever possible I try to use children's sensory profiles to plan specific sensory accommodations - very often these measures can help behavioural problems, anxiety and attention deficits. Lots of sensory issues are *heritable*; when investigating the sensory profile in one child, not infrequently Mum will see herself, her other kids or her husband as having similar sensory patterns. For these reasons we will take a chapter later in the book to explore sensory concepts in more detail.

For now I'd like to introduce four concepts and terms that I have found helpful:

1) **Praxis** means imagining, planning and then carrying out a muscle movement, especially a new movement. To successfully complete even a simple movement, such as picking up a pencil, an individual depends on smooth coordination of messages coming from *proprioception* (where muscles and joints are located with respect to other parts of the body), *vestibular* (where is the body with respect to gravity - i.e. is it tilted to the left or right or leaning back?), *touch* receptors and feedback from *vision*. So even basic activities such as moving eyes across a page when reading or writing require putting together input from at least four different sensory systems, all working in harmony!

2) To have **balance** it is necessary to have intact systems of *at least two out of three of the following:* Vision, Proprioception and Vestibular. Many people with FASD have problems in vestibular perception, which this causes movement and balance problems, especially if they also have problems in visual perception. Get folks to close their eyes. Now that they are down to only vestibular and proprioception; those with vestibular issues will demonstrate severe balance problems.

3) Finding optometrists who understand **eye movement issues** (which are common in FASD) is difficult. Children might describe words "bouncing around the page," find it hard to find their place in their notes if they look up to the board or simply are slow readers. Specialists trained in developmental optometry are more likely than other eye professionals to

be able to assist people who have difficulty with smooth eye movement. A "finder service" is provided on the College of Optometry in Visual Development website.

4) Testing hearing in a sound-proof booth, listening to pure tones in one ear at a time (the usual way hearing is tested) does not assess ability to hear the teacher or the parent when there are background (distracting) noises. *Some* audiologists are able to assess this skill, which is called **auditory *figure-ground discrimination***. Understanding a conversation (or lesson) despite background noise may be a more relevant skill for real-world functioning than what can be recognized by "usual" hearing tests. In FASD, auditory discrimination, accurately hearing one person or a particular sound in the presence of background noise is often profoundly impaired.

Sensory Filtering

Ideally, sensory perceptions *that are not needed* for functioning (e.g. pants rubbing on the legs when we are walking) should be filtered out so attention can be paid to what is important (e.g. the hornet that just landed on your shoulder!) The cerebellum, located just beneath the vision center at the back of the brain, helps to filter incoming sensory messages. If any of our eight senses are not properly filtered, a lot of distraction can result, leading to decreased attention and decreased learning. If there is *less* filtering, the input from any source is *less clear* and so learning is impaired. If there is *poorly coordinated filtering* children receive muddled, unclear, ambiguous sensory messages; interpreting these signals becomes difficult or impossible. If these muddled signals include your teacher's voice, learning can be severely compromised.

Figure 3. Cerebellum - a partial sensory filter

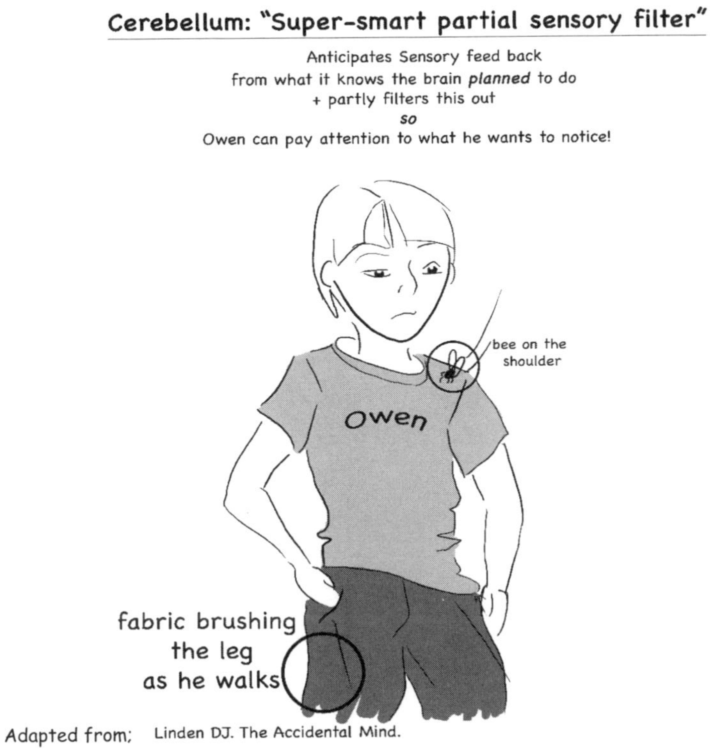

Figure 3. Notes:

If you were Owen you'd like your cerebellum to filter unwanted and distracting signals. You want to know about the bee that landed on your shoulder even though the bee's weight is negligible and your perception of it touching your shoulder is much less than your perception of your feet contacting the ground. Without efficient sensory filtering, Owen does not know what to pay attention to; he is bombarded with sensations.

I have asked kids with FASD whether they could tickle themselves. Often they can. This represents a reduction in the cerebellum's usual filtering power for sensory feedback from movements that the child initiated him or herself.

Accommodations/strategies for sensory processing difficulties

If children *have* to move (vestibular and/or proprioception input seeking), let them sit on a therapy ball or a blow-up cushion on their seat. If fluorescent lights are hard to tolerate, get a softer type of light or allow baseball caps or visors. If body signals such as perceiving the need to pee are confusing, create a schedule, for example, use the washroom at regular intervals rather than depending on unreliable perceptions to time these activities. If children have an aversion to loud noises, various types of hearing protection are available. An FM system in the classroom can be helpful if students have poor auditory discrimination; amplifying the teacher's voice helps students to hear the lesson and disregard distracting background noise. "Acoustic startle," which is hyper-responsivity especially to *unexpected* sounds, is often observed in people who were born prematurely, have alcohol exposure damage, or have Post-traumatic stress disorder (PTSD). Prior warning of loud sounds ("I'm going to start the blender - plug your ears!") allows anticipation, which can greatly lessen the startle. If oversensitivity to smell is an issue (e.g. if math class is next to the chef-training classroom and the smell of the baking bread is distracting) masking this with a different smell like lavender can be a successful strategy. If smell perception is decreased, the individual may lack an awareness of body odor. Showering on a regular schedule can be a useful adaption. If certain foods cannot be tolerated, usually these can be avoided. If brushing teeth is impossible, this can be harder to deal with. One trick is to eat cheese after any meal. Cheese coats teeth in healthy bacteria that can reduce the cavity forming bacteria. Proprioception and vestibular problems? Forcing clumsy people into team sports needlessly batters their self-esteem. Why not encourage individual physical activities such as walking or weight lifting? Heavy work activities like stacking chairs, pushing a broom, clearing snow, wheelbarrow walking, or pushing weights are often calming and grounding and so need to be included in the daily schedule. Many people can't stand the touch of certain things on their skin. They dislike being jostled in crowds, so should plan travel times and routes to avoid congested areas.

Every person, affected by prenatal exposure to alcohol or not, has a unique *sensory profile* or pattern of perceptual likes and dislikes. For example, I cannot sleep if there are ticking clocks. Unexpected touch startles many people. The goal is to become aware of your own unique sensory profile and learn how to work with it. Often children with FASD have enough over- or under-reactivity to certain perceptions that these issues affect *their ability to function.* Problems of this magnitude are called *Sensory Processing Disorder (SPD).* Like FAS, SPD is currently a "condition proposed by outside sources" for possible inclusion in DSM-5.

Memory Impairment

Figure 4: Memory

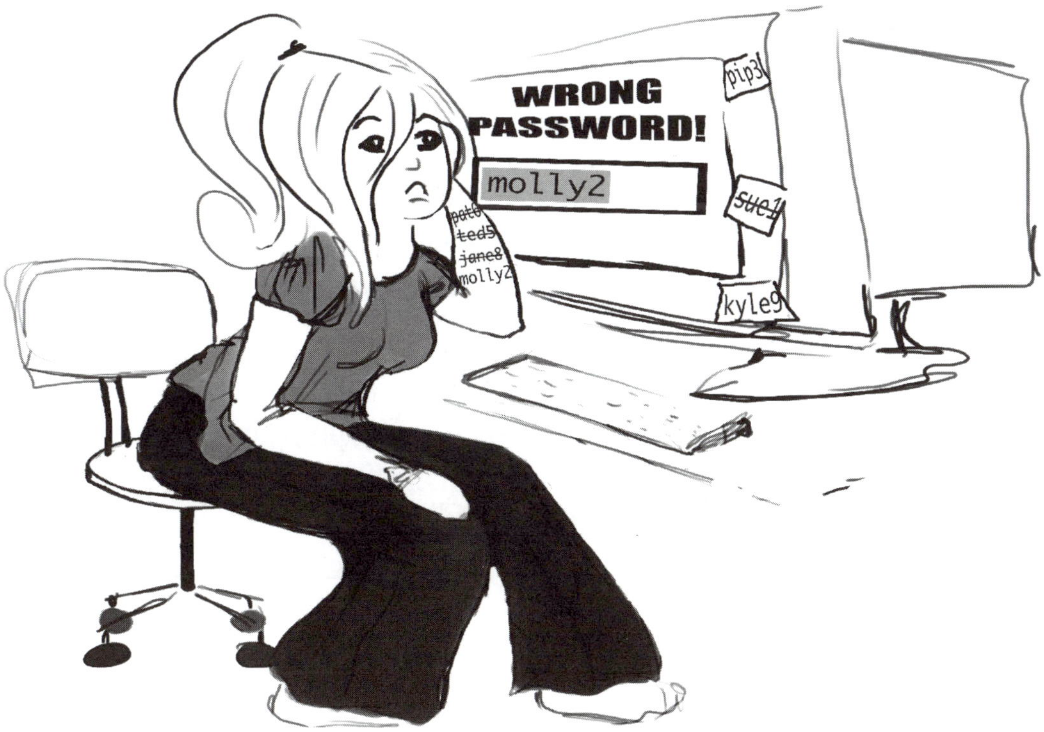

The hippocampus, an area located on the inside part of the left and right temporal lobes, is where new memories for facts and events are *encoded* (initially laid down). An encoded memory is stored there for up to a year or two and is then transferred to the adjacent temporal lobe for storage. Each day two thousand new nerve cells grow in the hippocampus; their job is to augment new memories that are being held in this structure. New memories in the hippocampus are augmented by 2000 new nerve cells that grow there each day. Magnetoencephalography (MEG) brain studies show that kids with FASD grow approximately twenty percent of the number of new nerve cells that age-matched controls do. Not surprisingly, study subjects with prenatal alcohol exposure will recall less after two hours - about fifteen percent of what was initially encoded - than non-exposed people, who can retain about ninety percent two hours later. (Sutherland, 2003)

Strategies to address this memory issue include repetitions, hands-on kinesthetic learning, using a computer for repetitive teaching assignments such as spelling (rather than getting irritated because "we've already been over this five times!") and especially avoiding loss of temper by caregivers. Memory, already profoundly impaired, is further *sabotaged* by fear and stress suggests Dr. Robert Sutherland, from University of Lethbridge. He also described the hippocampal memory functions as "exquisitely" sensitive to stress. (Sutherland, 2003)

Memory for facts and events is important, but even more critical for academic success are *procedural* memories (how to do things) such as *rules* of grammar, how to sound out a word, and how to write an "s" or a "b." Most language skills are rule-based, for example: discriminating word-sounds, correctly articulating and pronouncing words, segmenting words into sounds, phonics, writing conventions such as punctuation and capitalization, motor rules for forming letters the same way when writing, and spacing evenly between words. Arithmetic rule-based skills such as carrying over, and long division are also learned in procedural memory circuits. (Eide, 2010) Procedural memory circuits involve the cerebellum - an area often damaged by prenatal alcohol exposure. Drs. Eide say that the cerebellum *is the most commonly affected area of the brain* in a wide variety of conditions associated with learning challenges. (Eide, 2010) Children with procedural learning difficulties must focus more intently to perform the same assignments as other children - this overloads their working memory leaving less capacity available to attend to the task at hand. Children with procedural learning difficulties need accommodations such as use of a dictation device, assignment of a scribe or use of assistive technology. Assistive technologies recommended for specific learning difficulties by Drs. Eide include word and spelling prediction softwear, report writers such as Co:Writer 6, speech to text programmes such as Dragon Dictate, Iphone/Ipod Touch Apps for Dyslexia, and context-sensitive grammar programmes. More ideas for resources can be viewed at the Dyslexic Advantage website created by Drs. Brock and Fernette Eide.

Slower speed of thought/ emotional/language processing

Slower processing of brain signals is the result of prenatal exposure to alcohol reducing the number of neurons an individual has, the number of interconnections between them and the speed that a message (electrical signal) can travel along a nerve. Axons are projections, which usually take electrical signals from the nerve cell body *to* the next cell. Dendrites are projections that usually bring electrical signals from adjacent cells *into* the nerve cell body. The sheath around axons is called white matter. It is made up of a chemical called myelin. Myelin is reduced in those affected by FASD and seems to relate to lower levels of a chemical called choline. (Norman, 2009) If axons have less myelin in their surrounding sheath, the speed that an electrical message can travel down that axon is much slower. Myelin is very important - without good levels of myelin, nerve function is very impaired. Multiple Sclerosis (MS) is a condition in which damage to the nerves' myelin sheath causes slower transmission of a message down the nerve - and thus creates problems for the muscles that nerves are telling to relax or contract. Alcohol can damage both *the genes* that regulate myelination (growth of white matter) and *the proteins* that those genes make. (LeStrat, 2008) I have a patient with FASD who recently suffered a very serious attack of MS. I searched medical literature search to try to determine if a correlation between likelihood of MS attacks and FASD existed and could not find any articles on this subject.

Processing speed affects social situations. Imagine that you were a teenage girl with slow processing ability trying to figure out the facial expressions and meanings of this conversation with your 13-year-old girlfriends, "Awesome. That's crap!

So-o-much cow. Like, whatever. Such a prep. Sweet. Oh that's lame!" Chances are you'd be busy trying to figure out where someone pooed ("That's crap!") and your friends would already be on to the next topic. Situations like this happen all the time. To avoid social ostracism many kids learn to be adept at *faking that they are following* a conversation, yet often they do not understand the gist of what their friends really mean. Jump ahead a couple of years and consider the trouble that could result from faking that you understand an important conversation with your spouse, or a policeman or a judge.

In FASD-affected individuals, when language, thoughts (or sensory or emotional processing circuits) move information from one set of nerves to the next set of nerves (via synaptic transmission) the *transfer* of information is slower. For example, when *listening* to your dad say, "let's go to gramma's," auditory input (which might be muddled) needs to be sent to the temporal lobe language centers for translation of raw data (sound) into words. Subsequently, words are retrieved from memory, associations with those words ("gramma always makes warm scones!") are considered as the meaning of the message is discerned, these interpretations are moved to working memory areas, the data is considered in "association cortex" areas, an appropriate response is decided on, and then a message goes to the part of your brain which makes your lips move and you say your response ("let's go right now!") Due to slow processing speed, by the time you respond your dad's conversation has moved on to about the sixth topic past whether you want to go to gramma's place.

Intervention: (from one of my favourite teachers regarding a boy in her grade 7 class) Stand *right in front* of the child (this gives him a signal, "it is your turn!") if you want him to answer the *next* question. This intervention provides *a non-shaming work-around for slow processing speed.* See figure 2.

Executive function

I used to think that executive functions occurred in the prefrontal cortex (the very front part of the frontal lobe), but other areas are also involved. Working memory areas of the prefrontal cortex are damaged by alcohol, but so are projections from that area to a structure called the caudate in the basal ganglion (in the middle, deeper part of the brain), projections *from* the caudate to the prefrontal cortex and the caudate itself. Message: interconnections with important deeper structures, not just activity in the prefrontal cortex, are required for executive function and working memory. Executive function is like the manager in an office: If the boss is away the troops are at play! Deadlines, goal setting, long-term planning, seeing the big picture, knowing if you're off track, knowing how to get back on track, and pacing are all affected.

People with FASD can have damage to any part of the executive function system, but 1) working memory areas, 2) sequencing and 3) areas responsible for "cognitive estimation" may be more severely affected. Cognitive estimation (I find the term "silly guesses" easier to remember) might be related to a primary problem with number sense. Silly guesses often appear as follows: (True story - as all are in this book!) "How tall is that man?" the teacher asked. "Forty feet", came the reply. (The *number* is wrong, but the *units* are right.) The teacher said "no" and the next attempt arrived, "Hundred feet." "No." "Nine thousand feet." So the guesses are quite random and seem to be offered without an overall concept or over-arching strategy to guide the problem solving. Sequencing is a huge issue. In life's daily activities, *order is everything*. Think about trying to make your breakfast this morning, or getting to work on time, or getting an assignment in on time. What would happen if you did the steps of these tasks in the wrong order?

Suggestion: Sequencing issues need coaching (and perhaps visual cues such as pictures of what steps, in order, need to be followed) and caregivers must *expect* that sequencing is going to be a problem. Sometimes "lazy" really means, "not sure which order to do the steps in so I cannot get started."

Working memory

There are several types of working memory, and these are located in various parts of the brain as well as the frontal lobes. Subtypes of working memory include spatial working memory, arithmetic working memory, and social interaction working memory, to name a few. Working memory allows us to retrieve some idea and hold it "online" while we puzzle it over and make a decision. An easy way to understand working memory deficits in FASD-affected individuals is to think of a bank machine. My child, who has FAS, can easily go to the ATM, type in the right numbers and get money out of it. These tasks are all rote. For this to actually be a *functional skill*, however, a *lot* more information must be considered. When I go to the ATM I am thinking, "This is the 7th of January, I don't get paid until the 14th, I have $300 in my account, I have a bill coming up which is for almost that much, oh I'd better only take out $50." All that behind-the-scenes thinking is accomplished by working memory. *Quickness* of typing PIN numbers into the bank machine is *not a functional skill* if you take too much money out!

What does it take to answer a question *logically*? Planning ahead, flexibility in *shifting* attention from one thought to another more important thought, inhibiting unwanted urges or distractions and being able to form concepts allow the kind of sequential thinking that underpins logic. Psychologists often test concept formation by asking Twenty Questions. Let's try it: I can answer "yes" or "no." You might start by asking, "Is it alive?" Answer: "Yes." "Is it a plant?" Answer: "No." Your good concept formation ability then leads you to ask: "Is it an animal?" Answer: "Yes." "Is it a mammal?" "Answer: Yes." "Does it have fur?" Answer – Yes. You have narrowed down your questions by a logical process. Those affected by FASD often just take random guesses without a logical flow to structure of their answers. "Is it a car?" "Is it a plant?" "Is it my mother?" "Is it Tarzan?" etc.

Perhaps associated with sequencing issues is a poor sense of time. Poor sequencing abilities and a poor sense of time impair planning and organizing.

The working memory areas that are located in the prefrontal cortex also communicate with an area called the *insula*, which is a deep cortex structure located between the temporal and the frontal lobes. Dr Malisza's (2005) study used functional MRI imaging to examine brain activation in tasks of attention, memories of where objects are located in space, and working memory. In an easy task, those with FASD showed more activity in their prefrontal cortexes' working memory areas, meaning they had to work a lot harder than the non-affected folks to do the task. There was *less* activity, however, in the FASD-affected individuals' insula. This means they were less able *to integrate and make sense of body information* - for example, "I've got to pee." The insula, located at the deepest levels of the groove between the temporal lobe (below) and the frontal and parietal lobes (above), is an area of *integration* where sensory information from the body comes together with language from the temporal lobes and sensations from parietal lobes. The insula is an area where one *selects a response or inhibits an impulse.* As described in comments regarding the simulation (above), when subjects were asked to do a harder task, those with FASD showed very little increase in prefrontal cortex activity. This area was already maxed out - in FASD-affected individuals there is less reserve. Those not affected by FASD could ratchet up activity in the prefrontal cortex to meet the increased demand.

Question re: *Giving up*: What is going on if the child gives up?

Answer: Giving up might actually be smart because he or she might be already maxing out the brain's ability to try to accomplish a task - trying even harder might not improve function.

Flexibility

Flexibility involves a shifting smoothly from one task to the next, or perhaps from one emotion to the next. The frontal cortex cingulate area, which is the bottom part of the middle of the frontal lobes, and the caudate nucleus (in the basal ganglion or mid-brain) are all involved in this. Please note that we know now in 2011 that it is silly to talk about a given function as belonging to one specific brain area, because almost every brain process has to do with *circuits*. We know that the cingulate, the caudate and the working memory areas in the frontal cortex *and the pathways that connect these areas* are affected by FASD. So, is it any wonder that flexibility might be an issue? Inflexibility leads to meltdowns...

Meltdowns - rule of thumb

In FASD, one or more of the following situations may cause really outrageous behaviour, such as violence or out-of-the-blue aggression; understanding the cause often leads to effective interventions:

1. Does the child feel *cornered* emotionally or physically?
   Idea: Don't corner.
2. Is the child *over-stimulated*?
   Idea: Reduce sensory over-stimulation.
3. Is the child *surprised* (i.e. unprepared for a transition)?
   Idea: Plan transitions.
4. Does the child have a *perception of being abandone*d by a social attachment? Idea: don't abandon the child even if you are mad because your buttons have been pushed.

This is tricky. I have found Gordon Neufeld's ideas on "Discipline Without Dividing" (from the DVD series *Power to Parent Part 1)* to be practical guidelines and very empowering to burned out caregivers, including me. All Dr. Neufeld's DVD's are available from his website which is listed in the appendix.

5. *Out-of-the-blue* aggression? It may be wise to consider an undiagnosed traumatic head injury or temporal lobe epilepsy in this situation. (This section, FASD 101, is not really designed for psychiatry/ primary care professionals - nevertheless, I'd like to comment about a *potentially treatable* and very common issue I see working with people who have FASD: *Traumatic Brain Injury (TBI)*. Aggression, "time sense" problems, impulsivity and emotional volatility are often found in TBI. These symptoms disrupt patient's lives but can be successfully treated. Treatment can involve a mood stabilizer medication such as lamotrigine or valproic acid. One patient, Mrs. A., just out of prison, came to the clinic literally vibrating and seething about her landlord. "I know I'm going to hit him," she said, looking at the floor. I started her on 25 mg. of lamotrigine daily - eventual dose 100 mg daily. After 3 weeks she reported her thinking was much clearer, and was especially pleased that she could handle the strong emotions of the most recent dispute with her landlord, "I know I would have spazzed out at him and yelled and gotten into trouble before taking this stuff!" Her husband separated from her due to her volatility, yet he still was very much in the picture, wanting to help her with daily routines of grocery shopping, food prep, etc. Last I heard he was planning to move back in. Justifiably, many concerns regarding side effects of psychiatric drugs exist - it is wise to be cautious - but Mrs. A.'s is a situation where careful, targeted drug use, at very modest doses, improved function and actually changed a life for the better.

"Bookends"

Kids affected by FASD rarely know *when and how to start* and *when they are finished* a project or assignment. They need help with the executive function tasks called the "bookends" (getting started and understanding that they have finished).

Can we intervene to help executive function?

Although some parents and experts on FASD have criticized me ("There he goes, trying to *change the kid*!") I do think there are useful ideas from traumatic brain injury literature on how to help our kids' develop executive and adaptive functions *to an optimal degree*. I especially admire the brain injury rehabilitation work of Drs. Mark Ylvisaker and Tim Feeney. The gist of their approach is "roll-up-your-sleeves collaboration/coaching" on topics of "everyday, common, practical relevance" such as getting books and assignments to school or getting to work on time. They emphasize the importance of reducing unstructured time for FASD-affected individuals.

The philosophy behind provision of comprehensive sensory integration interventions in autism, I believe, serves children with FASD also: Make activities fun and interesting, don't push to the point of distress but don't let kids stay in a restrictive box; always help them extend themselves *just a little bit but not to the point of overwhelm*. Growth happens when we push ourselves just a bit, but not to the level of distress. As for my critics - I don't really know what brain science will tell us ten or twenty years from now, but somehow accepting that the function of important brain circuits cannot be improved does not seem logical. And, in the words of one of the adoptive dads that I have worked with, "We (caregivers) *live by hope, don't deprive us of hope*." Of course don't shame, blame or put down, but to ignore possibilities of improved function through neuroplastic changes (nerves and nerves circuits continuing to grow and remodel themselves - well into adulthood and even old age) simply sets aside recent science. (Doige, 2007)

Speech and language issues

Kids affected by FASD may be fluent speakers but have reduced comprehension, especially in understanding *how a story fits together*, (its cohesion) and what the *gist of the story* is (its coherency). Damage in the left temporal lobe (Wernicke's area) and corresponding parts of the right temporal lobe lead to comprehension difficulties.

Intervention - *please* don't assume "they got it" *if they can repeat it*. Comprehending what a story means is a very different skill than repeating the story.

Example: In 2000, Diane Fast and Julianne Conry released their book *Fetal Alcohol Syndrome and the Criminal Justice System*. Part of the book release involved a workshop on legal issues surrounding FASD, which I attended. This is a story from the workshop: Judge: "Do you know what you did wrong?" Defendant: "Yes, your honor, I violated clause (whatever it was) from the Criminal Code of Canada that states (whatever it stated)." Satisfied that the defendant understood his crime, the judge imposed a light sentence, only to be exasperated when, before long, the defendant re-appeared charged with the same crime. (Lesson: *his ability to state his crime did not mean that he understood it or that this knowledge would translate into the appropriate action of avoiding the same mistake* in judgment when faced with the same temptations later on.)

Connecting words such as "if", "only if", "before", and "after" are often overlooked and when this happens what a phrase means can be misunderstood.

Being able to put yourself in the shoes of another is just one important *social language skill* that depends on smooth function of the parts of the brain, including mirror neurons, which are responsible for "theory of mind." As previously discussed, these areas may be damaged by prenatal exposure to alcohol. Theory of mind refers to a person's understanding that his or her perspective is different from others. (i.e. what he or she knows is different from what another person knows.) It is very difficult for an individual with an underdeveloped theory of mind to understand others' points of view. Other types of disabilities, such as autism and Tourette's, have core problems with theory of mind also.

A *mirror neuron* is a nerve cell that fires when a person *observes an action* performed by another *or observes an emotion* shown by another. The bottom part of the parietal lobes, an area often damaged by prenatal exposure to alcohol, and the premotor cortex both contain mirror neurons. The firing of electrical impulses in mirror neurons is understood to underlie at least parts of empathy or subconscious, automatic awareness of the mental states of others. In FASD, we often see difficulties *putting yourself in the shoes of the other person and understanding body language or non-verbal communication.* Problematic mirror neuron function may explain these difficulties but I can't prove this because to date, I have not seen specific scientific articles regarding mirror neuron activity in FASD.

Example: Last year I assessed a grade 10 girl, who was prenatally exposed to alcohol. A fluent speaker, she seemed to be doing okay in school but terribly socially. It was easy to develop a good rapport with her because she and her family knew me quite well. One day I asked her, "Who is your favourite singer?" "Gwen Stefani, of course!"

She then went on to tell me all about her favourite songs, the names of Gwen's kids and so on. I then asked her *what it would be like to be Gwen, and why Gwen would say or do a certain thing.* In spite of trying hard to answer, being a great fan of Gwen's and knowing all kinds of details about Gwen's life, my patient had no idea how to even begin to answer these questions.

Probably, in part, related to processing speed issues: *receptive comprehension (understanding* what is heard or read) can be an area of great difficulty. Often, kids will say, "Too many words." *We should simplify and slow things down.*

I hope readers will become interested in the more precise assessment of visual skills (that can be done by developmental optometrists) for kids they care for because I find a lot of positive responses since I have started asking the right questions (do words bounce around on the page, is it hard to find your place in the book after you have looked up to the board, do you need to re-read a paragraph four or five times to make sense out of it?) Visual problems that therapy can alleviate may underlie *written comprehension issues.*

Since many students cannot pay attention to everything at once, test skills one at a time. When testing *comprehension* of a given topic do not overload students by insisting that they must write perfectly, spell accurately, use correct grammar and so on. In school or college, if students with FASD, ADHD or other similar issues are trying to do an assignment to show they understand a certain topic, it is wise to mark that assignment *on content* and not spelling, grammar or neatness, because to try to attend to *all* of these functions *simultaneously* can be over the top. (Attending to all these tasks *at once* requires precise divided attention and fully functional working memory skills) To write accurate notes from a fast-paced lecture is almost impossible for many who have FASD. Often it is hard to listen and write at the same time - patients tell me, "If I am writing, then I can't listen."

Rant Number Two: "Picky" Marking

If the goal is assess spelling, of course accurate spelling needs to be checked; however, picky marking and correcting of spelling, grammar, neatness and delivery style when the goal is to assess comprehension of course content sabotages momentum and is unfair, discriminatory and stifling to those with working memory "hardware" problems. A compromised working memory system is every bit as genuine and physical a problem as the muscle dysfunction in Cerebral Palsy - insisting that someone with FASD pay attention to *all* aspects of composition writing *at the same time* is similar nonsense to insisting someone with Cerebral Palsy take an unmodified Physical Education curriculum - ridiculous!

Helpful interventions for speech, language processing speed, and comprehension issues include use of audio or video recorders and arranging for an in-class scribe to provide disabled students with a good set of notes. The devil is in the details with such accommodations. Schools or colleges may feel that once they have permitted a video recorder or a note taker that the plan will happen. Not quite. How these best made plans might unravel, in my experience, often involves educators making *an assumption that the student with FASD will intuit a certain problem solving strategy* - and the student doesn't. This is not related to IQ or effort. A young man with FASD, who had a high IQ (115), was doing well on a university course but then was told he'd flunked because he did not turn in an all-important term paper. His dad was away for a few days and the student had finished the paper, but the printer ran out of ink and he did not intuit a "fix," which would have involved getting a new cartridge. He did not tell anyone about the issue, either. (He might have the hard to get started "bookends" issue discussed above.) His dad returned and the issue was resolved. The student got a B+ on the paper after the reasons for its lateness were explained. Issues like this seldom have a happy ending because advocates that understands these disabilities in "smart" people are rare, and allowing those advocates to be close enough to understand why certain parts of assignments are not understood is also rare. To the uninitiated (in FASD caregiving), attentive parental involvement looks like "that dad is too intrusive and nosey and should back off - give the kid some space so they can succeed." The initiated, on the other hand, understand that dad, by replacing printer cartridges and anticipating a thousand other roadblocks, *allows his kid to succeed.*

Out of the box thinking to be sure but I suggest *society, as a whole should be intrusive enough to allow our kids to succeed.* As a dad how can I say anything else?

The corpus callosum

The corpus callosum is a large tract of (possibly 800 million - but who could count 'em?) axons that link the left and right brain hemispheres. Our right side is always talking to our left side and vice versa; "four *billion* messages cross back and forth *every second,*" says neuroscientist Charles Wesson. The right hemisphere of the brain *cortex* (cortex refers to the top or outer layer) picks up body language and nonverbal communication, and this information *helps to temper* the left side - that is, if it can cross over to the left side via the corpus callosum. The left side has an "always-on storytelling/narrative centre." Sometimes it is really necessary to temper, calm down, or put a lid on this never-shuts-up storytelling area!

Every one of us has a bit of insight into what it is like to have an impaired corpus callosum, because this area does not work very well just as we emerge from sleep. Readers may recall wonderful, expansive, untempered thoughts and ideas upon awakening (when the corpus callosum is at half-power) which lose some luster later in the day when examined by logic or common sense. Traffic through the corpus callosum allows right-left and left-right transfer of information, including tempering the left side language centre. This traffic increases *after waking up*, especially when we are in a state of calm focus, and decreases with stress and anger. Not surprisingly, Tibetan monks who practice meditation are the Olympic Athletes of good corpus callosum function. The Dalai Lama graciously allowed fMRI study of some of his monks. When the monks were upset, information transfer across the corpus callosum went down; when the monks were calm and meditating information transfer greatly increased and a *state of calm focus* was achieved. Wouldn't a state of calm focus be lovely for kids with FASD and their caregivers? Numerous studies have shown damage to the corpus callosum by prenatal alcohol.

"Split-brain" patients: their experience can tell us much about corpus callosum damage.

Surgeons divided the corpus callosum in a desperate attempt to literally save the lives of some patients who had intractable seizures that were not responding to medications. This drastic measure worked - it did save some lives. Amazingly, these "split brain" patients *seemed* to do really well in *most* daily activities. However, researchers have observed some more subtle patterns of impaired function that are relevant for anyone with impaired corpus callosal activity, whether callosal damage is caused by surgery or prenatal alcohol damage or other factors. The language centre is in the left hemisphere. Studies were conducted in which the patient with a damaged corpus collosum was shown a sign reading "Get Up" in his or her *right* visual field. This information is analyzed in the *left* brain, which is where the language centre is. If such patients start to get up and the experimenter stops them, asking, "What are you doing?" most patients correctly respond, "I read the sign, I'm getting up." When the same patients perceive the "Get Up" sign in their *left* visual field, they analyze the message in their *right* brain - this side has only *rudimentary* understanding of language. Remember, the language centre is on the other side, the left side. Unconsciously, patients can interpret some simple words with the right hemisphere's rudimentary language skills, so they will start to get up. Again, the experimenters stop them and ask, "What are you doing?" The correct answer is, "My language centre is not on the part of my brain that saw the sign, so I have no sweet clue what I'm doing," but patients with split brains don't say this! *They make up a story.* "Oh, I have to pee" or "Oh, I've sat too long."

"Getting stuck," not being able to switch to a more adaptive idea, perseveration

Inflexibility may be caused by damage to circuits that include the caudate nucleus, its connections to the frontal lobe, and the cingulate. (The cingulate is a deep midline part of the frontal lobe.) Recent magnetic resonance spectroscopy (MRS) work by Susan Astley at the University of Washington confirms a low amount of the important neurotransmitter chemical, acetylcholine, in the basal ganglion (caudate) and the areas that caudate cells project to, i.e., the frontal cortex. Dr. Astley's findings confirm that the function of the caudate and the areas it connects to are impaired in FASD. (Astley, 2009)

Our (caregiver's) response to inflexibility should be to decrease coercion and stress when kids are getting stuck. *Diversion* is a lot smarter than trying to convince Granny (who has Alzheimer's) that today is actually Sunday not Tuesday. The same part of her brain (cingulate and connections to it) is damaged. Nathan Ory, a psychologist based in Victoria, B.C. helpfully adds that kids with FASD *live in the moment*. So if "the moment" is not working out very well and is headed "deep south" into confrontation and "head-butting" Nathan suggests, "just change the situation." Trying to talk your way out of potentially explosive situations with upset people usually doesn't work. (Ory, 2007) Bruce Perry would add that as people become more upset, stressed and threatened their language processing becomes increasingly impaired. (Cont'd pg 40)

Figure 5: "Lying"

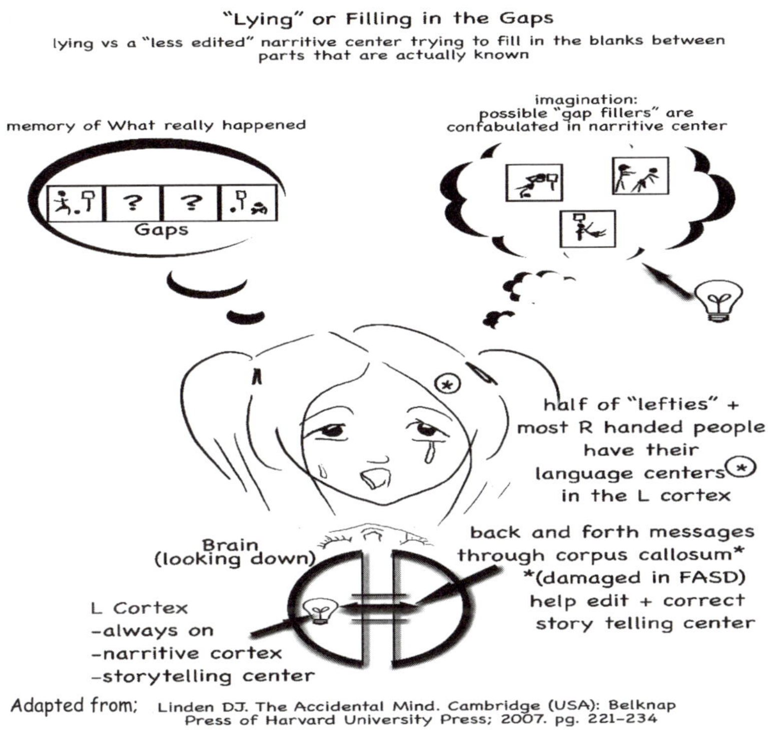

Figure 5. notes: If the corpus callosum is not working very well, there is less left-right communication and the left-sided narrative centre spins out yarns. Anyone who works with kids who have FASD might be saying, "OooLalahh" or "Aha!" I believe that it is usually inaccurate to say that folks who have FASD "lie." Rather, they remember certain episodes of reality (<u>spotty memory</u>) and then <u>spin a story</u>, retroactively - using their excellent narrative centers - <u>between those bits of reality</u>. (Linden, 2007) I like Dr. Gordon Neufeld's term for "filling in the blanks" in this manner: he refers to the process as <u>cognitive backfill</u>. David Linden's book, <u>The Accidental Mind</u>, is a playful, entirely readable romp through how important brain functions work; I highly recommend it. A brief example: he calls the brain, weighing two percent of total body weight and using twenty percent of its energy, the "Hummer H2 of the body."

Order Book: "Accidental Mind" by David Linden

In our family, foosball has calmed more upset feelings and "upset at life" issues than talk therapy. We'd better get it out again! Foosball is great because if you or your kids come home "all wound up and ready to kill" you don't have to say *anything*! Just pour all that venom into beating your foosball opponent and before you know it, you'll both be laughing. Magic! In our family we have *found that when parents or kids were getting stuck, usually the answer was doing something physical, not thinking about harder about the problem.*

Paying attention and maintaining attention – ADHD

ADHD involves *inattention*, impulsivity and hyperactivity. DSM diagnoses such as ADHD are simply "symptom collections" - ADHD is six or more inattention symptoms or six or more *impulsivity/hyperactivity* symptoms that were present since before age seven and cause impaired function in several life situations, for example at school and at home (these criteria will be updated in the new DSM-5). Attention Deficit Hyperactivity Disorder (ADHD) would more accurately be called "Trouble Paying Attention To Stuff That Bores The Crud Outta You" (but who would be able to remember the acronym: TPATSTBTCOY).

Rant Number Three: "Professionals" that don't know what they don't know are a menace!

Understanding the TPATSTBTCOY concept would have helped the vice principal of a prestigious West Vancouver High School who witheringly hissed at me, "Don't give me that 'ADHD stuff,' Dr. Densmore - *he can concentrate just fine if he* wants *to* - he runs around *all lunch hour* with a street hockey stick!" This ill-informed, judgmental administrator was poisoning the school environment for my patient. She did not understand that anyone of any age who has ADHD could pay attention to engaging topics that capture their interest and passion for hours. It's the more mundane or boring parts that are really hard to stay focused on - and willpower cannot "fix" this medical condition. Gordon Neufeld explains that caregivers must create "a place of rest" and acceptance for the kids that we look after in order to set the stage for optimal development - this harsh vice principal created the opposite situation and took *invalidation* to a whole new level.

I wonder if my patient dropped out of school; he did want to quit. My patient's only hope would be to disregard, to set aside, any toxic stuff coming from this administrator - and what kid, or weary parent, can muster enough confidence to do that? Why *should* a kid have to do that? Approximately five to seven percent of this vice principal's school population has ADHD - teachers and students! Since the vice-principal is in charge of "disciplinary matters," most likely, she would see a higher ADHD prevalence than seven percent in the students that she dealt with most. I hope she's now better informed - a great place to start for ADHD is accessing materials prepared by CADDRA, the Canadian Attention Deficit Hyperactivity Disorder Resource Alliance. CADDRA's website is listed in the appendix.

ADHD (Continued)

To be fair, the best thinking possible when DSM-4 was created over a decade ago went into designing ADHD symptom criteria; however, these criteria are *not based on a specific neurobiology or genetics of ADHD*. In other words, several different brain conditions could give rise to these symptoms and thus be diagnosable as ADHD. Patients I have seen that fit ADHD diagnostic criteria include those with traumatic brain injuries, FASD, and Sensory Processing Disorder - to name but a few causes of underlying brain neurologic dysfunction.

Irish psychiatrist, Kieran O'Malley edited the book *ADHD and Fetal Alcohol Spectrum Disorders* in 2007. I know this is not really FASD 101, but I suspect some readers will want to know how Kieran distinguishes between "ADHD caused by FASD" and "pure ADHD." Dr. O'Malley suggests that pure ADHD involves more problems with *focusing* and *sustaining attention*; at the brain biology level, it involves an imbalance in the "fronto-nigro-striatal" dopamine pathways (which is where methylphenidate [Ritalin] works). ADHD caused by FASD involves more problems with *encoding* (laying down of new memories in the hippocampus) and *shifting* attention from one topic to the next in a well-coordinated way (which depends on the caudate, cingulate and prefrontal cortex). At the brain biology level, there are more problems with the dopamine 1 receptors in the "mesolimbic" area (which is where dextroamphetamine [Dexedrine] works). Attention problems in FASD (as opposed to pure ADHD) are more likely to have an *earlier* onset. Some of the kids with FASD can be diagnosed as having a regulatory disorder as infants or toddlers. Kids who have attention problems due to FASD, rather than pure ADHD, are *harder to treat* - many experience *more side effects* and find medications, especially Ritalin to

Ritalin

ADHD r FASD

FASD + ADHD Harder to Treat

be *less effective*. Dextroamphetamine is generally a better choice for people who have FASD. People with FASD that have characteristics of ADHD also have more associated learning disabilities, especially in mathematics and higher order language problems such as social understanding. They are also more commonly diagnosed with psychiatric problems, including explosiveness, depression, anxiety and temporal lobe epilepsy (O'Malley, 2007).

Cerebellum helps coordinate the attention system

Paying attention requires smooth functioning in many areas, including the cerebellum, which we know are damaged in FASD. The cerebellum is an amazing little structure tucked in just underneath the back part of our cortex. We usually think of the cerebellum as a coordinator of muscle activity but it also functions like a "quarterback" for the brain's attention system. It coordinates the actions of the brainstem arousal centers, hippocampus, working memory areas and caudate.

To maintain attention, (1) *we have to be awake enough*. Wakefulness depends on noradrenaline. Kim Barthel, an occupational therapist from Victoria, B.C. points out that sensory input channels (hearing, touch, vision, etc) run in the brainstem very close to our arousal center. Sensory input helps wake up the arousal center. Some kids are like Eeyore the donkey - they need more sensory input to wake up, so they rock or spin or fidget or bite their lip to seek this sensory input. *Insisting that such individuals keep still will sabotage their ability to pay attention*. Parents are usually surprised when I offer my "spinney" office chair to these kids, but quite often I can have a very focused conversation with the child *once he can move* and isn't going nuts trying to sit still.

(2) *We also have to be able to focus*. This depends on dopamine. The cerebellum coordinates both the "awake-enough/ arousal" and the "focus" parts of our attention system. The cerebellum is often damaged in FASD - it is smaller, especially the anterior vermis bodies I through V (an evolutionarily older, central part of the cerebellum).

Another factor relevant to attention in FASD is *slower processing*. This leads to *less comprehension*, especially in time-limited tasks (like answering a question on a timed test). When topics *are incompletely understood they are much less interesting* so focus decreases and it is easier to get distracted and off the topic.

Some interesting work in Down Syndrome involves the use of memantadine (Ebixa). This is an Alzheimer medication and is thought to improve the signal-to-noise ratio, which means being able to pay attention to the message (the signal) and suffer less distraction from irrelevant background sounds and sights (the noise). I have not seen studies about the use of this medication for FASD, but it is tempting to try it for some folks when distractibility interferes with attention.

Emotional regulation

In part, emotional regulation depends on a balance between the calming effects of the hippocampus (and frontal lobe) and the "fear, fight/flight, freeze" circuitry in the amygdala and its surrounding structures. "Hippocampus," a big word, is hard to remember; I prefer hippycampus - what do hippies say? "Don't worry, be happy, Peace man!" What happens on a campus? You learn (or at least you are supposed to learn!) Thus, the two main functions of the "hippycampus:" learning (encoding new information plus short term storage of these memories) and calming. I'd also like to suggest a way to remember the amygdala. What do 14 -year-old daughters say coming out of the mall? "Oh my God, Oh my God." This is often abbreviated "OMG" - so one can say, "OMG, OMG, OMyGdala" - which might help us to recall that the "omygdala" is, amongst other things, "fear central." Unfortunately, in FASD, we know that the size and activity of the (calming) "hippycampus" is reduced and the reactivity of the ("OMG!") "omygdala" to stress increases. The result: lots more "freaking out" and less ability to "be cool" in response to a given amount of stress. Those wishing more posh terminology (as the British would say) could put it this way: In FASD, emotional regulation is impaired by kindling of the amygdala, leading to hyper-responsitivity to stressful stimuli, coupled with diminished "self-soothing" due to hypo-responsivity of hippocampal/ prefrontal cortex circuits.

To make matters worse, in FASD-affected individuals, the stress response system called the Hypothalamus, Pituitary, Adrenal (HPA) axis is hyper-responsive to perceived threats. HPA over-activation is a huge topic in mental health. It has major implications for stress reactivity, difficulties in controlling emotions, predisposition to addictions such as alcoholism, depression, and learning problems - in part because of reduced hippocampal memory. The *whole HPA axis is hyper-responsive to stress* in the offspring of rats that were fed alcohol in pregnancy. (Glaves, 2007) Prenatal alcohol exposure has been linked to *persistent impairment in hippocampal neurogenesis* (read: damage to the "new learning" and "calm down" centers). (Klintsona, 2007) Parents and caregivers know about over-reactivity to stress, correction, re-direction or even *very* gently applied discipline.

Epilepsy - also related to the hippocampus

Sorry to skip to the topic of epilepsy - but there is a reason. We are discussing the hippocampus and its importance to new learning, self-calming and stress regulation. Citing his group's very recent work, neurologist Peter Carlen says the hippocampus is also one brain area of focus for genesis of seizures. Peter described a retrospective chart review study of 425 patients with FASD. Almost 18% had some form of seizures - a high prevalence this seasoned neurology researcher described as "staggering." (Bell, 2010) Dr. Carlen's group then studied abnormally hyperexcitable circuits in the hippocampus of alcohol-exposed guinea pigs. He found that the unusual pattern of brain hyperexcitability relates to enhanced "GAP junctional" mechanisms in FASD. Usual ways to block seizure activity - such as blocking neurotransmitter-mediated (GABA and glutamate-mediated) synaptic transmission - *did not stop seizure activity in alcohol-exposed hippocampal cells.* Blocking the GAP junction connections between hippocampal neurons *did stop the seizure activity.* One drug used to stop GAP junction hyperexcitability (and resulting seizures) was carbenoxolone - the active ingredient in licorice!

Why am I torturing readers of FASD 101 with this "doctor-talk?" Dr. Carlen's group thinks that epilepsy is so common that *anyone diagnosed with FASD should have a diagnostic EEG test done to screen for epilepsy*. Dr. Carlen notes that many people have subclinical seizures and can be treated successfully. Further, Carlen questions, "Could seizures be a manifestation of *underlying hyperexcitable brain circuitry in FASD, seen even in those without a history of seizures, which could predispose to ADHD and other psychopathologies?"* This is a whole new approach to causes of mental health problems in FASD. I hope that soon, we may be able to offer hope for treatment-resistant problems - possibly by the use of GAP junction blockers in combination with standard seizure medicines such as valproic acid. (Sutarjono, et al., 2010)

Crisis Management

Our kids often lurch from crisis to crisis - in other words, they go from being overstressed in one way to overstressed in another. I think that Gordon Neufeld provides a useful model for crisis management in (see Neufeld, 2010)

1. Do not try to fix anything in the middle of the crisis.
2. Make it priority, even in the midst of a crisis, to try to hold on to the relationship. After all, it is only through the connection made possible by the relationship that you can communicate with and influence with the child.
3. "Throw the infraction flag down" if you've got an audience and you have to. "This just isn't working today" is all you need to say. That way, onlookers such as siblings can't whine, "that's not fair - he didn't get into trouble!"
4. Let the situation cool down, but not by shunning or shaming or blaming. If someone needs a time out, take it yourself so you can cool down enough to not be too reactive.
5. When the timing is right (tempers have cooled down) and *after* you've got the eye and attention of the child later, if something needs to be said, go ahead.

"Silly, you're just enabling a manipulative child," you say. Please think about it. If you send a child to his room, expect him to think about his "sin," make an internal pledge to not misbehave again, and remember his newfound pledge the next time he is tempted or overstressed, then I ask you to check these assumptions - for *any* kid (or adult!), let alone one with FASD who has stress system and self-regulation hardware issues such as those described above.

"But she can't spazz out this way with her future husband - she'll never stay married - I *have* to teach her right from wrong," you say. Absolutely. These ideas are not about sanctioning or enabling dysfunctional behaviour; they are about trying not to "teach a lesson" or correct kids when they are so overwhelmed that nothing will be learned and all that will happen is they will think you are mean and withdraw. Disciplining a reactive, withdrawn or "ready to take your head off" child is really hard work; I am definitely on a learning curve also. I have repeatedly handled emotionally upsetting situations with family members in ways that could be described as "clumsy and dumb." We can

(continued) →

look to some wise folks for guidance. "Be the change you want to see in the world," said Ghandi. "Failure is only the opportunity to begin again more intelligently" said Henry Ford. You become what you think, attract what you feel, create what you imagine. So be careful what you think, feel and imagine. Caregivers do have choices - be intelligent, think about Dr. Neufeld's ideas for crises and apologize when you blow it. Another Neufeld pearl is not to make criticism or correction of your child *personal* - try "this is just not working" rather than, "you need to stop misbehaving." If the child is upset, just touch the contentious topic gently and then get out of there! *Don't try to teach in the midst of a crisis, wait until things are calmer and you have a good connection with the child - see if you have their eyes and a smile - now they will be receptive to your ideas."*

Having FASD is draining, exhausting and very stressful at times. Our kids need to gradually become experts at management of their own stress. Trying to be an effective caregiver for a child who has FASD can also be draining, exhausting and stressful - as caregivers learn better ways to manage their stress, they can help model useful ideas for their kids too.

Alexithymia (means "no words for emotions" and is common in FASD)

To process emotions we need be able to perceive them, recognize them and name them. Difficulty interpreting facial expressions creates problems at the most basic levels of "perception of emotions." How can we read body language without facial [expression] perception?

We know that alexithymia is common in alcoholism and FASD. A study of fifty alcoholic patients (in recovery) showed more problems with understanding facial expression than control subjects; abstinence does not improve accuracy of understanding the emotions behind others' facial expressions. Those who could not remain abstinent had more problems with understanding facial expression. Thus, those who have troubles understanding negative facial emotions need more help to maintain sobriety. (Foisy, 2007)

Dr. Kim Kerns at the University of Victoria Psychology Department is working with a group of kids who are affected by FASD. She is hoping that direct work on teaching what facial expressions mean may help.

Self-regulation of emotions for adults means not spazzing out when your landlord is mean, and not yelling at your kid if he yells at you; for children it means not hitting your sister if she gets something first, staying in school even if you hate math, and not always needing to get your way.

Mentalization

Once we can start to 1) self-regulate our emotions and 2) focus our attention, then life gets really interesting, because these two skills allows us to develop curiosity about what's on other people's minds, as well as the ability to stand back and consider what our own thoughts are. *Mentalization* is the term Peter Fonagy uses for "knowing what is on your mind and others' minds." Mentalization forms the basis for empathy, accurate interpretation of body language, impulse control and understanding boundaries (accurately figuring out "this is me/this is mine" and "that is you/that is yours"). Dr. Fonagy says that it is by the reflections of an attuned caregiver, usually mum, that baby *learns to control his emotions*. Firstly, mum reads what is going on in her child - "well…I just fed him and burped him so I guess this crying just means he wants a cuddle." Secondly, she mirrors this back to baby in a kindly way - "hey kid, don't worry, it'll be okay, you just need a hug and cuddle." Thirdly, baby, who is born with few ways to moderate his emotions, starts to develop a *core psychological self* initially, by attuning to mum and letting her bring him down from his upset, which in some "pre-language way" tells the child that upset does not need to go on forever, *I can depend on mum to help me solve upsetting problems and eventually even help me relax; being calm is possible.*

Consider mum. She cannot really provide this attentive feedback for her child (she cannot accurately mentalize what is on baby's mind) if she's worried about her own safety because of domestic abuse or is preoccupied with caring for 3 toddlers as well as baby. But if we believe Dr. Fonagy, hers is the most important job in the world - to actually grow the core of her baby's ability to self regulate emotions, recognize himself as separate from her, and eventually to learn to respect boundaries and take responsibility for himself. (Fonagy, 2009) Mentalization is at the very core of our humanity. Extended family looking after her other kids so she can devote more energy to the baby, getting grandpa to help, good daycares to care for baby, treating her postpartum depression or PTSD - *whatever it takes - let's support mums enough so they can grow their children's brains.*

Coping with kids who don't do as they are told can be very draining - off-the-wall humor sometimes helps. I have found that not very far under the surface of political correctness many folks working in this area have a quirky, sometimes slightly dark sense of humor. These little zingers have helped me: "If you're going through hell, keep going," said Winston Churchill. "What will you do if all your problems aren't solved by the time you die?" questioned an unknown source. "Young psychologists can find a 'natural consequence' for anything; then they have kids. Old psychologists are all developmentalists," says Gordon Neufeld. My favourite is "For every expert, there is an equal and opposite expert" by Arthur C. Clark.

Working with kids affected by FASD grows us (the caregivers and professionals) up also! "How FASD forces parents to confront strategies and ways of thinking that don't work and modify them would be a good book to write - if I had time," said Dr. Stirling Clarren a few years ago at a conference in Regina. Compliance by coercion doesn't work. Gramma's advice seldom works. People who say, "That (mis) behaviour never occurs at my house, I don't know what you are doing wrong" should probably be "beaten away with a stick," as comic writer Dave Berry puts it. Unfortunately, FASD is not usually an important part of training curricula for psychologists, psychiatrists, primary care doctors, nurses, social workers, early childhood professionals, teachers, police, judges, lawyers or many other people who interact with our kids on a daily basis. I hope this book can be used to support such curriculum development. Most lessons from this book apply to kids and adults with *any* developmental disability, especially head injuries (traumatic brain injuries). However, understanding nuances of how prenatal alcohol exposure changes the brain can lead to better intervention strategies and that is why FASD brain differences are discussed in some detail.

Eye problems

Eye problems can be extensive, probably affect at least thirty to forty percent of kids who have FASD, and are usually not diagnosed. FASD-affected children often have fewer nerves in their retinas (optic nerve hypoplasia), reduced clarity of vision (poor acuity), and difficulty *moving* their eyes together in a coordinated way (conjugate gaze problems). Eye globe size is often reduced. This affects the clearness of their vision. Squint is a common problem. Coordination of gaze is very important for fluent reading (and understanding of content). (Stromland, 1996)

Standard optometry or ophthalmology visits may not assess or treat these issues. Although access to ***developmental optometrists*** is not always easy, I believe that seeing these folks is worth the trip. I live in rural British Columbia, half way between Vancouver and Calgary - the closest developmental optometrist is a four-hour drive away. One mum said, "after struggling for his first five school years, and several pairs of glasses not helping, my son is finally making some progress" (after doing a series of eye muscle exercises that the developmental optometrist suggested). Interested readers are advised to access developmental optometry websites such as those listed in the appendix.

Muscle coordination

Damage to the parietal lobe and cerebellum (two areas we know are harmed by prenatal exposure to alcohol) affects the quality of both fine motor and gross motor movements. Fine motor movements include writing, smooth coordination of eye muscles (oculo-motor tasks), and well-organized chewing, swallowing and tongue movements (oral motor tasks). Picky eaters often have *major problems with coordination of their mouth muscles.* Pediatric gastroenterologists (gut specialists) work with occupational therapists (O.T.s) trained in sensory integration to help kids with swallowing and other eating problems. Suitable accommodations for *eye muscle coordination* problems include: allowing of extra time for writing and reading, assigning a note-taker for a student, or providing a computer with voice recognition software. Anticipation of the movement of objects in space sounds like an austere "doctory" concept - nope! This *prediction* of movements over time - for instance, "will that car hit me?" - depends on coordinated eye movements, sequencing and the brain's accurate representation of where the car will be in the future. We know these prediction skills can be poor in some people with FASD. Traffic safety must be taught with these issues in mind. Gross motor problems often involve clumsiness; in this situation it is wise to avoid team sports in favour of individual exercise/leisure activities that can be enjoyed later in life, such as swimming and bowling. On the other hand, exuberant physicality is often a strength, a great way to blow off steam and self-regulate - kids need to be encouraged to do all the sports/activities that they can. Remember your helmet!! Kids with FASD already have one brain injury and sure don't need another.

Learning problems

IQ is largely a function of the back part of your brain. *Adaptive function* mostly relates to the front part of your brain. Average IQ for those with FASD is in the low 80s. About 15% of those with FASD have an IQ below 70, which is considered the intellectually disabled range. There is a much larger problem, though, with adaptive function. Diane Russell is a psychologist in Nanaimo, B.C. who has tested *more than a hundred* children who have FASD and found *only two* that had adaptive function scores (measured by such tests as Scales of Independent Behavior-Revised (SIBR) or Vineland) as high as their IQ. Usually, there is a very large gap - average adaptive function is in the 60s or below, which is more than twenty points lower than average IQ scores. *Adaptive function is a more accurate predictor of ability to live independently than IQ.* IQ lets you pass tests in school. Dr. Sterling Clarren has suggested that often kids with FASD can pass tests yet flunk life.

Sensory issues make it harder for kids to get a clear signal from what they are trying to see or hear. Importantly, a *muddled or ambiguous* sensory input is really *hard to remember*. Coping strategies for this problem include teaching topics using hands-on kinesthetic experiences and making sure that distractions are minimized. Poor memory due to hippocampal damage is also seen in FASD. We know that the hippocampus contains less "brain fertilizer" (called BDNF) after prenatal exposure to alcohol. BDNF helps grow new nerve cells in the hippocampus that are required for retaining memory. The cerebellum, another area often damaged in FASD, coordinates attention. Of course, we can only learn what we can pay attention to. In FASD, learning is often *context specific.* I have seen students learn where middle C is when playing a particular piece of piano music, but the same students are *unable* to locate middle C on the next page! They must re-learn where middle C is in the new piece (the new context). Teachers, parents and bosses assume lessons learned in one situation to be generalized to another, similar situation. If only this assumption was true life would be so much easier for those with FASD! Possible strategies for problems with generalization include teaching in different contexts, role playing and making learning situations as realistic as possible. As previously mentioned, mathematics/arithmetic and higher order (e.g. social use of language) language learning disabilities are common.

Learning from mistakes

How do we learn important *life lessons*? At least one way is to learn from our mistakes. This requires us to accept that we have made a mistake (which is a *vulnerable* position - a place anyone who had been traumatized would avoid) and openness to trying another solution (which requires cognitive *flexibility* - a skill often damaged in FASD). When we are wrong, we need to realize it and, instead of clinging to our position, direct problem-solving energy in a different direction, i.e., to try something different. None of us could lower our guard enough to try new solutions if we were too defended or hardened or armored because we felt unsafe or overly vulnerable. Tragically, often children with FASD have lived very chaotic, hard lives - being defended and "invulnerable" is often a necessary survival strategy. Few of us could emerge from abusive early family experiences without being guarded and suspicious. Suppressing skills that defend against harm in dangerous situations (hyper-alert vigilance and defensiveness) is never a goal. However, gradually understanding that there *are also safe circumstances* where it is reasonable to allow vulnerability and be open to others' influence can *allow* learning!

"Defendedness" can help protect us in abusive circumstances.

"I wish I had not prescribed a sedative without first asking him if he was in a safe place," a psychiatrist told me. She was responding to disabling sleep deprivation affecting a desperate young man. His abusive uncle later molested the young man - this has haunted the psychiatrist since. She worries that the lowering of her patient's guard, caused by the sedatives she prescribed, contributed to the sexual assault. She wishes she'd helped the young man access safe housing *first* and *then* treated the sleep deprivation.

Possible intervention for defensive, guarded people

Focus on safety in the relationship. Interested readers wanting additional ideas for understanding traumatized children could obtain a copy of Dave Zeigler's book, *Raising Children Who Refuse to be Raised.* (Zeigler, 2000) Ziegler points out that developing the trust of traumatized people often takes years. Once working relationships are achieved, kids, especially older kids, can be scripted to take up a relationship with their own thinking difficulties. Children's self-advocacy might sound like this:

- » Those instructions are too fast for me.
- » It would help if you could write them down, please.
- » I am not making much progress on this right now. I will come back to it in about ten minutes.

Self-advocacy

I don't know a better self-advocate than Myles Himmelreich, and I recommend that readers look at his interview in the DVD included with this book or the *FASD Relationships* website.

Abstract thought

Abstract thinking is often difficult for kids with FASD. That is why in Grade five or so, when long division is introduced, and in Grade eight or nine, when algebra is introduced, kids typically struggle more.

Missing "little things"

Psychologists can test this by making a very large "D" out of a bunch of little "Y"s. The right brain sees the big picture, the big D. The left side sees the little details, the little "Y"s. As we have discussed, the right-left communication channel (corpus callosum) is often damaged in FASD, so putting the big picture together with the little details can be slow. Kids with FAS have great trouble with this test - they often copy the big D but miss the little Y. Aside from the corpus callosum, I do not know where the exact site(s) of damage are. However, obviously, if kids cannot pay attention to the little things they may not get the gist of something that is complex.

Sleep - it's *supposed* to be an oasis of restoration

Melatonin, made by the pineal gland in the middle of the brain in response to darkness, is a wonderful hormone. Amongst its numerous actions (including antioxidant activity and enhancing the immune system) melatonin binding to its receptors helps to bring on sleep. Prenatal alcohol and other toxins can damage the pineal gland (Jan, 2007) and lower levels of melatonin can be found in children with FASD. (Jan, 2010) Melatonin levels *ought to rise* when a person is exposed to very dim light. Recent work in Toronto has revealed fragmented sleep patterns (including delayed sleep onset) possibly related to reduced ability to make melatonin in response to dim light in children with FASD. (Goril, 2010)

In a Seattle study up to 50% of kids with prenatal alcohol exposure had sleep problems, primarily too little sleep.

Fragmented sleep and sleep apnea were also observed. Investigators suggested that sleep problems contributed to extreme daytime hyperactivity. (Bonthius, 2006) A study of 325 Canadian children with FASD confirmed shorter sleep duration and also showed delayed sleep onset. Other problems identified included night terrors (74 children), sleep-walking (10 children), and waking more than twice during the night (169 children). (Stade, 2010)

Neurologist James Jan and his colleagues recently published "Sleep Health Issues for Children with FASD: Clinical Considerations" This comprehensive review notes medical issues such as allergies, obstructive sleep apnea, esophageal reflux and chronic pain that interfere with sleep. Children's comprehension/memory problems and caregiver exhaustion can limit success of any "sleep hygiene" (rituals of predictable bedtime wind-down) interventions. Melatonin pills can be a very helpful intervention. (Jan, 2010) I particularly recommend caregivers download a copy of "Recommendations for Sleep Health" from Dr. Jan's article. (Jan, 2010)

Clinically, many kids with FASD are very restless sleepers. Family members complain, "she kicks off all her covers and if we go camping no one wants to sleep next to her - they'd wake up black and blue!" Video recordings that confirm excessive limb movement are starting to raise the question of whether restless legs syndrome or similar nocturnal movement disorders could be more common in FASD. (Chan, 2010) Recently, I have identified several patients with FASD who have obstructive sleep apnea symptoms (breath-holding, loud snoring and daytime sleepiness) and possible restless legs syndrome (involuntary leg movements at rest often associated with unpleasant tingling or "pins and needles" sensations). These patients have been referred to sleep clinics for definitive diagnosis. Since both obstructive sleep apnea and restless legs syndrome have many evidence-based treatments I am optimistic that I can offer some help for these patients' sleep disruptions soon. At present, I do not think there are any published studies of specific techniques to address sleep apnea or restless legs in persons affected by FASD.

To summarize, children's sleep disruptions may impair daytime attention, learning, and behaviour and contribute to daytime hyperactivity. Caregivers can try Dr. Jan's sleep hygiene measures and also give their children supplemental melatoinin. Sleep apnea and restless legs syndrome should be treated if kids have symptoms of either.

Yes, sleep deprivation can result in grouchy kids and weary, exhausted parents but psychologist Ellen Frank suggests disrupted routines can cause mental health problems. She says we are all rhythmic creatures; sleep-wake cycles, menstrual cycles, and cortisol cycles are just a few examples of the many biological rhythms that are *the foundation* of how we maintain our equilibrium. Disruptions in *social rhythms* (for example, time of waking, time we first talk with another person in the morning, time of eating, time of sleep onset) change biological cycles enough to predispose vulnerable individuals to mania and/or depression. Restoration of these social rhythms to a more normal pattern is the focus Dr. Frank's 2005 book *Treating Bipolar Disorder: A Clinician's Guide to Interpersonal and Social Rhythm Therapy* and is an effective treatment for not only manic symptoms but also depression, especially in teens and young adults. (Frank, 2010)

Many of my patients live in chaos; life is a series of disruptions and threats caused by poverty, violence, evictions and homelessness. I believe Dr. Franks ideas offer a partial explanation of why so many decompensate after yet another disruptive crisis. For example, a middle-aged lady (who has FASD, seizures and traumatic brain injuries) had managed to maintain a good balance for years by adhering to rigid routines: Monday-laundry, then the shelter for lunch, then busk at the mall; Tuesday-bath, then lunch at a different shelter, then sing with friends in the afternoon, Wednesday-doctor appointment and get this week's pills, lunch at the clubhouse, etc. She carried around a book with all appointments written in it and many songs written out - all in her favourite keys, with all the chords and melodies. Music is her passion and is sustaining for her; she's a great accordion player and a good singer. Someone bought her some beer, she went home drunk which violated the landlord's rules so she was evicted. Someone stole her accordion in the shelter, so she took off and lived on the street. Her book got soaked with rain, she forgot her doctor's appointments and forgot about her pills. She got mad, tried to commit suicide, was briefly hospitalized, released after 2 days, and as she walked out of the hospital she started banging on a car. Soon she'll be in front of a judge (again)...imagine the cost to society and how battered this lady's self-esteem is. I think she "lost it" because, predictably, her social routines became chaotic after she was evicted. Her body's biological rhythms soon were massively disrupted and she became irritable, violent, depressed and lost control. Society's legal response is off the mark - she needs stable housing so she can get back into her predictable routines - these are her lifeblood. In my experience, Dr. Frank's concept (that mental health depends on maintenance of the social rhythms that, in turn, stabilize biologic rhythms) is even more important for those affected by FASD. Interventions that do not enhance predictable social rhythms are counterproductive.

More research is needed to definitively confirm whether an association between prenatal alcohol exposure and sudden infant death syndrome (SIDS) exists. On a theoretical basis, this association is likely because prenatal alcohol reduces the number and activity of serotonin neurons in critical areas of the brainstem (chemoceptors) that recognize low oxygen and high carbon dioxide levels from reduced breathing during sleep and immediately signal brainstem arousal centers to wake up the person before lack of oxygen causes death. (Zhou, 2005) A 1990 study of 2143 infants born to mothers recently treated for substance abuse problems in Los Angles showed the incidence of SIDS to be increased by *7.4 times*. (Ward, 1990) Tobacco use contributes towards the increased incidence of SIDS in children born to recovering drug-addicted mothers (Koren, 2010) but I suspect that prenatal alcohol exposure is also a significant risk factor.

If they believe the risk of SIDS is elevated, caregiver's main concern is what can be done to reduce the danger. Children who die of SIDS have less of a certain kind of serotonin receptor (serotonin 1A receptor) in their brainstem chemoceptor (oxygen and carbon dioxide monitoring) areas. Growing more 1A receptors would help but I don't think even animal researchers are close to discovering how to do that. Caregivers can avoid known risk factors by not swaddling, or placing blankets over a child's head, removing sheepskin pads and polystyrene bead pillows from where the baby sleeps, and not bed-sharing with infants. Caregivers should also keep the bedroom temperature at 18 degrees Celsius or less, *room-share* with infants up to five or six months of age and use a pacifier after age one month because these measures are protective factors. (Corwin, 2007)

Part Two: "Secondary Disabilities," brain differences that develop later - after a child has been exposed to environmental stressors

Current understanding suggests that if appropriate supports are not in place, a child may develop what we call secondary disabilities. Diane Malbin points out that chronic frustration results when kids with FASD are not able to meet society's (unrealistic) expectations. This frustration can result in secondary disabilities, which include:

1. Disrupted school experiences (defined as being expelled, suspended or dropping out)
2. Trouble with the law (defined as being charged or convicted of a crime, arrested or otherwise in trouble with the law)
3. Mental health problems
4. Alcohol and drug abuse or dependency
5. Inappropriate sexual behaviour (defined as inappropriate sexual advances, sexual touching or promiscuity)
6. Confinement to inpatient psychiatric care, inpatient drug dependency programs or incarcerated.

Adult patients may have two additional secondary disabilities:

7. Dependent living (living with family or friends, group home or some sort of assisted living)
8. Problems with employment (defined as requiring ongoing job training or coaching, not being able to keep a job, or unemployment.) (Streissguth, 1997)

Secondary disabilities are a parent's, teacher's and government official's nightmare. They are costly to deal with and destroy lives.

Diane Malbin has found that it is possible to reduce these secondary disabilities by training those who are involved in an FASD-affected individual's life to ensure that environmental expectations are appropriate.

Since 1996 we have known that the following are all **universal protective factors** against developing secondary disabilities:

1. Living is a stable nurturing home over 72% of life

2. *Early* diagnosis (prior to age 6)
3. Safety (never having experienced violence against oneself)
4. Stability (staying in each living situation at least 2.8 years)
5. Experiencing a good quality home in middle childhood (age 8-12)
6. Access to supportive services designed for developmentally disabled persons
7. Paradoxically, being diagnosed with Fetal Alcohol Syndrome rather than partial Fetal Alcohol Syndrome
8. Having basic needs met for at least 13% of life (Streissguth, 1996)

The potency of these **protective factors** *can* give hope to caregivers and policy direction ideas to health care planners:

- Odds of disrupted school experiences, mental health problems, and inappropriate sexual behavior are reduced by all 8 universal protective factors
- Trouble with the law is reduced by all universal protective factors but especially by eligibility for supportive services designed for developmentally disabled persons
- Confinement is reduced by all universal protective factors but especially by living in a stable, nurturing environment and early diagnosis
- Alcohol and drug problems are reduced by all universal protective factors but also by an additional factor: having lived with an alcohol abuser for a shorter time (i.e. less than 30% of life)

Streissguth, et al. have identified that the percentage of time spent in a stable, nurturing home environment is *the most influential protective factor,* reducing the odds of occurrence of most secondary disabilities by three- or four-fold. (Streissguth, 2004)

How often do family support services ensure that enough support is available for families that protective measures are achieved? I have lived the reality of having a diagnosed child in my family for sixteen years, so I can answer this question: Not as often as we'd all like. Our family, even in crisis, was never offered case management or respite services. Most cases of FASD are unrecognized, undiagnosed and untreated. What are the odds of planners of family support services ensuring that these protective factors are offered to those families? Even smaller.

A stable, nurturing home can be the result *if* caregivers are empowered and equipped.

I believe that that if caregivers and professionals looking after kids who have FASD can understand a bit about *why* problems occur, *which* part of the brain is affected and *how*, we will be better able to address problems, experience less tension with our kids, and have happier kids and encouraged parents. *Empowered parents are the key to their kid's success*. How else could kids access the stable, nurturing home that is such a powerful protective factor?

There are "Mum and Dad" (for a general audience) parts of this book and "Doctor" (for Health Professionals) parts. I hope that the "Mum and Dad" parts help parents, teachers and other non-medically trained stakeholders. The "Doctor" parts are designed to help health professionals understand more about FASD and how to assist families. I expect that a parole officer in Saskatoon is going to pick up this book, turn *immediately* to the "Genetics in FASD Doctor" part, and then hiss at me for talking about single nucleotide polymorphisms (SNPs). Beware! I will hiss back, "You were warned to stay outta there buddy!"

None Medical Professional!

WARNING! —

Psychologists and doctors *should* hiss at me if I *don't* talk about the SNPs that relate to alcoholism - that's why I discuss SNPs *in their part of the book*! Remember, kids will benefit if both caregivers and professionals get interested and learn more about FASD *so just know your place and don't hiss at me*, Mr. Parole Officer! (Just kidding)

This book's modules could be adapted for curricula development. I'd like that because I sense a need. As of 2010, the psychiatric residents* I spoke with at recent Canadian and American Psychiatric Association meetings did *not* have didactic teaching about FASD (or Sensory Processing Disorder) in their training. This is a shame, a barrier to FASD becoming more widely recognized, and part of why I wrote the "Health Professional" parts of this book.

Shame!

*Psychiatric Residents: The only lingo this "prove it to me mister" crew seem to understand is the tedious world of "level A evidence in placebo controlled, randomized clinical trials" so, out-of-necessity, "Doctor" parts of the book will "talk Dr. lingo."

Genetics and Secondary Disabilities (summary for Dads - and Mums)

"This is FASD 101," you protest, "don't talk about SNPs." Okay you win. Keeners will want to look at the health professional's version of Genetics and FASD, but we can summarize some useful recent information and still keep the lingo civilized.

We each have 46 chromosomes of genetic material (half from mum and half from dad) arranged in 23 pairs. We each have 25,000 genes. We now know *where* each gene is located and how genes can *vary*. Even more important information is the question of **epigenetics**: how to *turn off* or *turn on* any given gene. (Cloud, 2010) Genes causing increased risk for alcoholism are better understood than genes that cause increased risk of most other mental health issues. This is partly due to studies that have analyzed the genes of thousands of family members of alcoholics (see Family study, NIAAA in the appendix) and partly due to dumb luck. (The poor guys researching which genes increase the risk of manic depression tried the same methods - analyze all the genes of at-risk family members, see which genes show up more commonly and figure out what those genes do - and on their "fishing trip" they've been skunked - ouch!!)

No one wants to change a gene. The name of the genetics research game is to 1) understand the risk factors which produce a problem, 2) find the genes associated with those risk factors and 3) understand the mechanisms through which those genes work. The better we understand risks, genes and mechanisms, the better we should be able to provide early identification and prevention of any disorder, FASD included. (Schuckit, 2009)

In 2010, we know about half the genes that increase risk of problems from alcohol

Any one gene only increases risk by a small amount. For example, a certain type of the **GABRA2** gene increases risk of alcohol dependence by twenty percent. Genes affecting the risk of alcohol dependency may also affect other conditions. For example, that same type of GABRA2 gene discussed above increases the risk of social problems (chances of being *able to stay married* are reduced *six times*.) Recognizing a profound issue with alcoholism in a patient's family, I described more details of what has been recently understood about GABRA2 to a healthy young professional lady who drinks "one or two glasses of wine per day." People with GABRA2 are more likely to be dependent on *both* alcohol *and* drugs,

20%

begin drinking heavily at a younger age, go on larger binges, and experience more profound withdrawal symptoms. They are also more likely to have mental health issues, such as conduct disorder as a child or antisocial personality disorder as adults, and are more likely to have accidents due to risk-taking behaviour. "Crap!" this young woman exclaimed, *"That's my family!* Dad's in jail, Uncle Bob is too, Bob's kid is hard to get along with and threatens her sisters, everyone has hangovers from hell, everyone binges big time. I've *never* had just one 'social' drink. I am worried about my son!" Giving some literature extolling abstinence to her 14 year-old son who has this level of genetic risk is like tossing a copy of the Canada Food Guide at the obese daughter of a 30-year-old poorly controlled diabetic. These examples are not minor risk factor levels for trivial disease; both deserve ongoing *aggressive* intervention efforts. The mum decided she'd get her son more involved in youth group activities and a jazz band, hoping that would help him avoid the heavy-drinking peers that he was starting to hang out with. She sent him on a Sail and Life Training Society (SALTS) (website: www.salts.ca/) trip to help him see that fun and interesting people don't all drink and that great activities need not involve alcohol. She sent him to Uncle Joe's in Calgary - Joe has a woodworking shop and her son wants to learn to use the lathe. What's the result so far? Her son is 16 and not very interested in booze-- he thinks it's "kinda lame" - and he's *nuts* about a girl he met at SALTS. She does not like alcohol. Bottom line: If you've got a high genetic risk, don't just think about doing something some day; really "get off the can" and *robustly change your environment*. Be passive and this level of genetic risk could clobber you and your family.

Example

FASD, as we've seen, involves many different behaviours and traits. What genes could my child inherit that might put him or her at risk for problems, especially the secondary disabilities? parents ask.

This is the list of genetic conditions I discussed recently at the 2010 Alberta FASD Conference in my *Genetics and FASD* Workshop:

» Sensory Processing Disorder: Oversensitivity to sound and touch has about 50% heritability. (Goldsmith, 2006)

» Impulsivity has an overall heritability of up to 75%. This trait is associated with early and risky sexual behaviour, including lower rates of condom and contraception use, which increases sexually transmitted disease, unintended pregnancy and prenatal exposure to alcohol. (Cavazos- Rehg, 2008)

» Emotional lability or "dyscontrol" is a little harder to study than the impulsivity trait but has about 50% heritability. (Paris, 2003)

» There are several categories of genes that increase risk for alcohol problems. Mark Schuckit has developed models that show that a *family history* of alcoholism predicts that a person (of any age) will have a low level of response (it takes a lot of alcohol before he or she feels tipsy). In turn, the *low level of response predicts alcohol problems in 40-year-olds, their 17- year-old kids, and even a sample of 13-year-olds who were just at the earliest stages of drinking.* Dr. Schuckitt says that low level of response is a genetic trait and pointed out many of the genes that increase risk of this trait. (Schuckitt, 2009)

Different mental health issues have varying degrees of heritability: manic depression (bipolar disorder) is up to 70% heritable, (Stovall, 2009)), ADHD may have up to 76% heritability, alcohol dependence has a 50-60% heritability (Gelernter, 2009), borderline personality disorder is thought to be about 69% heritable, (Paris, 2003) and heritability of "externalizing" behaviours (predisposition to conduct disorder, antisocial personality disorder and a substance abuse) is up to 80%. (Gelernter and Kranzler, 2009)

A Preliminary List of how Heritable Conditions influence Secondary Disabilities

(Heritability figures for various risk factors or mental health issues are in parentheses.)

» Disrupted school experiences *might be related* to emotional lability (50%), externalizing behaviour (80%), ADHD/ impulsivity (76%), oversensitivity to sound and touch (50%), or problem drinking (50-60%).

» Trouble with the law *is often associated with* externalizing behaviours (80%), ADHD/ impulsivity (76%), alcohol problems (50-60%), and *may be related to* emotional dyscontrol (50%).

» Mental health problems include bipolar disorder (up to 70%), borderline personality disorder

(69%), ADHD (76%), substance abuse/dependence (50-60%) and antisocial personality disorder/ externalizing symptoms (80%).

- Alcohol and drug abuse or dependency is 50-60% heritable.
- Inappropriate sexual behaviour may be influenced by impulsivity (75%), substance abuse (50%)or mental health problems (heritability of 30-70% depending on the diagnosis)
- Confinement to inpatient psychiatric care, inpatient drug dependency programs or incarcerated is influenced by mental health issues (30-70%), impulsivity (75%), and substance abuse (50-60%)
- Dependent living is influenced by impulsivity (75%), mental health issues (30-70%) and substance abuse (50-60%)
- Problems with employment are impacted by impulsivity (75%), mental health issues (30-70%), substance abuse (50-60%), and startle responses to unexpected touch or noise (50%)

Others who are more familiar with the heritability of learning disorders, behavioural problems and problems of social attachment such as reactive attachment disorder could add to this list.

I'd like to see our present concept of secondary disabilities updated to include recent understandings of genetics. People with FASD *are born with* a genetic predisposition to develop what we now call secondary disabilities. It is a bit radical for "a little old rural G.P." to want to "tweak" a paradigm. However, there is a payoff, I believe. If we could shift our focus to the study of the risky genes our kids carry and learn how to help them *not express* those genetic tendencies, the world would be a better place indeed. That's my dream and it is possible.

Rant Number Four: Blaming Parents

I'd like to see an end to parents being blamed (and especially blaming themselves) for adverse outcomes their kids might have. You bet - try to do the best job you can, but then get off your own case, because up to eighty percent of a bad outcome is heritable anyways. The real quest is helping kids who carry big-league genetic predispositions to nasty problems *avoid expressing those genes*. Shame and blame has no room in this quest - we are too busy for that destructive crud. So BE RADICAL ----AND EXPLOIT THE MEASLEY TWENTY TO FIFTY PERCENT THAT YOU CAN INFLUENCE FOR ALL IT'S

WORTH! Then go have a nice nap! Don't let yourself get reactive and grouchy - you'll export those attitudes onto your kids and that'll make life harder.

Read Bruce Perry's *Born to Love: Why Empathy is Essential - and Endangered* and Lucy Jane Miller's *Sensational Kids: Hope and Help for Children with Sensory Processing Disorder.* Both of these books explain therapies that have successfully re-wired the brains of kids who have been exposed to trauma or damaging substances, or those who were born prematurely. Re-wiring is not scary, it is constructive; Bruce Perry would say it is the foundation for success. If you are not sure where to begin (and the situation is complex: abuse, head injury, FASD, chaotic life, sensory problems) read Dave Ziegler's *Raising Children who Refuse to be Raised.* Start with safety for yourself and the child.

Being a parent of a child with FASD is a whole lot like being a primary care doctor. Last week, in one morning, I saw two kids with learning problems caused by FASD, an elderly fellow who has widespread colon cancer, a lady with PTSD, a little boy with abdominal pain, a man worried about his wife's depression and declining memory, a man trying to deal with chronic pain from a pelvic fracture and a lady with restless leg syndrome - its an *infinite* job - there is no way I can be expert with each of these issues; I could worry myself into ill health trying! So…in order to *be as effective as I can be* I need to let go of any illusions of absolute control I might have - try to keep up to date at least as well as the guy whose office is down the street and relax and have a good sleep. It's the same with parenting a child who has FASD. It's an infinite job. Nobody can do it perfectly. There's a ton to learn but if we worry too much we'll become too wound up to learn. The best option is to do what we can and then put our feet up and have a good snooze - with a clear conscience and peace of mind. Tomorrow needs us!

3) Caregiver Distress

The extent of caregiver distress

I have come to understand the deep level of commitment and - unfortunately - the level of distress of primary caregivers. I have adapted Dr. Betsy Robinson's Caregiver Strain Index. (Robinson, 1983) This was originally developed to assess stress in Alzheimer caregivers. It has twelve questions, answered "yes" or "no," and a score of *7 or above* indicates enough strain that the caregiver is likely to suffer physical illness.

Questions include:

1. Is sleep disturbed because your child is in and out of bed or wanders around at night?
2. Is the time spent helping your child an inconvenience for you?
3. Has the effort and concentration required to look after your child become a physical strain?
4. Is the restriction of your free time due to looking after your child confining?
5. Have there been family adjustments due to lack of privacy or because helping your child has disrupted routines?
6. Has looking after your child caused changes to personal plans, such as not being able to go on a vacation, having to turn down a job, etc.?
7. Has looking after your child placed other demands on your time, such as attending to additional concerns of other family members?
8. Has some of your child's behaviour been upsetting - for example, "taking" things?
9. Have there been emotional adjustments, for instance because of severe arguments?
10. Have there been work adjustments, for instance having to take time off work?
11. Has looking after your child caused financial strain?
12. Have you felt completely overwhelmed, for instance because of worry about your child, concerns about how you will manage or worry about the future?

The first group of thirty parents I did this assessment with had an average score of *10.5/12*. A much bigger group of almost 300 had similar scores. Remember that a score of *7 or above* indicates enough strain that the caregiver is likely to suffer physical illness. Recent work by Dr. Heather Carmichael Olson's group in Seattle has used the Parenting Stress Inventory (PSI) as a measure of parental distress. Several years ago, Dr. Carmichael Olson told me the PSI assessment tool was designed for families with kids who had physical (not behavioural/cognitive) difficulties and that it was difficult to capture the level of distress that caregivers of FASD-affected individuals experience with the PSI. I recommend readers look at her recent publication: *Family Matters. Restoring Hope: Empowering caregivers raising children who have FASD* (Olson, 2009)

One of the most helpful parts of Dr. Carmichael Olsen's *Family Matters* article is the list of "Top Unmet Important Family Needs of Caregivers Raising children with FASD and Behavior Problems." By now, readers will appreciate that I find Dr. Gordon Neufeld's DVD parenting courses helpful; I have undertaken the training to become a facilitator of these courses. The last dozen or so caregivers who have taken Dr Neufeld's "*Vital Connection*" course which I facilitated provided feedback. Larger numbers would be required to conduct a scientific study and to *prove* my hypothesis (that this Vital Connection course is effective in combating parental stress); a control group that did not receive the parenting course would need to show significantly less improvement than course participants to prove effectiveness. Participants included eight parents/grandparents looking after a total of twelve kids who have FASD, plus three other parents looking after seven kids who do not have FASD but have been affected by family strife and disruptions. The DVD course is taught in eight sessions, two and a half hours each. Topics include: stages of attachment, how attachments with parents and other caregivers are meant to develop; what keeps a child from developing/ maintaining deep relationships with adults who care for him/her; how to connect with children even when they are drawing away from us; how to address the roots of aggression; how we can maintain strong links with our children when they are subjected to huge forces from competing attachments such as peers or manipulative ex-spouses; and how to discipline in ways that do not divide. I find the content of this course to be relevant and practical; I also like to make caregivers of kids with FASD aware of some relevant aspects of the brain biology of FASD. In each session, the DVD lasts an hour and then there is extensive time for discussion.

I find that too many courses on FASD deliver a huge amount of information in too short a time, at break-neck speed, with hard-to-decipher powerpoints! The facilitated Neufeld DVD course is a very different model - equipping participants with practical skills they understand and actually use right away - that is why I've wanted to teach and understand this approach.

Figure 6

Parental Need/Desire	# Responding	Before course	After course
Sense of being able to cope with behaviours*	7	1.9	3.4
Being able to share feelings about parenting with someone who has gone through similar experiences*	7	2.9	3.7
Ability to understand child's thoughts and behaviours*	11	2.2	3.7
Ability to have realistic expectations re: behaviour and thinking of child*	5	2.5	4.0
Ideas that help if your child is upset or acting strange*	7	2.6	3.4
Ability to modify your response to the child's behaviour	4	2.0	2.9
Sense of effectiveness as a parent	9	2.5	3.6
Sense of confidence as a parent/grandparent	11	2.4	3.4
Feeling empowered as a parent/ grandparent	11	2.2	3.4
Peace of mind	4	1.3	2.5

Scale: 1=very low 2=low 3= OK 4=optimal

*Figure 6. notes: The first five Parental Needs/Desires (marked *) are from Dr. Heather Carmichael Olsen's list of "Unmet Important Family Needs from Caregivers Raising children with FASD and Behavior Problems." (Olson, 2009) The next five Parental Needs/Desires, situated lower in figure 6, are goals that Dr. Gordon Neufeld hopes his DVD courses can meet. These preliminary data suggest some progress towards addressing unmet caregiver needs can be attained with this initiative.*

I presented this information as Poster 6: Restoring hope: an adapted attachment-parenting DVD series empowers caregivers of children who have FASD at the September 14, 2010 Fetal Alcohol Canadian Expertise (FACE) meeting in Vancouver. (Densmore, 2010) The abstract my poster presentation can be viewed at the Journal of Population Therapeutics and Clinical Pharmacology website listed in the appendix.

Figure 6: Results of the Vital Connection course I facilitated for parents/grandparents - the facilitation involved discussion of how to adapt Dr. Neufeld's concepts for children with the types of brain differences of FASD

Difficulties finding accurate parental stress assessment tools aside, parenting a child with FASD has pushed my personal mental health and financial resources to the limit (and past) many times. My wife is a Pediatric O.T. with extensive training in early childhood development and sensory integration. Often, we have been stumped because we didn't know how to solve or even think about a problem. Often, despite having huge networks of knowledgeable colleagues, we have not been able to address important problems that affected our whole family. Work places *can* be supportive. Many are the opposite. Readers might think that other doctors who have been involved in care of my family might be understanding of my child's FASD, or at least open to some information about it - some have been and I am very grateful to them. Others have been the opposite. Sigh. If you get the picture that parenting can be a costly, lonely, harrowing, isolating, lonely, tiring road for the likes of me, you got it! Now think of parents with less money, educational resources or family support - and shudder!

Good models for supporting the caregivers of children who have FASD are elusive in medical literature (aside from Dr. Olsen's article referenced above) but if one looks to the area of children who have an acquired brain injury and their families, one can find some very helpful ideas. Dr. George Singer and others authored a book called *Children With Acquired Brain Injury*. (Singer, 1996) The *whole* book has been a wonderful source of helpful ideas for our family. One study, however, really caught my eye. Success for kids affected by brain injury was measured as being able to live on your own (albeit with supports), being able to function in a job (albeit with support) and, a "cute" criteria was being able to manage a chequing account (albeit with supports). The factors that predicted success, as measured by the above criteria, were very interesting. Logically, readers might think that information such as how long a child was in coma, how bad the child's head injury was, how low his or her Glasgow Coma Scale was, etc., would predict whether or not that child would be successful, but, in fact, the strength of the parents' marriage and how well the parents could problem solve, i.e., *parental adaptive function*, predicted their kid's success *better* than any of the other factors! Supportive, adaptive parents were the key for their kids' success. Doesn't this sound a lot like Anne Streissguth's concept that the percentage of time spent in a stable, nurturing home environment is *the most influential factor* to protect against secondary disabilities? Please advocate for respite provided by FASD-savvy respite workers and other robust ways to support parents such as access to sensory assessment and programming. These programmes are not easy to set up, but they can bring hope and restoration to an exhausted set of parents - and success for the kids.

Caring, ongoing supportive relationships are *the* key to optimal success for our kids - that is why this book is called *FASD Relationships.*

4) Children Affected by FASD: Some final ideas

Books to read, experts to follow

Jan Lutke, Tina Antrobus and other FASD caregivers have created FASD Connections. The goal of this initiative is to build "a community in which adolescents and adults with Fetal Alcohol Spectrum Disorder are included and encouraged and where their desire and potential is supported; where the experience of families is understood, acknowledged, and accepted; and where systems are equipped to respond in an informed, compassionate and responsible way." One way FASD Connections realizes this goal is by constantly updating a series of articles on virtually all aspects of FASD. FASD Connections' website is listed in the appendix.

Fetal Alcohol Syndrome Diagnostic and Prevention Network (FAS DPN) is "Mecca" in the FASD world. This group of clinics situated in Washington State has done diagnostic evaluations for FASD for more than twenty years. FAS DPN has created the 4-digit diagnostic code for FASD and has published extensive research including surveillance, intervention, and neuro-imaging of individuals with FASD. The FAS DPN website is included in the appendix.

Motherisk, an organization at Toronto's Hospital for Sick Children offers "research and counseling on reproductive risk of drugs, chemicals and maternal disease in pregnancy." Motherisk has a website listed in the appendix and also has the Fetal Alcohol Research website (also listed). The Fetal Alcohol Canadian Expertise (FACE) Research Roundtable Webcasts (accessed through Motherisk's Fetal Alcohol Research website) are a "course on FASD" in themselves.

Diane Malbin, a social worker (and mother of adult children who have FASD) from Portland, does wonderful work in effectively supporting those who have FASD and their caregiver networks. I recommend her three-day training to anyone interested. Diane's organization is called Fetal Alcohol Syndrome Consultation, Education and Training Services, Inc. (FASCETS) Her website is listed in the appendix. The essence of her dream is to have a more inclusive society, one that accepts differences in *all* people. If we consider folks with FASD, practical extensions of Diane's work play out in many ways: accurate diagnosis leading to appropriate school programs, appropriate interventions and support and, above all, seeing behavioural and cognitive differences are based on brain problems not willful defiance.

My wife and I have found that *Tanya Helton*, MSc., who grew up with two siblings that have FAS, offers resources and counseling services that were most helpful. Her organization provides telephone consultation and mentoring for parents of kids with attachment difficulties. Her organization is called "Forest Cottage Centre: Helping Parents of Challenging Children" and her website is listed in the appendix.

Figure 7.

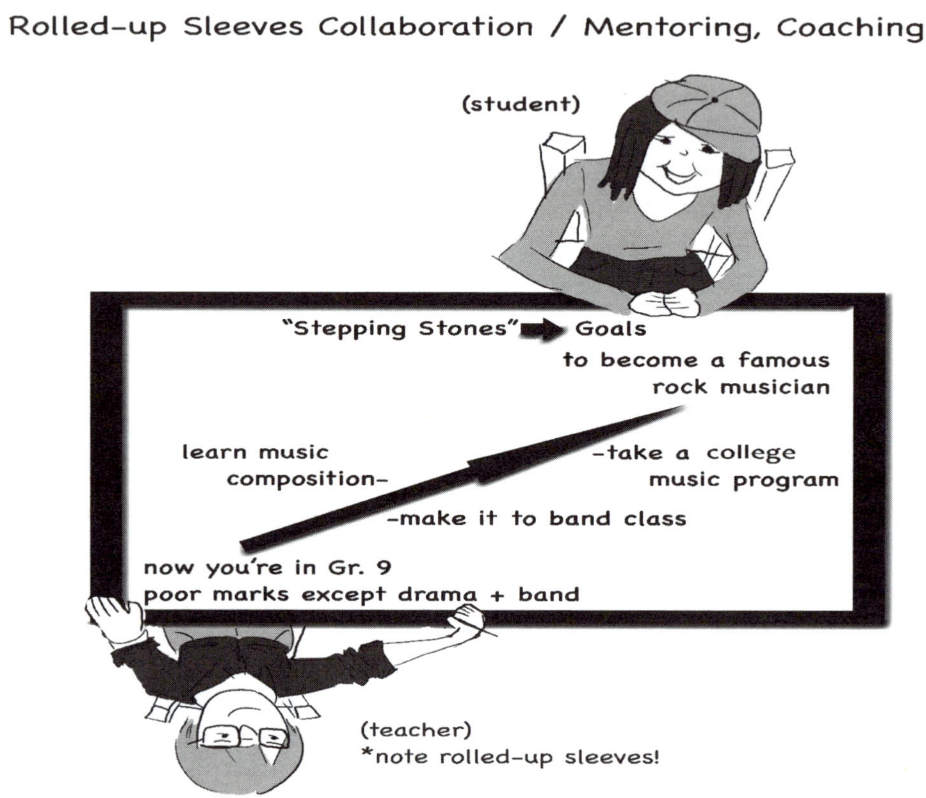

I think we should be using Tim Feeney's and Mark Ylvisaker's strategies (see figure 7 above) to optimally develop executive functions. Remember, their model is that we are all roll-up-your-sleeves collaborators, and the subject matter is to coach and assist the kids on their every day chores: getting their books to school, getting to the youth group, how to deal with a critical youth group leader, etc. A conversation with Mark can be viewed at the International Brain Injury Association website listed in the appendix.

Up-to-date approaches pediatricians use in dealing with children with complex brain injuries and their families is well described in *Treating Neurodevelopmental Disabilities: Clinical Research and Practice.* (Farmer, 2006) On page 150 of this book there are some important statements that ought to pertain to FASD programmes. Starting in 1997, accreditation examiners of organizations ("that serve children and adolescents with significant functional limitations as the result of congenital or acquired impairments and aim to prevent further impairments, reduce activity limitations, and minimize participation restrictions, while maximizing growth and development") have reviewed the programmes of those organizations to see if their practice follows the *eight Principles of Pediatric Family-centered Rehabilitation.*

This is a paraphrase of the principles:

» Programmes and personnel who work in those programmes are transient. *The family* is the biggest constant in children's lives.

» Teamwork between the family and health care professionals is a priority always.

» Complete, unbiased information is shared with families in an appropriate and supportive way.

» Support for the emotional and financial needs of the families are priorities for programme design.

» There is respect for the family's culture, coping mechanisms and unique strengths.

» The developmental needs of children and their families are appreciated and built into interventions.

» Parent-to-parent support is encouraged and facilitated.

» Rehabilitation systems are flexible, accessible and responsive to families.

Clearly, current *standards of care* for dealing with challenges in complex, developmentally delayed children involve respecting, including, and working with caregivers. Parents, if you are not made to feel welcome and included in the decision-making at your next meeting with professionals, *they, not you, are "doing it wrong."*

Adoptive parents (or other parents) who have experienced infertility have stress levels beyond what they or the professionals who work with them anticipate

Recent work in Boston at the Harvard's Benson-Henry Institute for Mind Body Medicine shows that their *most* stressed patient groups are 1) those with AIDS, 2) Cancer and 3) Infertile women. Much harm could be avoided if professionals realized that this extreme level of caregiver distress also appears in families where infertility has been encountered. This Harvard institute has studied stress medicine since the mid 1970's; their website is listed in the appendix.

Regrettably, I have heard one adoptive mum falsely described as having "Munchausen by Proxy Syndrome" (this diagnosis means that a caregiver is deliberately misleading doctors into thinking something is wrong with a child by lying about and exaggerating symptoms). This (incorrect, misleading, and damning) diagnosis was suggested, no - *declared* - by a non-physician during a family planning conference. This is abuse of a patient - the adoptive mum. This abuse absolutely violates the generally accepted principles of pediatric rehabilitation listed above. By all means, if there are safety concerns do an investigation, but don't be slinging such terms around - especially when you are not qualified to make such a diagnosis! (The more accurate diagnosis was: unsupported, desperate adoptive parents that were confronted with uncontrolled destructive behaviour and pleaded for respite, counseling and other help more than six times to no avail. They were not coping very well - neither would you!) The correct approach would have involved investigation and support, not labeling. This Neanderthal way of dealing with stressed-out parents violates the most basic principle of "do no harm." Offer no support, wait until they yell or do some silly thing and then blame them - callous and ethically bankrupt as "blame the parents, especially the mum" thinking is, in 2011 I cannot tell you this destructive concept is dead and buried. Too bad.

A Long and Silly Habit of "Professionals" Blaming Parents (I know, this is a continuation of Rant Number Four!)

There is a long tradition of so-called professionals exporting blame for a child's misbehaviour or psychiatric symptoms onto parents. Kasanin and Fromm-Reichmann proposed a few zingers in the 1930s and 40s: that "maternal rejection or overprotection were influential in causing schizophrenia" and that "the schizophrenic is painfully distrustful and resentful of other people due to the severe early warp and rejection he encountered in important people in his infancy and childhood, as a rule mainly the schizophrenogenic mother." (Keitner, 2010) Dumb follows dumb, I guess - the 1950s and 60s brought forth the "Refrigerator Mother" whose coolness and non-responsiveness apparently caused autism. The common denominator of these wrong-headed examples is bullying of parents, especially mothers, by so-called professionals. In 2011 we know enough about bullying to put an end to all this.

If having lost my patience to the point of saying and doing some really stupid things means that I am an unfit father, then I am guilty. If I had been pushed a millimeter more would I have swatted my kid? Probably. Should I be allowed to swat my kid? Absolutely not. If I had swatted my kid should I be forced to confront that and forced to undertake counseling and educational measures to address the concern? Yes. Should I be allowed to argue my way out of such measures? No way! At the time, would I have accepted such interventions willingly? Maybe, but probably not. Should I be monitored by a programme that had enough teeth in it to intervene if I kept on swatting my kid? Absolutely. If my child's situation looks destructive to child welfare personnel, should they err on the side of caution and place my child in another home? Absolutely.

Birth Parents, or any other caregivers, and "Inconsolable Crying"

Birth parents are also at high risk for over-the-top levels of stress *especially* in the infant's peak "inconsolable crying period," which occurs when the child is six to ten weeks old but may last until much later than that in children who have FASD. Often it is hard to settle newborns that have FASD - they may be hard to feed, have disrupted sleep and be very fussy. Indeed, as Dr. Kieran O'Malley points out, these children can be so hard to comfort and so difficult to settle that pediatric psychiatrists could diagnose *regulatory disorder of infancy*. No reader that has not personally dealt with a colicky baby will really understand how draining, frustrating and exhausting that condition can be to new parents. Regulatory disorder of infancy? Think "colicky baby times two."

Sensory processing problems–especially "acoustic startle," which means that loud, unexpected noises can really throw you off - are quite common in traumatized women. If these women are parents and are also dealing with their own depression, addictions, and other mental health challenges at the same time as the squalling baby there is a real risk of child abuse including Shaken Baby Syndrome. Peak incidence for Shaken Baby Syndrome is 10-12 weeks. The National Center on Shaken Baby Syndrome maintains a very informative website (listed in the appendix) readers can access for more information and resources.

One of the coolest ideas I have seen to address at-risk newborns is from France. *Prenatally*, mums and dads attended video-facilitated classes that talked about fussy babies, how to change the baby, how to hold him and calm him, newborn care, seeing the doctor if you might have post-partum depression and so on. *The same people* that facilitated the class were available on the phone *postnatally* to help trouble-shoot "before problems build up." This meant stressed young parents could call up their old buddy who taught the class to de-escalate a situation - I am sure it lowered barriers to reaching for help. Smart guys, those French!

Don't overlook "harm reduction"

My family doctor worked for many years at an alcohol treatment centre. One of his patients with FASD, last seen at age 16, haunted my doc because this young man took off to Vancouver's harsh East Hastings Street area, once again succumbed to uncontrolled drinking and eventually committed suicide. My colleague's regret was that he did not do all he could in the area of harm reduction. Being connected to an adult that cares about you and takes an interest in you is one of the main ways to reduce harm. My colleague had a great working relationship with this young man. He regrets not asking him to come in more often and not connecting him with some responsible caregivers - even a friendly doctor that worked with patients in East Vancouver - when the patient moved. In other words, *he regrets not taking a more active, hands-on approach*. In hindsight, tragically, my friend the G.P. was the first responsible adult who had an ongoing, caring connection with this young man. The young man's dad was in jail, his mum sold drugs, and he had no extended family in B.C. He had been out of school for years. Sometimes, one-on-one relationships with a parole officer, therapist, social worker, physician, etc., do not work very well, but when they do it is wise to see them as *very* valuable and do all that is possible to maintain the links with these people who care and have a vital connection with the young person.

Supervision is necessary for kids with FASD. When they won't take direct advice from parents, it is wise to connect them with other adults and get them involved in groups such as Cubs, Scouts or youth groups, after school programs, bowling, etc. They should keep busy. Unstructured time can be very difficult. Weekends and summer can be hell. We have resorted some summers to sending our child to a number of summer camps. During the school year, youth group activities are a blessing. The programme called "Staying in School/Staying on Track" at John Templeton Secondary School in Vancouver featured a full program of after school activities, weekend activities and summer activities. An updated version of this programme now exists at West Coast Alternative School. This school's website is listed in the appendix.

Linking your child with a doctor and nurse who can develop a relationship with the child is a good idea. Specifically, the medical person should advise kids on birth control, sexually transmitted diseases and create a welcoming "doctor-patient" relationship. Make sure the kids feel relaxed about being able to report *any* symptoms or ask *any* questions.

Rehearsal of plans such as what to do if in danger, what to say if in contact with the police, and how to get help if hurt or lost, might save a life. Having a phone card and knowing how to contact some key people can also save a life. Through all the clutter of information coming their way, which no doubt kids with FASD will say involves "too many words," they need to know that parents and other caring adults love them and think they are wonderful. Having an adult that cares about you deeply may be the *only* thing between kids with FASD and homelessness, trouble with the law, joblessness, sexually transmitted diseases and all the other secondary disabilities we have talked about.

Vaccinations, including hepatitis A and B, meningitis and human papilloma virus are a good idea - they might save a life.

The most shocking case of sexually transmitted disease (STD) I have seen was in a 15-year-old homeless pregnant girl from Vancouver. She had severe pelvic inflammatory disease - the bacterial infection had entered her blood stream. Her blood pressure was low. She needed I.V. antibiotics. She nearly died. Immaturity of the teen cervix predisposes to more severe STDs. The nurse and I that saw this young lady were shocked at her lack of basic understanding about contraceptive options or condom use, and her lack of awareness that she could seek help from a health care provider. If the barriers for her to seek medical help were lower, and her motivations to get contraception were higher maybe she could have gotten help sooner or even avoided her near-death experience.

Motivators and Barriers to obtaining contraception

Young women using reliable birth control is at least part of FASD prevention. Recent information helps clarify options for women and helps programme planners understand which barriers must be addressed to increase birth control effectiveness. Sexually active young people are more likely to seek contraception if they *have been* pregnant or *thought* they were, *don't want* to get pregnant, have friends that use contraception, plan to *stay in school* and continue education after high school, or are older. Both men and women need to become more comfortable with carrying and always using condoms. Use increases once people are *not embarrassed* to use them, view AIDS as "*something that could happen to me*" and understand that condoms can *prevent AIDS*. Young people don't really know that what they discuss with the doctor or nurse stays private. Specifically tell young patients that *what they discuss will remain confidential* except in unusual circumstances, such as having thoughts of suicide or harming others - in these unusual situations health care providers *are required* to inform the relevant authorities in order to ensure public safety.

Young women naturally approach the idea of having a pelvic examination with a degree of apprehension. "The first pelvic examination is a milestone for the adolescent. It needs to be a positive experience to foster communication on sensitive topics between the adolescent and her health care providers" says adolescent medical specialist Dr. Mariam Chacko in her review. (Chacko, 2010.) One way to help build trust and make the experience positive can be to delay the examination for a few months - a reasonable option if there are no acute issues such as abnormal vaginal discharge, itch, odor, etc. Choice builds trust. Women are concerned about these possible side effects of contraceptives: weight gain, blood clots, risk of birth defects, infertility and loss of bone mass (risk of osteoporosis).

Dr. Chacko says estrogen-progestin ("The Pill") and progestin-alone options ("Depo" or "Mirena IUD") have not been shown to cause weight gain, infertility or birth defects. Depot medroxyprogesterone acetate (Depo-Provera) reduces bone mass (by up to 1.8% in a study of its use in adolescents. *Recovery* of bone mass that was lost when using Depo-Provera was complete within 12 months of discontinuation of Depo. Readers should note that pregnancy reduces bone mass by 2 to 8% and breastfeeding reduces bone mass by 3-5%.) (Kaunitz, 2010) With low estrogen dose oral contraceptives the risk of blood clots is very low but not zero - progestin only options are better if a woman has a personal or family risk of clots (i.e. pulmonary embolism, leg clots, or stroke).

The intra-uterine device (IUD) offers a reliable and practical option for birth control, especially since the levonorgestrel (Mirena) device (which actually decreases cramping, pain and period flow) has become available.

Dr. Roey Malleson's "Contraception: What do Women Want?" review was the most helpful information that I've seen recently on this topic. (Malleson, 2010) Dr. Malleson suggests that the ideal contraceptive must be effective, reversible, *and forgettable!* She then introduced the concept of *continuation rates*: if you don't keep using a method, it won't work. Because of *discontinuation*, effective contraceptives like "the pill" have poor "first year failure rates" in real-world use...8% for typical users. I wonder if failure rates would be closer to 10 or 15% for women with distractibility from ADHD, memory issues from depression, or focus issues from sleeplessness if they are not in a safe living situation or if they are having to feed a baby at night or keep an aggressive roaming five-year-old from hurting her sister in the middle of the night. Real world first year pregnancy rates for Depo-provera are 3%, 0.8% for copper IUD (NovaT) and 0.1% for progestin IUD (Mirena). Women with current cervical infection, uterine infection, and some uterine abnormalities cannot use an IUD - others can. In the past, women who had not been pregnant before, had heavy painful periods, or had a history of ectopic pregnancy, multiple partners or previous STDs were advised not to use an IUD. Recent evidence allays these concerns. Serious pelvic infection (PID) is increased only in the first 3 weeks after IUD insertion and is related to active infection of the cervix at the time of insertion - so don't insert if there is active infection; treat the infection then have the patient return for insertion. If a woman develops PID, results of treatment are equally favorable whether the IUD is removed or not. IUDs actually *reduce* the risk of ectopic pregnancy. (1.2-1.6% of sexually active women have an ectopic pregnancy per year, 0.25% of women using NovaT have an ectopic per year and 0.02% of Mirena users have an ectopic in a given year.)

To summarize contraception comments, society needs to make IUDs and Depo-provera more readily available. (In B.C. Mirena costs about $350, NovaT about $170, Depo between $40 and $80 [depending on availability of generic forms] and birth control pills about $20 per month. Mirena lasts 5 years [$5.83 per month], NovaT lasts *a maximum* of 30 months [approx. $6.00 per month] and Depo shots last 3 months [$14-$27 per month]). Very clear information about options needs to be available for all women and their partners - this means educational resources must be provided for women with impaired literacy or other learning problems. Provision of a non-judgmental advocate to help homeless or otherwise marginalized people who attend a clinic may be required, or some won't be able to access contraception. Also, clinics must be welcoming - stigma-free and shame/blame-free zones!

5) Who are the Birth Mums?

I think birth mums are just like the rest of us, trying to bumble along through life as best they possibly can in today's world. Birth mums certainly have been dealt a number of cards that make their path difficult. Birth mums are absolutely anyone; they could be your neighbor, your friend or your cousin. The group of birth mums studied a decade ago in Seattle were an average age of 27 when their FASD-affected child was born (21 when their first child was born) and had an average number of three kids. (Astley, 2000) Most were not married. Most lived in poverty, with an annual household income of less than $10,000, but there were some with a much higher income. Talking informally with a group of psychologists from Northern Alberta I first learned the term "Fort McMurray Syndrome." This refers a certain lifestyle that had been observed in some people employed in highly paid oil-sector jobs this northern "boom town." "Big job, big money, play hard, party hearty, drink hard, work hard" would be a fitting mantra for men and women who live this way; women would add, "I can do anything that the guys can do." This lifestyle might explain some people in the higher income group, but "hip" urban professionals who like to party are also at risk.

Story from the Isle of Skye

My daughter and I were in the line up for the bridge that leads to the Isle of Skye in Scotland several summers ago. I began talking with a fit-looking 60ish-year-old fellow in the next car. He was a recently retired social worker from Manchester who described his daughter, a 30-year-old psychologist. I am always talking about Fetal Alcohol issues ("I hadn't noticed that," you say!) The social worker was mortified about the risk to kids who will become his grandchildren. He said his daughter was *typical of her peers*: she was often intoxicated, "wasted" for a night or two most weekends; she had lots of party action, lots of money and lots of boyfriends.

Continuing the **Seattle birth mother study** discussion, the average birth mum had five DSM-4 psychiatric diagnoses. Some had ten! *This is a huge burden of mental health problems.* Few were diagnosed and fewer were appropriately treated. 95% had been sexually and/or physically abused. Abuse trauma commonly leads to PTSD and addictions. Most common mental health problems (more than a third of the women had experienced these) were alcohol abuse (86%), posttraumatic stress (77%), depression (60%), simple phobia (44%), social phobia (43%), antisocial personality (39%), agoraphobia (37%) and generalized anxiety disorder (34%). Bipolar (21%) and panic disorder (20%) were also common. In May of 2009 I attended the American Psychiatric Meeting in San Francisco. There was much discussion at this meeting on how under-diagnosed, common and destructive (untreated) borderline personality disorder is. I believe that if the Seattle study investigators had been looking for borderline symptoms that, likely, these would also have been common. Traumatic brain injury was not assessed in the study either; likely it would not be rare.

Post-Traumatic Stress Disorder (PTSD)

You cannot understand birth mums (or dads) without thinking about *their genetics* - emotional lability, impulsivity, bipolar, externalizing symptoms, and substance use problems all carry significant heritability. Birth parent's *environmental stress, their gifts/ interests* and support networks (or lack thereof) are also very relevant risk or resilience factors. A young lady I saw last year comes to mind: 22, single mum, 4 year old son who is usually looked after by gramma, boyfriend in jail, probably has

FASD herself but has not been diagnosed, trying to go to college to complete her high school diploma, depressed (suicidal), anxious, disrupted sleep and nightmares of childhood sexual abuse and physical abuse, startles easily when her son shrieks (which he does often!), various addiction issues with crack and alcohol, "clean and sober" for the last few months. Before considering early retirement because you as a caregiver or clinician have no clue how to begin to help this mum, consider Dr. Dave Ziegler's ideas from an adoption course he taught in 2000. "Always start with the trauma," Dave explained. Many patients I have seen over the last decade would agree with Dr. Ziegler, because getting a handle on some parts of the trauma can give hope and some degree of positive momentum to their lives. (Ziegler, 2000)

So, PTSD is important to recognize and deal with - what follows are some tools I have found helpful for my patients. *All* these ideas are based on this incredibly helpful reference: *Effective Treatments for PTSD, Second Edition.* (Foa, 2009)

This is the **"Psychoeducation re: PTSD"** (learning about your mental health issue) teaching module that I like to go over for patients who have PTSD. Please feel free to share it with any of your clients:

PTSD can happen to *anyone*; just apply enough stress. Anyone has his or her limit and can be pushed past the breaking point. Consider (Canadian) Lt-Gen. Romeo Dallaire, a tough, experienced soldier from a family of tough experienced soldiers. When confronted by AK-47 wielding thugs literally hiding behind pregnant teenagers as they shot at General Dallaire's U.N. peacekeepers in the early days of the Rwanadan genocide, what was he to do? Die or shoot back? To save the lives of his peacekeepers and the Tutsis they were protecting he shot back - and it haunts him to this day. An inert U.N. hierarchy refused to send reinforcements despite General Dallaire's repeated pleas - the Canadian Army sent a small group of officers and enlisted soldiers to help. Most of these officers returned home with PTSD. Several have committed suicide. General Dallaire himself nearly committed suicide. These guys are tough, well-trained, disciplined, super-fit, well supported professionals - they could teach the most macho mountain climber or extreme elite athlete a lot about being cool under pressure. These guys are the polar opposite of sissies. Take any notion you might have of PTSD being a condition brought on by weakness of will or lack of character strength and bury it - because it is not true!

Any traumatic event - combat, incest, assault, car accident, a cancer diagnosis - that involves witnessing or experiencing death or serious injury or threat to physical integrity of self or others could lead to PTSD. 40-90% of us experience such trauma. If the initial response to trauma is one of horror, helplessness or fear and symptoms last more than 30 days, a diagnosis of PTSD is possible. Symptoms of PTSD come in three categories:

1. Re-experiencing - nightmares, flashbacks, intrusive recollections, inability to get the trauma out of one's mind - these are the most common symptoms.

2. Hypervigilance - constantly on the watch, jumpy, easily startled.

3. Numbing or avoiding - avoids going out on his or her own, unable to feel sad or happy, avoids certain activities - this last group of symptoms is the most specific to PTSD (versus other anxiety disorders) and, if severe, tends to predict more difficulties in treatment. Other symptoms include depersonalization, which is a feeling that somehow some part of life is occurring outside of oneself. One patient describes this: "it is like I am watching my life unfold on a T.V. - I am there but it feels like I am outside looking in on myself."

Resiliency factors that help reduce the likelihood of PTSD after exposure to trauma include having:

1. An "internal locus of control" ("It's hard, but *I can do something about this traumatic event*") instead of an "external locus of control"("It's all her/his fault")

2. Long-standing optimism

3. A sense of humor

4. A religious affiliation

5. A higher socio-economic situation (Panda, 2009)

Prevention or early intervention strategies vary depending on the situation. Refugees after a natural disaster such as a hurricane or earthquake find themselves living in a crowded fishbowl - there is no privacy in the "tent city." Privacy is needed *at times* but there is also a tendency to isolate and that makes things worse. Refugees have no power or control - wise administrators will organize a "village council" within the disaster camp that promotes a sense of self-efficacy. This sense of agency (I *can* have some control over my destiny even in this mess!) is healing.

A rape victim might benefit from ventilation (sharing their experience with a supportive listener) *if it does not inflame*, exposure therapy such as taping a narrative of the trauma and playing the tape *while doing relaxation exercises such as progressive muscle relaxation*, and use of medications such as the beta blocker propranolol or the alpha blocker prazosin to reduce nightmares and flashbacks and help block the consolidation of the traumatic memory. This is pretty exciting: there is evidence that we can help prevent a traumatic memory from sticking into the long-term memory storage in such a "hard-to-dislodge or extinguish" way by using early interventions such as prazosin.

Key points *required* for recovery include:

1. Realization that recovery is *not* passive
2. Appreciation that recovery involves *learning* that old fears do not fit new (unthreatening) situations. The goal is for the "calm down" parts of the brain (frontal lobe and hippocampus) to talk the "fight and flight" parts of the brain (amygdala) out of excessive wind-up.

In PTSD, the brain acts like one is in danger *all the time*. The middle, inner part of the frontal lobe (anterior cingulate) shows *less* activation in PTSD patients. This area is an emotional clutch--when it works well, it interrupts emotional stimuli for long enough to *process* a response. One does not *have to* respond immediately as if being pushed around by emotions; thinking about a wise response is possible. The speech production area (Broca's area) can be suppressed in PTSD, which explains why some patients experience speechless terror.

A problem in approaching PTSD is that many of the traumatic memories are held in non-verbal, hard to talk about (*deeper than the cortex*), layers of the brain, such as where smells or feelings of touch or recollections of certain sounds (e.g. footsteps) are held. Yet our main tools to help extinguish such traumatic memories are the verbal and symbolic representations *in the cortex*. Darn, eh? Nevertheless, as Dr. Kosten stated this in a recent workshop: "your only hope is your cortex when you have PTSD--you've GOT to get it re-engaged." (Kosten, 2009)

Thus, if your only hope is learning, it is *essential to not impair learning*! What this means, on a practical basis, is not to use benzodiazepine medications in PTSD because these impair learning. Many patients are using diazepam (Valium), lorazepam (Ativan), clonazepam and other benzodiazepines - and are reluctant to give them up because they do help settle angst - but if we are serious about evidence-based practice, better alternatives need to be used.

I have found the *PTSD Checklist--Civilian Version (PCL-C)* to be an easy-to-use and helpful clinical tool. (Weathers, 1991) Symptom questions are answered using a severity scale of "up to 5" on each. Questions include: are you bothered by repeated disturbing images or dreams of a stressful experience? do you avoid thinking about the stressful experience? do you feel distant or "cut off" from others? do you feel emotionally numb? are you jumpy or easily startled? The maximum score is 85 (a score of 5 on each of the 17 questions). (50 or above suggests the possibility of PTSD). I have seen scores of 78 - this represents a crushing burden of symptomatology. The PTSD checklist is just a screening questionnaire, diagnosing PTSD requires a more detailed assessment.

Medications I have found helpful for PTSD symptoms

Logically, it makes sense for trauma to cause flashbacks, nightmares, edginess or anxiety and other brain-based symptoms. However, *muscle and body tension* due to excessive adrenaline and other stress hormone activity seems to mediate a significant part of these *mental* symptoms. The mind gets tense because the body is tense. Blocking this adrenaline-based body tension alleviates significant mental distress. Prazosin (Minipress), propranolol (Inderal), and clonidine (Dixarit) have proven their effectiveness in reducing PTSD symptoms. I use these three meds commonly and often find them to be very effective in reducing symptoms of PTSD. I don't want to be irreverent to medication governing bodies (such as the pharmacists at Pharmacare in B.C.), but to attend a course and learn some exciting way of helping a patient who is really having terrible symptoms, and then not be able to use that method because "that drug is not funded by Pharmacare" can be incredibly frustrating. Prazosin, propranolol and clonidine are all old and cheap *blood pressure* drugs that most drug plans cover financially. However, Pharmacare did not want to fund prazosin prescriptions for some of my patients in 2010. Some patients do not like the idea of using brain drugs such as antidepressants, but find the idea of using an "anti-excessive adrenaline blood pressure drug" not only acceptable but also kind of intriguing.

Prazosin, propranolol and clonidine block excessive adrenaline wind-up, but do so using slightly different mechanisms, because they each belong to a different medication category. I usually explain to patients that the goal is to see if a small amount of one would assist in stress reduction without causing side effects. All of these drugs can cause some sedation, lightheadedness or "spaceyness". Usually these side effects are very minor and become insignificant after a day or two. I always start with tiny doses such as 0.5 mg of prazosin at night for a few nights, then twice a day for a few days then three times a day for a few days. Prazosin is really interesting because there are also some recent studies about its effectiveness in reducing excessive drinking. In the last 3-4 months I have used prazosin for over thirty patients - one was over-sedated on just 0.5 mg so we switched to propranolol and that was well tolerated. Three could not continue to use prazosin because they noticed their sinuses were congested when they were on this med. Several who are easily tolerating moderate doses (4 to 5 mg two or three times a day with no significant drop in their blood pressure) have told me this is the first time in their adult lives they have not been consumed by a pervasive desire to seek and drink alcohol. "I've never felt this way in thirty-five years," one lady explained... "for the first time I can remember, I can take it or leave it when it comes to booze."

A patient with a harrowing history of incest as a child at an Indian Residential School and physical abuse as an adult started with a PCL-C score of 69. She is now using 5 mg of prazosin twice a day (very gradual increase to this dose over 5 weeks); her current PCL-C score is 35. She says, "I don't *ever* remember feeling this good." An even more precise measure is my terrific medical office assistant's analysis when she sees this patient's new appearance and attitude: "Wow!"

The lady with a score of 78 ended up with 40 mg of propranolol twice a day - her score is now 38 and she says, "The monster is off my back! I've been to counselors before - they are nice people and welcome me but I didn't get much from the counseling - now I am better able to listen and work with my counselor."

Since all three of these drugs are used to medicate blood pressure, obviously blood pressure and pulse need to be checked before using any of them or increasing a dose. Propranolol *cannot* used for patients with asthma or severe allergy reactions. Sleep issues, especially nightmares and intrusive recollections of the trauma, seem to be the first things that these meds improve. Interestingly, both of the above patients had engaged in counseling previously, but without making much progress. Now that their symptoms are down to a dull roar, both are really interested in further talk therapy. The reason I am giving significant detail to drug doses in this section is not because I am hoping all readers will now want to be pharmacologists or doctors - I just want to describe how an evidence-based but very low-tech approach can be used in a rural setting to achieve (so far) very encouraging results. Most primary care doctors have patients on propranolol and clonidine; prazosin is not a difficult medication to prescribe, especially if one starts with very low doses.

Psychotherapy (talk therapy) for PTSD has also been rigorously evaluated for effectiveness. Two approaches seem particularly helpful for patients I see. Psychologist Lisa M. Najavits has developed a treatment manual called *Seeking Safety*. This approach, designed to reduce both PTSD and Substance Abuse symptoms, has proven effective for men, women and adolescents diagnosed with PTSD. Even sub-threshold patients - that is, patients who do not show enough symptoms of sufficient severity to reach the "diagnostic threshold" for PTSD - can be disabled by their illness; *Seeking Safety* also significantly reduces symptoms for this sub-threshold group. Interested readers can learn more at the Seeking Safety website listed in the appendix.

Interapy is an evidence-based on-line treatment for PTSD. One of my patients lives in a tiny town of two thousand where access to a psychologist or counselor is not possible. She wondered about on-line resources so I asked Brett Litz, Ph.D. (a professor at Boston U. School of Medicine and staff member of the USA National Centre for PTSD) what he'd recommend. Dr. Litz himself had developed an internet-based treatment and written about it in Dr Foa's *Effective Treatments of PTSD* book described in previous sections. This is his reply: "There is an evidence-based online treatment that I do recommend and it is called Interapy. I know this group and they are excellent." Interapy's website is listed in the appendix.

Story: Self-medicating with Alcohol

At a course several years ago, a pleasant forty-year-old mother of two children shared her story. When she was in her twenties, she became interested in psychology and pursued a Master's degree at the University of Washington. She had a one-hour commute each morning. She was very fuzzyheaded when she woke up. It took one or two drinks before she could concentrate enough to face the day. She would then get in her car, drive across town, attend her Masters of Psychology classes, complete her home work in the library and drive home at night. She became pregnant. Her two kids have FAS. Likely, she has ADHD. The alcohol was used as a self-medication to try to deal with early morning focus issues. She would have more safely and more effectively been treated with standard ADHD meds.

Story: But for Grace

Dr. Val Massey, neuropsychologist, conducted an FASD educational event in 2003. I think I was the only primary care doctor in a room full of child psychiatrists and psychologists. Val asked these questions:

» How many of you have gone to college?

» Have you ever had a party after exams to blow off steam?

» Have you ever drank a bit too much?

» Have you ever had sex about that time?

Lesson:

But for grace, there would be a lot more FASD.

Story: Blame and shame predictably cause the urge, "I'll show you!"

Dr. Stirling Clarren recently alerted attendees at an FASD conference: "We blame and shame the mothers despite their mental health burdens. This further alienates them... the most attention they get from the mental health system and the health care system is when they are pregnant, and then the child is often removed. Not surprisingly, the result of this practice is 'I'll show you' and they become pregnant again."

Why drink in pregnancy?

In the study *Alcohol use in pregnant and non-pregnant Russian women* almost 900 women of childbearing age in St. Petersburg, Russia were investigated. (Kristjanson, 2007) Almost 96% had consumed alcohol in the last twelve months and of the non-pregnant women drinkers, almost 8% drank more than 30 ml of absolute alcohol per day, which is an extreme amount. 18% had binged (had five or more drinks in one sitting) at least once. Of the pregnant women, nearly all drank in the year prior to the pregnancy. 60% drank when they knew they were pregnant. 90% of the pregnant and non-pregnant women believed that alcohol had a harmful effect on the fetus.

So, why does this disconnect exist? Why, if they are aware that alcohol can harm the baby, do some women continue to drink?

Answer: Dr. Christina Loock, a Vancouver-based Developmental Pediatrician, has proposed a model involving **primary, secondary and tertiary prevention strategies**.

In *primary prevention*, people just need a little bit of a reminder, like some posters emphasizing the use of folic acid, abstinence from alcohol, and good nutrition if one is contemplating pregnancy.

Secondary prevention: Some people who are prone to a more dangerous drinking pattern may need specific interventions. Actually, even hearing their primary care health providers specifically say "do not drink in pregnancy" and receiving some counseling and information on the issue significantly reduces this group's consumption of alcohol while pregnant. Labels on liquor bottles warning against dangers for pregnancy help both primary and secondary prevention. There are twenty-four countries now with alcohol-does-not-mix-with-pregnancy beverage warning labels, including France (where all that nice wine comes from and where "the norm" is supposedly for older kids to have at least a few sips at dinner)! Yet our government in Ottawa defeated a recent motion to put warning labels on liquor bottles. I really cannot understand why Stephen Harper's government voted this way - their decision appears to be at odds with their recent focus on child and maternal health at the 2010 G-8 Summit.

Tertiary prevention involves hands-on programs for women who drink a lot despite having alcohol-related health problems and suffering adverse consequences from their drinking. There are numerous examples of these programs. Vancouver has "Sheway" which operates on the downtown east side. (see Sheway in references) Seattle has P-CAP. (see P-CAP in references) "P-CAP" stands for the Parent Child Assistance Program. To the uninitiated, such programs may look invasive.

When folks do not make appointments, often the counselors go to them or arrange for transportation, child care and other barriers to be overcome to allow the meetings to occur. These programmes follow a harm reduction model. There is no place for judgmental attitudes or simplistic strategies like "three strikes you're out." It is appreciated that a third of birth mothers in such programs could well have FAS or FASD themselves. Sheway supports families from the time of a child's birth until that index child turns three. A flaw in many such programs is that when an index child turns three, his or her mum "ages out" of the intensive support network which has helped maintain recovery from addiction, treatment for mental health issues, improved parenting/child care skills, improved self esteem, and birth control. Do I have to suggest that "backsliding" is often found when services are withdrawn? You'd guessed that already, right?

I am sorry I cannot locate the reference but in discussing one such program a few years ago, this question was posed at a conference: "What is easier - to help women take regular birth control or to abstain from alcohol since both 'ingredients' (the alcohol and the lack of effective birth control) are needed to have a child that is affected by FASD?" The speaker suggested it was easier to get people to abstain from drinking than it was to get them to use regular birth control.

Barriers to reducing drinking

The most common barriers to reducing drinking, which participants shared in the Seattle Birth Mother study, included: alcohol use for coping with stress (94%), a lack of desire to give up alcohol (87%), depression (79%), discomfort about having a problem with alcohol (75%), involvement in an abusive or violent relationship (72%), the belief that alcohol dependency was not a problem (60%), the belief that reducing alcohol consumption wouldn't help, (44%), fear (the belief that seeking help with alcohol would mean) that her children would be taken away from her (42%), a lack of adequate childcare while the mother attended a treatment program (39%), and a boyfriend/husband/partner who did not want her to attend a treatment program (39%).

Good planning can overcome many of these barriers. I know many readers are now rolling their eyes and thinking that I am in dreamland and that the "bean counters" in their health systems would never fully support comprehensive (and sometimes life-long) systems of support for birth mums. Here's a useful question: if your local bean counters *really are* wanting to make the best of their scarce health care dollars, why don't they consider the *total* cost of supporting FASD? A lack of excellent prevention work costs at least 1-2 *million* dollars per child with FASD. (Stade, 2007) "Let's cut the program when the kids get to age 3 because we don't have enough money" might be the wrong decision, not just for humane reasons, but also on the basis of the strictest cost-effectiveness analysis.

"Tough Love"

Why is the tough love/boot camp approach ("shape up or your kids will be removed") almost completely useless?

Possible answer: Maybe a third or more of clients in birth mum support programs have FASD, and that can make it difficult to link cause and effect. More importantly, all clients of these programs, I think rather naturally, are hardened and defensive towards yet another put-down or negative judgment. *How many of us respond well to coercion?* Enlightened programmes such as *Behavioural Treatment for Substance Abuse in People with a Serious and Persistent Mental Illness* (Bellack, 2007) have no room for "shame and blame." This book is a surprise - a didactic handbook of sorts, very little theory and lots of "here is exactly what we say and do" when working with a most profoundly impaired population. Guess what the results (for this supportive, validating, relationship-based programme) are with respect to lessening use of substances? As good as the results of addiction programmes for patients who do not have other serious mental health problems!

Out of chaos

I have met many birth mums in my clinical work and continue to be shocked that so many have *so seldom* been supported by links to caring family or friends. How can *anyone* care *when he or she has not been cared for*? Despite very harsh backgrounds, most birth mums I have worked with have a huge heart for and desire to do right for their kids. "Courageous, determined, spunky, and really caring about their kids" are ways I think about birth mums that I have met. Systems of care need to harness and foster this wellspring of positive intent and energy. Even if *daily* care of kids is beyond what a mum can do, honouring her by a welcome invitation - allowing her involvement (inasmuch as she is able) - does much to prevent the despair that leads to further substance abuse and more alcohol-exposed pregnancies.

Dr. Lori Vitale Cox works in a small First Nations community in Atlantic Canada. She has described methods of inclusion for disabled birth mums in her community. These mums, though not able to provide full-time care for their kids, were respected and as involved as they could be in school and community activities. (Cox, 2007)

Amounts of alcohol consumed prenatally

The study *Alcohol Consumption During Pregnancy in Non-Indigenous Western Australian Women* interviewed about 10% of *all* non-indigenous women who gave birth between 1995 and 1997. (Colvin, 2007) This involved 4800 women. 47% had *not* planned their pregnancy (only ½ of the pregnancies being planned is a typical result in most populations!), 80% drank alcohol in the three months prior to their pregnancy (I think this is a bit higher than in North America), 59% drank alcohol in at least the first trimester (ouch), 19% drank at least two standard drinks per occasion in the first trimester (ouch), and 4.3% consumed five or more drinks on a typical drinking occasion at least in the first trimester (it would be hard to assume that these children would be undamaged). Conclusion: (this study is typical of many populations) *many* children are prenatally exposed to alcohol.

Is there a "safe" dose of alcohol during pregnancy?

It is unethical to do human experiments, obviously. Pregnant mice were given a relatively small amount of alcohol so their blood alcohol concentration *just* approached the "legal" limit of 0.08%. Offspring were tested in a "Morris water task" (spatial processing and memory test). Alcohol-exposed offspring performed very poorly in this test of spatial memory (they got lost and could not remember where they wanted to go). A separate study giving *less than a third* of this amount of alcohol to pregnant mice ensued - these offspring also performed poorly in tests of spatial ability. Mice, like it or not, are pretty similar to humans genetically! If a small dose of alcohol (which results in blood levels *one third* as high as what we consider "impaired") measurably harms offspring of our genetic "cousins,"(Sutherland, 2003), what logic could possibly be used to endorse "safe" drinking in pregnancy?

When does a woman know she is pregnant?

Answer: Usually at five to six weeks after the last period, due to a combination of late period, breast tenderness, tiredness, etc. Pregnancy tests can be sensitive enough to show a "positive" at just about the time of the missing period if a woman is pregnant, though this could be a bit later if her ovulation was late.

When can alcohol damage the brain and face?

Answer: At day 19 to 21 of gestation the facial changes found in more severe types of FASD can occur when the fetus is exposed to alcohol. At this stage of pregnancy a woman may not yet know that she has conceived.

Concerns: How many women have irregular periods, which would make it hard to know if the period was late? (Answer: lots.) How many women at high risk of having a child with fetal alcohol problems have a well-tuned awareness of signals their body is giving them? (I often see this as a concern in my clinical work, but am not aware of any studies that look at difficulties clearly interpreting body signals in children affected by prenatal exposure alcohol or their parents.)

Alcoholics Anonymous (AA)

AA or another structured support group can often play a role in recovery. An alcohol counselor once explained to me "be sure your patients know there are some AA groups that might not work well for them and some that will. Shop around till you feel at home," she advises. AA began with a now-famous encounter between "Bill" and Carl Jung in which Dr. Jung said, "You will recover from substance abuse only if you find your way back to God." Soon after, Bill, who was a stockbroker, and an alcoholic doctor friend of his, formed Alcoholics Anonymous. Some of the keys to success for this often-copied group include: high levels of support with weekly meetings and 24/7 availability of a sponsor, "surrendering individual illusions" and admitting that the love of drink is stronger than your will and depending on a "higher power" to get you through.

Comment:

For some, AA may be the first time they have ever experienced a "place of rest" and support. Accountability to the group is another feature of AA. Group members might attempt to spin an elaborate yarn about why they had to drink but, likely, no one will buy it. There is a nice balance in good AA groups of being able to tolerate "no B.S.," but not belittle or ridicule.

Comment:

This is a lot like Dr. Gordon Neufeld's picture of being an "agent of futility" (you can't fool me with the story, you're just trying to rationalize; quit fooling yourself) and at the same time an "angel of mercy" (you do not have to make excuses, you're OK, you've got this group to support you, you'll be all right, in fact you'll be better without these excuses).

Impulsivity

Birth mums, and the rest of us, possess some personality traits that are highly heritable. Impulsivity is associated with reduced frontal lobe activity and is an important contributor to many psychiatric problems, including substance abuse. Impulsivity is defined as "action without planning" or "behavior that is prematurely executed and has maladaptive consequences" (acting without thinking). It appears to be associated with difficulty controlling urges and a compromised ability to consider implications of impending acts (forecasting and predicting the future). [Rod's note: Forecasting is likely a working memory and sequencing issue.]

In the study *Reduced Frontal Lobe Activity in Subjects With High Impulsivity and Alcoholism* (Cheng, 2007) patients' brain electrical activity was assessed. Researchers found that alcohol dependent subjects had a higher score on the Barratt Scale for impulsiveness and had less activation of P300 electrical signals in the cingulate (inner central), medial (central) and superior (upper) frontal lobes. P300 is a type of electrical signal in the brain - the better the P300 signal, the better the processing and understanding of touch, sound, visual and other perceptions. Reduced P300 signals mean the brain does not perceive sensations very well - how can you pay attention to that which is not perceived accurately? If you had problems paying attention, you'd be more impulsive.

Interested in more detail? Keeners might like to know that, specifically, alcoholic patients were found to have less activation of event-related potential P300 scores (brain activations from processing auditory input [listening to a conversation] in five regions of their frontal lobes that are called Broadman's areas 6, 8, 24, 32 and 33).

Take-home point: The part of the brain that should have sorted out what a conversation meant was not working very well. Less of the frontal lobe was available to figure out what was being said. If you couldn't figure out what was said, and had less activity in the "now wait a second and let's think about that" part of your brain, you'd be more impulsive.

Impulsive Suicide - what can we learn from an expert?

Dr. Joel Paris' work since 1972 in Montreal has focused on impulsivity and emotional lability in studies of hundreds of patients for over thirty-five years. (Paris, 2003)

I think a lot of Dr. Paris' comments about suicide and suicidal behaviour are relevant for both birth mums and their kids. I am sorry I do not remember the reference but have certainly heard a number of times the nature of suicide attempts in those affected by FASD can be a bit different. Attempts are a little less likely to be the result of a continuous downhill course into worse and worse states of depression, and a bit more likely to be impulsive when the FASD-affected person feels "cornered."

Through working with his population of patients who suffered huge burdens of depressive thoughts, anxiety, impulsivity and emotional lability, Dr. Paris has developed the following ideas about suicide and self-harm:

-He says that developing a secure, caring relationship with the patient is key. The relationship must be safe, predictable and stable. It is dangerous and counter-productive to fire a patient, despite what might be alienating behavior from the patient. Never abandon the patient, even though you may find yourself "walking on egg shells." Suicide is very common in anxious, depressed, emotionally labile impulsive people and any threats or attempts must be taken very seriously.

-Suicidal threats, overdoses and self-mutilation *all communicate distress*. In addition to "standard assessments of suicide, causes and attempts"(assessment of level of depression, seriousness of suicidal intent, access to a weapon, etc.) it is essential to *treat the episode as a cry for help - listen to what the distress is and provide help or the patient might assume that their cry was not heard and escalate their behaviour until their cry is heard and responded to.*

-Empathize but provide structure. Perhaps unexpectedly, Dr. Paris suggests that we *can* expect long-term success with such patients, especially if they have a social support system in place. Ideally, that should involve *long-term relationships* with their family and with their doctor and other mental health providers. These relationships need to provide safety, (emotionally) a place of rest, and unconditional acceptance. Success is more likely if patients can find a purpose in life and can gradually feel more comfortable with themselves. This helps in their formation of identity/sense of self.

-Those who complete a suicide are more likely to be male, older, avoid treatment, use more lethal methods and die on the first attempt. Those who attempt but do not complete suicide tend to be female, younger, use less lethal methods and be discovered, but mistakes can happen - "Russian roulette" can end in death. 1/3 of chronic suicide attempters meet borderline personality disorder diagnostic criteria.

- In a 1994 study of youth who committed suicide, 1/3 met the criteria for borderline personality disorder. Very few had ever been diagnosed or treated. Less than ½ had seen mental health workers in the previous year and 1/3 had never ever been evaluated. Dr. Paris says we need to involve family. We should inform patients early in their treatment that their families will be contacted if they are seen to be at risk and that a therapist treating chronically suicidal patients should make a point of talking to relatives and significant others at an early stage. This practice need not involve any breach of confidentiality.

-Self-mutilation is very common in borderline personality disorder and is usually repetitive. It can be addictive. Painful emotions are translated into a relieving flow of blood. Patients report they feel better after cutting. Cutting, they say relieves painful emotions, and they "feel less numb" and "more alive." External pain helps them feel less internal pain. See self-mutilation as communication of the patient's distress to others - it is also a plea for help. If no one understands their suffering *they turn up the volume*! To address this, try to understand what they are trying to communicate.

Dr. Paris tries to proceed this way with patients who self-harm:

1. Validate dysphoric feelings. Example: "You must have had really bad feelings to be so upset you wanted to hurt yourself."
2. Explore what brought on these feelings.
3. Implement ideas to reduce the intensity of the feelings. This is a problem solving venture and is very much different from the "all or none" thinking that often results in self-mutilation or a suicide attempt.

Mental health workers' goals are to reduce impulsivity first, because acting out impulsively prevents therapy from addressing any other goals (reflection and intuition are swamped by "crisis all the time" mode). Later, when patients are calm enough to work with therapists, there are efforts to try to modify the instability of emotions. One key is that when patients feel empowered they have no further need to choose death or self-mutilation. This essential work is often overlooked in the midst of a crisis. Gordon Neufeld says that social support is essential for prevention of suicidal behavior. He describes an increase in suicide risk by a factor of nine times in Inuit youth and correlates this to the disruption of their extended family social structure over the last couple of generations.

What comes first, depression or alcoholism?

Answer: Clinical depression (not just depressive symptoms) is often a precursor for alcohol abuse, especially in women. Researchers "have not ruled out that the link between alcohol consumption and depression could be due to a third factor causing both" (Graham, 2008).

Why do we drink?

Answer: In part to self-medicate internal angst, in part because of positive reinforcement - this refers to a positive feeling of well being that we might notice after a few drinks. This is caused by dopamine neuron excitation in an area called the reward center (ventral tegmental area [VTA]).

Causes of heavy drinking include:

- avoidance of the misery of severe withdrawal symptoms
- severe stress
- peers who drink heavily (a powerful influencer in teens)
- belief we might be sexier or more attractive or less inhibited or improved somehow with a few drinks
- PTSD or bipolar disorder or other conditions that are strongly associated with alcoholism
- unlucky genetics, especially a family history of low level of response (it takes a lot to feel tipsy - families with this trait suffer very high rates of alcoholism).

The study of the role of hormones in alcoholism is just coming into its own. Future research on the role of leptin (this is a satiety factor which tells us when we are full), ghrelin (this is secreted in the gut and tells us we are hungry and need to eat more), prolactin, melatonin and oxytocin may lead to some helpful therapies. All these hormone systems are affected by alcohol - and affect likelihood of problem drinking.

Who might be the spouse of someone who has alcohol dependence?

Answer: G.D. Grant, after surveying 6000 Australian twins commented that was that there was a modest effect of "like marries like." (Grant, 2007) This was important because if one gets genes for alcoholism from both parents it would increase genetic burden for the kids.

Birth Dads

"Not much has been reported about birth dads," says Susan Astley, "but we do have a little bit of data from our clinic's recent study." Birth dads accompanied their child to the diagnostic evaluation 8% of the time (versus 20% for birth mums). On average, birth dads were 29 years old at the time of birth of the child that was subsequently diagnosed with FASD. (Birth mums were 3 to 4 years younger.) 39% of birth dads did not finish high school, while 50% reportedly had learning disabilities. Of 1400 patients evaluated, the names of 765 of birth dads and 955 of birth mums were known. (Astley, 2010)

Future questions that I hope will inspire society to allocate adequate resources to effective support of individuals affected by FASD, including birth mums:

Birth mums deal with extreme degrees of mental distress from undiagnosed and inadequately treated psychiatric conditions. Society must come to realize the futility of punitive strategies for birth mums. We can understand something about the depth of impairment –and what to do about it if we consider BDNF. Brain derived neurotrophic factor (BDNF) is an important nerve growth factor - it tells nerves (like the memory-encoding neurons in our "hippycampus") to grow. The average level of BDNF in alcohol-dependent controls was *half* that of control subjects. Lower BDNF not only plays a role in alcohol dependence, it also helps us identify those who will need more help to recover from addictions and other mental health problems. "Low BDNF" sounds like some research scientist's obscure finding, but nothing could be further from the truth

- low BDNF means low "brain cell fertilizer," and this leads to loss of hippocampal cells (which help to calm us down an allow us to learn) and frontal cortex cells (which help calm us down, prioritize and think clearly). When unenlightened people say, "Those (homeless people, birth mums, mental health patients - take your pick) need to 'get with it' and try harder" what I hear is, "Let's *add* some invalidation, stress and frustration to the lives of people who already have stress-overwhelmed brains and trauma-compromised 'learning hardware' when we already know that stress will further impair their learning and sabotage their abilities to problem solve and adapt." Just who doesn't "get it" here? Can we accept judgmental attitudes? Heck no! If we want to be efficacious, respect and encouragement is the route to effective interventions. Don't believe me? Read this: Bellack et al's *Behavioural Treatment for Substance Abuse* and you'll *have* to change your mind.

One reason that we need to comprehensively understand birth mothers (and birth dads) is that obviously they will pass genetic traits along to their kids. Heritable traits are likely to show up in their kids even if abstinence has been observed during a given pregnancy. Character traits such as impulsivity and emotional lability are highly heritable.

When a birth mum is identified, society has a huge opportunity to step up to the plate with supportive and preventative programmes - we can help reduce the potentially multi-generational cycle of FASD. Model programmes of intensive support such as Sheway in Vancouver exist. *Sheway* is an effective programme, reducing the number of alcohol-exposed pregnancies - but why does it stop when the index child turns 3 years old?

As discussed, the level of mental health pathology (usually untreated) in birth mums is alarming. We saw that Stirling Clarren and Susan Astley published a study of 160 birth mothers in 2000. **Startlingly, several years after they had given birth to their children, 25% of these young women were missing or dead!** I don't know of types of cancer *or any other disease* with 25% *mortality* in 30 year-old women! Birth mums in this study had started life at all levels of society, but as adults most lived in poverty. There were nearly universal reports of lifetime experiences of extreme physical, sexual and emotional abuse and nearly all had longstanding battles with alcohol use and abuse. Life consisted of social isolation, very few friends, strained relationships with family and limited activities. Of 160 birth mothers, only 80 could be located. Researchers felt that about half of these women had FASD themselves. Their best chance to access resources for social benefits, housing, mental health and medical services was during pregnancy. As a society, we can do better - much better - in supporting birth mums. Let's do this so we can write a better epilogue to FASD 101 in a few years.

Thank you, readers, for taking the time to learn about FASD by looking through this chapter. Your efforts will help children like mine so I am most grateful to you,

Rod Densmore, M.D., Parent of a child who has FAS

References

Allen JG, Fonagy P, Bateman A. 2008. Mentalizing in Clinical Practice. Washington, DC: American Psychiatric Publishing.

Astley SJ, Bailey D, Talbot C, et al. 2000. Fetal Alcohol Syndrome (FAS) primary prevention through FAS diagnosis: II: A comprehensive profile of 80 birth mothers of children with FAS. Alcohol and Alcoholism: 35(5): 509-519

Astley SJ, Aylward E, Olson HC, et al. Magnetic resonance imaging outcomes from a comprehensive magnetic resonance study of children with fetal alcohol spectrum disorders. Alcoholism: Clinical and experimental research 33(10): 1-19

Astley S. 2010. Profiles of 1400 patients evaluated for FASD at the WA FAS DPN by interdisciplinary teams using the 4-digit code. (Conference presentation) 11th Annual Fetal Alcohol Canadian Expertise Research Roundtable (FACE) Sept 14, 2010 (available webcast at: http://www.motherisk.org/FAR/index.jsp)

Bell S, Stade BS, Reynolds JN, et al. 2010. The remarkably high prevalence of epilepsy in subjects with FASD. Alcoholism: Clinical and experimental research 34: 1-6

Bellack AS, Bennett ME, Gearson JS, et al. 2007. Behavioural Treatment for Substance Abuse in People with Serious and Persistent Mental Illness. New York: Routledge.

Bonthius DJ, Olson HC, Thomas JD. 2006. Proceedings of the 2006 Annual Meeting of the Fetal Alcohol Spectrum Disorders Study Group. Alcohol 40(1): 61-65

Brett-Green BA, Miller LJ. 2008 Multisensory Integration in Children: A Preliminary ERP Study. Brain Research 1242: 283-290

Cavazos-Rehg PA, Spitznagl EL, Bucholz KK, et al. 2008. Predictors of Sexual Debut at age 16 or younger [ISSN online 1573-2800]. Archives of Sexual Behavior. October 10, 2008.

Chan F, Barbosa AV, Vatikiotis-Bateson E, et al. 2010.Differentiating restless legs syndrome (RLS) as a cause of circadian sleep rhythm disorders (CSRD) in children with FASD: video studies in home setting – commercially available low-cost equipment. Poster presentation at: 2010 Fetal Alcohol Canadian Expertise (FACE) Research Roundtable. Abstract published: Journal of Population Therapeutics and Clinical Pharmacology 17(2): e284-e301; August 12, 2010.

Chacko MR. 2010. Contraception: Overview of issues specific to adolescents. UpToDate Desktop 18.1 Medical Reference DVD

Cheng, ACH, Porjesz B, Rangaswamy M, et al. 2007. Reduced Frontal Lobe Activity in Subjects With High Impulsivity and Alcoholism. Alcoholism: Clinical and Experimental Research 31(1): 156-165

Cloud J. 2010. Why your DNA isn't your destiny. Time. Jan 6, 2010. (Available at: http://www.time.com/time/health/article/0,8599,1951968,00.html)

Colvin L, Payne J, Parsons D, et al. 2007. Alcohol Consumption During Pregnancy in Non-Indigenous Western Australian Women. Alcoholism: Clinical and experimental research 31(2): 276-284

Corwin MJ. 2007. Sudden Infant Death Syndrome. UpToDate 15.3 (medical reference CD-ROM)

Cox LV. 2007. The Prevalence of FASD in a Maritime First Nation Community. (Conference presentation) 2007 Fetal Alcohol Canadian Expertise (FACE) Research Roundtable. (available webcast at: http://www.motherisk.org/fas6/webcast/index.html)

Densmore RJ. 2010. Restoring hope: an adapted attachment parenting DVD series empowers caregivers of children who have FASD. Poster presentation at: 2010 Fetal Alcohol Canadian Expertise (FACE) Research Roundtable. Abstract published: Journal of Population Therapeutics and Clinical Pharmacology 17(2): e284-e301; August 12, 2010. Also viewable at: http://www.cjcp.ca/pubmed.php?articleId=273 page e291

Doige N. 2007. The Brain that Changes Itself. New York: Penguin Books.

Eide B, Eide F. 2010. Common Learning Challenges in Sensory Processing Disorder. (Conference presentation) at Sensory Processing Disorder Foundation 11th International Symposium and Pre-Conference Institute. Bellevue, Washington. November 12, 2010.

Farmer JE, Donders J, Warschausky S. (Editors) 2006. Treating Neurodevelopmental Disabilities: Clinical Research and Practice. New York: Guilford Press.

Frank E, Young T. 2010. Biological Rhythms and Neuroplasticity: A Unified Approach to Understanding Mood. Conference presentation at: Canadian Psychiatric Association Annual Meeting. Toronto. September 25, 2010.

Foa EB, Kean TM, Friedman MJ, et al. 2009. Effective Treatments for PTSD, Second Edition: Practice Guidelines from the International Society for Traumatic Stress Studies. New York: The Guilford Press.

Foisy ML, Kornreich C, Fobe A, et al. 2007. Impaired Emotional Facial Expression Recognition in Alcohol Dependence. Alcoholism: Clinical and Experimental Research 31(3): 404-410

Fonagy P. 2009. Advances in Personality Disorders: Attachment and borderline personality disorder: a mentilization – based approach. (Conference presentation) American Psychiatric Association Meeting, San Francisco, May 16-21, 2009.

Gahagan S, Sharpe TT, Brimacombe M, et al. 2006. Pediatricians' Knowledge, Training, and Experience in the Care of Children With Fetal Alcohol Syndrome. Pediatrics 118: e657 - e668

Gelernter J. 2009. Symposium 70: Genetic vulnerabilities for drug use and co-morbid mental health disorders: Approaching comorbidity in addiction genetics. (Conference presentation) American Psychiatric Assoc. Annual Meeting. San Francisco. May 16-21, 2009.

Gelernter J, Kranzler HR. 2009.Genetics of alcohol dependence. Human Genetics 126: 91-99

Glaves MM, Ellis L, Yu WK, et al. 2007. Effects of Prenatal Ethanol Exposure on Basal Limbic-Hypothalamic-Pituitary-Adrenal Regulation. Alcoholism: Clinical and Experimental Research 31(9): 1598-1610

Goleman D. 2006. Social Intelligence: the new science of human relationships. New York: Bantam Books. p 231

Goldsmith HH, Van Hulle CA, Ameson CI, et al. 2006. A population-based twin study of parentally reported tactile and auditory defensiveness in young children. Journal of Abnormal Child Psychology 34(3): 378-392

Goril S, Shapiro CM. 2010. The prevalence and patterns of sleep disorders and circadian rhythm disruptions in children with Fetal Alcohol Spectrum Disorders (FASD). Poster presentation at 2010 Fetal Alcohol Canadian Expertise (FACE) research roundtable meeting published as: 2010 FACE Poster Competition Abstracts Supplement. Journal of Population Therapeutics and Clinical Pharmacology 17(2) Summer 2010: e284-e301

Graham K, Plant M, Plant M, et al. 2008. Alcohol Consumption and Depression. Alcoholism: Clinical and Experimental research 31(1): 78-88

Grant JD, Heath AC, Bucholz KK, et al. 2007. Spousal Concordance for Alcohol Dependence. Alcoholism; Clinical and Experimental Research 31(5): 717-728

Jan JE, Wasdel MB, Reiter RJ. 2007. Melatonin Therapy of Pediatric Sleep Disorders: Recent analysis, why it works, who are the candidates best to treat. Current pediatric reviews 3: 214-224

Jan JE, Asante KO, Conry JL, et al. 2010. Sleep health issues for children with FASD: Clinical considerations. International Journal of Pediatrics. Published online July 14, 2010. Retrieved from: http://www.ncbi.nlm.nih.gov/pmc/articles/PMC2913852/November 28, 2010.

Kapp ME, O'Malley K. 2001. Watch for the Rainbows; True Stories for Educators and Other Caregivers of Children With Fetal Alcohol Spectrum Disorders. Calgary, Alberta. Frances Kapp Education.

Kaunitz AM. 2010. Depot medroxyprogesterone acetate for contraception. UpToDate Desktop 18.1 Medical Reference DVD

Keitner GI, Heru AM, Glick ID. et al. 2010. Clinical Manual of Couples and Family Therapy. Washington, DC: American Psychiatric Press. p 43

Klintsona AY, Helfer JL, Lyngine H, et al. 2007. Persistent Impairment of Hippocampal Neurogenesis in Young Adult Rats Following Early Postnatal Alcohol Exposure. Alcoholism: Clinical and Experimental Research 31(12): 2073-2082

Koren G. 2010. Personal communication.

Kosten T. 2009. Neurobiologic determinants of the Comorbidity of PTSD and Substance Abuse. In: Symposium 35: PTSD and Alcoholism, emphasis on returning veterans. (Conference presentation) American Psychiatry Association Annual Meeting, San Francisco. May 16-21, 2009.

Kristjanson AF, Wilsnack SC, Zvartau E, et al. 2007. Alcohol use in pregnant and non-pregnant Russian women. Alcoholism: Clinical and Experimental Research 31(2): 299-307

Lebel C, et al. 2010. Brain Imaging and Neurocognitive Functioning in Children and Twins with FASD (Conference presentation) Alberta FASD Conference, Calgary. Feb 9, 2010.

LeStrat Y, Ramoz N, Schuman G, et al. 2008. Molecular Genetics of Alcohol Dependence and Related Endotypes. Current Genomics 9: 444-457

Linden DJ. 2007. The Accidental Mind: How Brain Evolution Has Given Us Love, Memory, Dreams and God. Cambridge, Massachusetts: Belknap Press.

Malbin D. 2002. Fetal Alcohol Spectrum Disorders: Trying Differently Rather Than Harder. Portland, Oregon: FASCETS, Inc.

Malisza KL, Allman A-A, Shiloff D, et al. 2005. Evaluation of spatial working memory function in children and adults with fetal alcohol spectrum disorders: a functional magnetic resonance imaging study. Pediatric Research 58: 1150-1157

Malleson R. 2010. Contraception: What do Women Want? (Conference presentation) 45th Annual Post Graduate Review in Family Medicine, University of British Columbia. March 4, 2010.

Neufeld G. 2010 Power to Parent, Volume 1: The Vital Connection DVD (Available from: http://www.gordonneufeld.com/)

Norman AL, Crocker N, Mattson SN, et al. 2009. Neuroimaging and Fetal Alcohol Spectrum Disorders. Developmental Disabilities Research Reviews 15: 209-217

Olson HC, Oti R, Gelo J, et al. 2009. "Family Matters:" Fetal Alcohol Spectrum Disorders and the Family. Developmental Disability Research Reviews 15: 235-249

Ory N, Dykstra T. 2007 Working With People With Challenging Behaviours: A Guide for Maintaining Positive Relationships (Spiral-bound). New Lenox, Illinois: High Tide Press.

O'Malley K. (editor) 2007. ADHD and Fetal Alcohol Spectrum Disorders (FASD) New York: Nova Science Publishers.

Panda A. 2009. PTSD and Disaster Psychiatry. (Conference presentation) American Psychiatric Association Annual Meeting. San Francisco. May 16-21, 2009.

Paris J. 2003. Personalities Over Time: Precursors, Course, and Outcome. Washington, DC: American Psychiatric Publishing Inc.

Perry B. 2010. Understanding the impact of trauma in the developing child: clinical implications and applications of neurodevelopmentally-informed treatment strategies. (Workshop) Justice Institute of British Columbia, New Westminster. June 2-3, 2010.

Robinson B. 1983. Caregiver Strain Index. Journal of Gerontology 38. pp 344-348

Schuckit MA. 2009. How Alcoholism Develops: Identification of Genetic and Environmental Influences in a 25-year Longitudinal Study. (Adolf Meyer Award Lecture) American Psychiatric Association Meeting. San Francisco. May 16-21, 2009.

Singer GHS, Glang A, Williams JN, editors. 1996. Children With Acquired Brain Injury. Baltimore: Paul H. Brookes Publishing.

Stade B, Ungar WJ, Stevens B, et al. 2007. Motherisk update: Cost of fetal alcohol spectrum disorder in Canada. Canadian Family Physician 53: 1303-1304

Stade B, Barozzino T, Bennett D, et al. 2010.The nature of sleep in Canadian children with Fetal Alcohol Spectrum Disorder. Poster presentation at: 2010 Fetal Alcohol Canadian Expertise (FACE) Research Roundtable. Abstract published: Journal of Population Therapeutics and Clinical Pharmacology 17(2): e284-e301; August 12, 2010.

Stovall J. 2009. Bipolar Disorder: Epidemiology and Diagnosis. UpToDate Desktop 17.1 CD-ROM Medical Reference

Stromland K, Hellstrom A. 1996. Fetal Alcohol Syndrome- an opthalmological and socioeducational prospective study. Pediatrics 97(6): 845-849

Streissguth AP, Barr HM, Kogan J, et al. 1996. Understanding the occurrence of secondary disabilities in clients with fetal alcohol syndrome (FAS) and fetal alcohol effects (FAE): Final report to the Centers for Disease Control and Prevention. Seattle. University of Washington, Fetal Alcohol and Drug Unit.

Streissguth AP. 1997. Fetal Alcohol Syndrome: A Guide for Families and Communities. Baltimore: Brookes Publishing.

Streissguth AP, Bookstein FL, Barr HM, et al. 2004. Risk factors for adverse life outcomes in fetal alcohol syndrome and fetal alcohol effects. Developmental Behavioral Pediatrics 25: 228-238

Sullivan AK. 2007. FASD in the Adult: Vulnerability, Disability or Diagnosis - a Psychodynamic Perspective. In: O'Malley KA, editor. ADHD and Fetal Alcohol Spectrum Disorders (FASD). New York: Nova Science.

Sutarjono B, Florez C, Brien JF, Reynolds JN, Kapur B, Carlen PL. 2010. Hippocampal excitability in young postnatal guinea pig following prenatal alcohol exposure. Cited in: Carlen PL. 2010. Fetal ethanol exposure and postnatal brain hyperexcitability: the tip of the neurobehavioural iceberg. (Conference presentation) 11th Annual Fetal Alcohol Canadian Expertise (FACE) Research Roundtable Sept 14, 2010 (available webcast at: http://www.motherisk.org/FAR/index.jsp)

Sutherland RJ. 2003. Prenatal alcohol exposure neuropathology and cognition: integrating behavioral and neural approaches in rats and humans. (Conference presentation) Fetal Alcohol Canadian Expertise (FACE) 2003 Research Roundtable. (available webcast at:http://www.knowledgenetwork.ca/fasii/index.html)

Ward SL, Bautista D, Chan L, et al. 1990. SIDS in infants of substance abusing mothers. Journal of Pediatrics 117(6): 876-881

Weathers FW, Huska JA, Keane TM. 1991. PLC-C for DSM-IV. Boston: National Center for PTSD - Behavioral Science Division

Weinberg J. 2007. Prenatal alcohol exposure in an animal model: fetal programming and implications for vulnerability in adulthood. (Keynote Address) 8th Annual Fetal Alcohol Canadian Expertise (FACE) 2007 Meeting. (available webcast at: http://www.motherisk.org/fas6/webcast/index.html)

Zhou FC, West JR, Blake CA, et al. 2005. General discussion at the Fetal Alcohol Syndrome Symposium. Experimental Biology and Medicine 230: 407-412

Ziegler D. 2000. Raising Children Who Refuse To Be Raised: Parenting Skills and Therapy Interventions for the Most Difficult Children. Phoenix, Arizona: Acacia Press.

Chapter Two

Interview with Myles Himmelreich

This chapter contains worksheets of the questions posed to Myles Himmelreich, and his answers. The interview is included in this book's DVD and may also be viewed at: fasdrelationships.ca I believe people affected by FASD and those that work with them need to discern what relative strengths and gifts an individual possesses and work within those. Thus, I also include worksheets noting some strengths and challenges Myles discusses in his answers. I encourage readers to add to this list as they listen to Myles.

Myles Interview: Questions

The following are the 20 questions asked over the interview:

1. What do you live for?
2. How have you become a spokesperson for FASD?
3. What is new in your message?
4. What are your ways to help others understand FASD better?
5. Why does focusing on negatives not work?
6. What happens when those in power are judgmental and unsupportive?
7. What worked well and what did not? (specifically teachers)
8. What about bullying?
9. What are your coping strategies as a teen?
10. Did you "need" to go through that stage?
11. How could you transcend overuse of drugs and alcohol?
12. Should young people who have FASD drink?
13. Has spirituality helped you?
14. How have sensory issues affected you?
15. Were there any accommodations made for your sensory issues?
16. Have you used simulation as a teaching tool?
17. New ideas discussed? (Consensus Development Conference on FASD/ Edmonton 2009) To see conclusions of the Consensus Conference view: http://fasd.statusfirm.com/index.php?video=2009-10-09-conclusion
18. What Vocational support ideas are useful?
19. Have you had mentors along the way?
20. What are your goals and dreams?

Myles Interview: Questions and Answers

The following are the 20 questions asked over the interview and some of the key points found in the answers given by Myles. The answers are in point form with the times they appear in the interview posted in front.

1. 1:57 - What do you live for?

- » 2:13 - getting up and having a good life (where he is in life now)
- » 2:25 – having a job, and his own place
- » 2:38 – feeling like he's "part of society"
- » 2:50 – enjoy having good friends, sports, and work

2. 3:25 –How have you become a spokesperson for FASD?

- » 3:39 –someone who had been helping him asked if he'd like to share his story at a conference
- » 4:17 –while speaking, Myles realized it was easier to just "speak from the heart"
- » 4:50 –realized that "this is what I'm supposed to do… what I've been searching for"
- » 4:58 –continued speaking at conferences and has been doing so ever since (5-6 years)

3. 5:28 - What is new in your message?

- » 6:00 –the story grows "and I grow"
- » 6:10 –FASD is a life long disability "I will always be learning from it and growing through the struggles"
- » 6:52 –being able to share those stories

4. 7:15 –What are your ways to help others understand FASD better?

- » 8:00 – introducing it to them while talking about what he does for a living
- » 8:28 – with professionals, discuss what methods work and what doesn't
- » 9:00 -"strength-based" is key to helping people with FASD

5. 10:13 –Why does focusing on negatives not work?

- » 9:25 –you can get lost in the negatives (discussed at the end of the previous question)

6. 11:00 –What happens when those in power are judgmental and unsupportive?

- » 11:47 –it's like there's an un-written plan for how you should live your life
- » 12:07 –people get scared and tend to stay away from people who stray or can't follow the ideal life style
- » 13:29 –is the point helping someone get through a math problem or supporting their strengths, for example: "piano player"

7. 14:57 –What worked well and what did not? (specifically teachers)

What didn't work:

- » 15:33 – teachers (and other professionals) need to realize what they don't know
- » 16:04 – as a student not being able to explain what the problem was
- » 16:07 – as a teacher not knowing/ understanding that sensory issues were a problem

What worked:

- 7:05 –keep them busy
- 17:10 –sweeping the floor -"see the results" and "easy steps to remember"
- 17:57 –attendance to the office -feel good for helping others

Involving parents (or guardians):

- 18:30 –teachers and parents teaching with different methods = confusion
- 19:00 –involve more communication between teachers and parents to develop one simple routine for problem solving

What could also help:

- 19:39 –asking "how can I help you?"
- 19:44 –understanding! it's not always going to work
- 20:04 –encouraging the student (something they don't get from their peers)

8. 20:35 –What about bullying?

- 21:20 not knowing why he acted the way he did
- 21:30 –maturity level is lower than what is considered normal for that age. Get picked on because of this
- 22:23 –invisible disability- no "visual aid" to point out disability. It's only explained by diagnosis
- 23:20 –not understanding why he was different or acted the way he did was worse than the bullying

9. 24:40 –What are your coping strategies as a teen?

- 25:05 –drugs and alcohol
- 25:20 "drink away my problems"
- 25:48 –finally being "accepted" so long as he bought the beer

10. 27:01 –Did you “need” to go through that stage?

» 27:25 –made him stronger, helped him get up to speak

» 27:33 – embracing everything that happened because it made him who he is today

» 28:58 – learning from it

» 29:25 - realizing what FASD really meant (especially in his personal situation) helped come out of depending on drugs and alcohol

11. 31:05 –How could you transcend overuse of drugs and alcohol?

» 31:36 – self-awareness

» 31:45 – finding something to replace it. What can I do instead? What do/ did I enjoy doing? for example: sports

» 32:41-stay busy, don’t leave time for drinks

12. 33:23 – Should young people who have FASD drink?

» 34:32 – controlled drinking with friends is all right as long as it’s not being depended on

» 35:51 – depends on individual needs

13. 36:39 – Has spirituality helped you?

» 37:34 –at a point that's all you have "okay, it's just you and me"

» 38:22 –gives life purpose

14. 39:32 –How have sensory issues affected you?

» 40:30 –not being able to work and learn in a classroom

» 40:54 –FASD can also lead to muscles and bones not growing properly, makes it difficult to participate

15. 15) 42:02 –Were there any accommodations made for your sensory issues?

» 42:12 –not while he was going to school

» 42:41 –not aware of anything for students now, difficult problem to work with

16. 43:22 -Have you used simulation as a teaching tool?

» 44:10 –use noisemakers and speak quietly

» 44:48 –they don't know the answer, just as he wouldn't have known the answer

17. 45:34 – Any new ideas discussed? (IHE Consensus Development Conference on FASD)

(in depth discussion on:)

- what is FASD
- how do you diagnose it
- what supports are out there
- Jury of 12 who received all presentations worked together to come up with a consensus manual

18. 48:31 – What vocational support ideas are useful?

- 48:43 – the 2 R's Routine and Repetition "get used to it and get good at it"
- 49:05 – employers being open to helping more than once (it doesn't "stick" easily)

19. 50:29 –Have you had mentors along the way?

- 50:47 – more now than when he was struggling
- 51:00 – he is a mentor now because he knows that would have helped

20. 52:39 – What are your goals and dreams?

- 52:50 – get married and have a family
- 52:56 – get license and a car
- 53:02 – keep a good job and continue public speaking
- 53:13 – complete biography
- 53:19 – keep going on a good path

Myles' Interview: Gifts/Strengths and Symptoms/Struggles (Answers 1-20)

Myles can teach us all much about transcendence of difficulties by working within one's strengths. The numbers represent the question each point comes after. As you watch the interview see if you can add to these lists of Strengths that Myles describes and the Symptoms of FASD that he has struggled with.

1. **Gifts/Strengths**

» Satisfied with life as it is

» Understands what he is good at

» Able to reflect on what happened in his life and learn from these experiences

» Appreciates (really savors) what he's got now because of past difficulties

2. **Gifts/Strengths**

» Confidence to make the transition from written notes to "speaking from the heart", willing to "put himself out there" (able to let himself be vulnerable - this may indicate the quality of his relationship with and trust in Liz, his colleague)

» Able to take advantage of opportunities (not "second guess" himself and hesitate until opportunities pass by)

» Natural public speaker, sees public speaking as a calling

» Interested in knowing self, on a quest to understand himself

3. **Gifts/Strengths**

» Sees failures/disappointments as inevitable, but is not defeated by them - strives to learn from these experiences - refuses to be "stuck" in a cycle of defeat and negativity, interested in sharing his ongoing life lessons with others

4. **Gifts/Strengths**

» Able to avoid resentment towards people in positions of power who may have made his life difficult because they did not understand FASD in the past

» "Honored" to share what it's like from a personal perspective

» Sees the futility of being negative - knows the benefit of looking for the positive

» Committed to strength-based ways of working through issues

5. This Section has no comments

6. Gifts/Strengths

» Able to gently (without anger) invite us to look at people's stories (e.g. the girl who gets pregnant) - and to suspend judgment

» Can help us to see the deep humanity and dignity in everyone's struggles even those who do not "follow the approved path"

» Points out that education can come also from seeking to understand your own life experiences vs. specific course curricula - "we can get lost in what our (real, most important) outcome is" - for eventual life satisfaction, skills like playing piano might be more helpful than learning to answer a math question

» Refuses to let struggles in learning defeat him - "you may have struggles but step back (and don't get stuck because a central goal of education is to) teach and help you learn how to find out who you really are"

Symptoms/Struggles

» School/academics were a struggle, got to grade 10-11

» Felt like he was not meeting expectations

» Thought, "I was a failure"

7. Gifts/Strengths

» Now knows what works in a learning environment and what doesn't

» Now able to recognize and adapt to some sensory distractions

» Now able to see "someone else's side" - the teacher "could not understand what's wrong if I did not tell them"

» Liked activities that might have been "unconventional" but 1) kept him busy, 2) gave him a feeling of accomplishment (sense of contributing, sense of "agency"), 3) often involved "heavy work activities" (like sweeping the floor in woodworking class) and 4) did not require a lot of sequential steps

» Now recognizes that the understanding and care of the student (by concerned adults) can give them hope - (often) "kids do not have hope and they don't get it from other students!" (Validation and support from teachers and other adults who are in a position of power is so important so very helpful.)

Symptoms/Struggles

- "I could not explain what was going on" - e.g. sensory issues like light sensitivity, irritation from tags in clothes and distraction from the noise of tapping pens
- Did not understand the effects of FASD
- Did not want to embarrass self especially as a teen
- Had much less self-awareness as a child than he has now
- Woodwork projects that involved lots of choices, a long sequence of steps, having to remember what those steps were over a long period of time and having to create a picture in your mind in order to understand were very difficult. (This suggests working memory, distractibility, attention, sequencing, ability to form representations and concept formation difficulties.)
- School academics were hard work - to have to do homework was a struggle especially if the way mum and dad explained how to do a problem at home was different from how the teacher explained it at school. Communication between parents and teachers can help address this problem.
- It was hard to understand the instructions - what was really meant
- If scared, nervous or "didn't know how to do it" Myles might have just sat there (versus asking the teacher for clarification and embarrassing himself). Myles points out how helpful it would have been if, at times like these, he'd been asked, "how can I help you?" (or, "lets see if we can get started")
- Variable ability (from one day to another) to perform academic tasks

8. Gifts/Strengths

- Now, as an adult, understands how "invisible" disability, made it so difficult for kids to be understood by peers, adults and themselves
- Now, as an adult, Myles is able to revisit even very painful feelings (not knowing why he acted the

way he did as a child and feelings of being bullied and alienated)

Symptoms/Struggles

» Really wanted to "fit in" but "it was not going to happen for me"

» Struggle to find a role, an identity - " I was the goofy, silly guy"

» "I knew I was different but I did not know why and I could not understand it and could not explain it to myself or others"

» Lower maturity level - "I was 13-14 and acting like a 7 yr. old" so Myles was bullied

» Poor self-awareness (as a child) - "Don't know why I acted like I did"

» Because FASD is not a (physically) "visible" disability nobody "cuts you some slack" or offers accommodations and also Myles, himself, did not see the disability when he looked in the mirror - not understanding why he was different or acted the way he did was even "worse than bullying"

9. Gifts/Strengths

» Knows now that drugs and alcohol don't solve problems - "at the end of it - they end up causing more pain"

» Knew (even at the time) that his "party-friends" weren't really friends

» Knows he had a need to be accepted

Symptoms/Struggles

» Anxiousness, frustration and weariness with ongoing struggles led to drugs, alcohol and partying as coping strategies - "it took away the pain if only for a night"

» Craving of companionship and acceptance led to hanging out with some people who were only there because of drugs and alcohol - "I even knew at the time they were not my friends".

10. Gifts/Strengths

» Able to learn from struggles and hardships –these sentiments are very powerful:

"Horrible stuff happened, I can see that now. I'm not lazy, I'm not stupid, it's not that I don't care, it's not that I can't do the school work, it's not that I can't keep a job, it's because of the FASD that I have these struggles but (the question is) what can I do to work on them? FASD is a hard road. Others (with FASD) have similar struggles and make similar choices, bad choices - that's ok - just learn from it!" "Don't be scared of FASD" (and the negativity and stigma surrounding the term FASD which is based on awkward feelings many people harbor towards those who drink during a pregnancy but extends also to those who have FASD). FASD is "part of who we are - I have FASD, I am not FASD. See it (the FASD) and work with it. Understand your FASD - what is really means for you - what parts cause issues and problems."

Symptoms/Struggles

» Addictions, times of "couch-surfing", times of homelessness

» Forgot to eat

» Troubles with time management

11. Gifts/Strengths

» Knew personal strengths and weaknesses, self-awareness, curious and motivated to understand FASD

» Understood he needed something positive to replace the alcohol

» Likes and is good at sports

» As he was emerging from addictions intentionally "kept busy" (and he had the opportunity to do so in a non-drug environment)

12. Gifts/Strengths

» Realizes one doesn't need the alcohol, that there are better things in life

» Able to get great enjoyment from being with his friends

» Can be with friends now without needing to have alcohol (I did not ask Myles but I suspect his present friends may drink less than some of his friends in the past)

» Notes that for some it is best not to drink at all

» For himself, using alcohol modestly and not as a coping mechanism is ok

(Rod's note: Problem drinking seems to have at least 5 "engines" which "keep it going" each of which relates to certain neurotransmitters and neurologic circuits in the brain: 1) "Priming dose" reinstatement of heavy drinking can occur in some folks who have a very rapid descent into alcohol dependence after just a small amount of alcohol. People with this pattern should avoid alcohol. 2) "Low level of response" to alcohol (it takes a lot to make one "feel it") is a very powerful predictor of problem drinking so people with this pattern should avoid alcohol. 3) "Stress –induced" reinstatement of heavy drinking could be avoided if there was less stress (which Myles was able to effect by doing more sports). 4) "Cue-related" heavy drinking changes when one changes friends and the situations in which one drinks (e.g. not drinking to "get drunk" but just having one or two when in a social situation). 5) "Alcohol withdrawal avoidance" is another reason for heavy drinking but is less likely if not enough alcohol is consumed to cause significant withdrawal symptoms. Summary: "Priming-dose inevitably leading to problem drinking" folks and "Low level of response" folks really are wise to not try to "drink just a little" because they will be wrestling with some awfully powerful biochemistry which is conspiring to drive them towards excessive consumption of alcohol.) References: 1) Schuckit MA. Adolf Meyer Award Lecture. How Alcoholism Develops: Identification of Genetic and Environmental Influences in a 25-year Longitudinal Study. American Psychiatric Association Meeting. 2009. San Francisco 2) Edwards G, Marshall EJ, Cook CCH. (2003) The Treatment of Drinking Problems: A Guide for the Helping Professions 4th Edition, Cambridge University Press, Cambridge, U.K.

13. Gifts/Strengths

- Sees talents as gifts and is thankful for talents and opportunities
- Comfortable in a belief there is a force beyond the "here and now", grateful for this source of support - "there was a point that's all I had. It might be a coping mechanism but it is a pretty good one!"
- At times calls on a spiritual being so is not all alone
- In part through spiritual belief has a sense of purpose and effectiveness

14. Gifts/Strengths

- Understands sensory issues- so can reduce distractions and issues from these, tries to work with his chronic knee and leg pain issues so he does not have to avoid sports

Symptoms/Struggles

- Leg/knee pain with exercise, visual hyper-responsivity (bright lights bother him), touch hyper-responsivity (tags on shirts bother him), auditory hyper-responsivity or discrimination issues (distracted by extraneous noises - makes it hard to hear what others are saying)

15. Symptoms/Struggles

» There really were no sensory accommodations made for Myles when he was at school as he recalls

16. Gifts/Strengths

» Realizes that "hands-on" learning works well for himself

Symptoms/Struggles

» There is variability in symptoms of FASD - "some days I have more struggles"

17. This Section has no comments

18. Gifts/Strengths

» Knows some effective techniques: "Have the same routine and the repetition of doing the same kind of thing so you can get used to it and understand it". Myles points out that jobs can energize you if you do them well and repetition can help you do them well.

» Aware of how important it is to ask employers for help, and to give them a "heads up" regarding some common problems and solutions

Symptoms/Struggles

» Variable performance of job skills from one day to the next

» Needs reminders

» Might need to relearn skills

19. Gifts/Strengths

» Despite not having mentors when he was younger Myles realizes how important they are and is moved to be a mentor to kids who have FASD

» Very appreciative of long-time support from his family and his friend, Liz

» It is not just all about struggle; it is great to celebrate successes with mentors and supporters too

20. Gifts/Strengths

» Myles aspires to be a husband and dad, to learn to drive, continue his meaningful work and complete a biography. As my daughter, Julia, notes, "Myles' goals and dreams are really the same as anybody else's".

Chapter Three

DVD Power Point Slides

This chapter contains power point slides from the seven lectures on this book's DVDs:

1. Genetics and FASD for a General Audience
2. Sensory Processing and FASD
3. Neurobiology of FASD for a General Audience
4. Neurobiology of Attachment
5. Our Brain
6. Genetics and FASD for Health Professionals
7. Neurobiology of FASD for Health Professionals

As part of lecture 2)—Sensory Processing and FASD—I have included Worksheets for sensory profiles of: D.L., C.R. and A.J. These worksheets offer a hands-on exercise for readers to develop a sensory profile and list of accommodations and strategies for patients D.L., C.R., and A.J.

The DVD lectures are designed to help learners move past knowing to understanding and using information. These Power Points are not about overwhelming readers with numerous slides; this hurried format seldom results in deep understanding. I encourage readers to use this chapter in this way:

Relax! Grab a coffee.

Stop, start, and review the DVD as often as you like,

and be unhurried but thorough about making notes on the parts of a topic that are directly relevant for you and the kids you care for.

Genetics and FASD
For a general audience

Dr. Rod Densmore

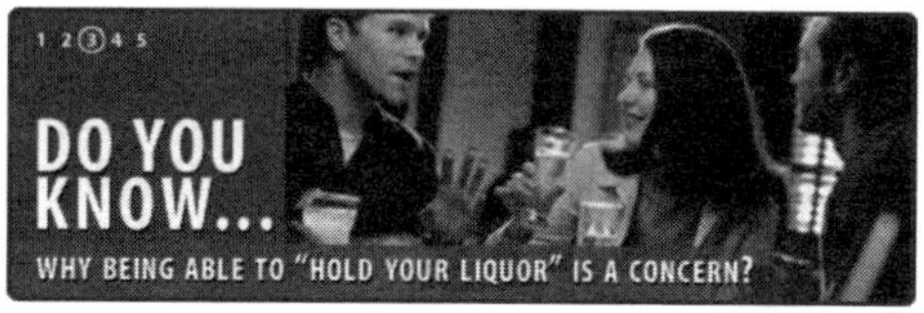
1 2 3 4 5
DO YOU KNOW...
WHY BEING ABLE TO "HOLD YOUR LIQUOR" IS A CONCERN?

http://rethinkingdrinking.niaaa.nih.gov/

Genes

46 Chromosomes

½ from mum ½ from dad

Arranged in 23 pairs

25 000 genes – where the genes are and how DNA sequence varies

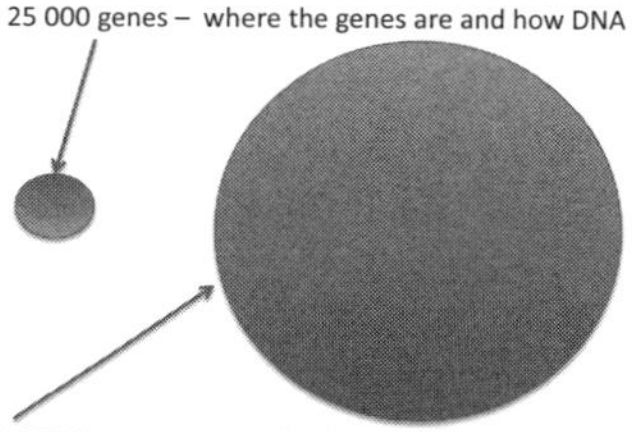

Cloud J. 2010. Why your DNA isn't your destiny. Time. Jan 6, 2010. Available at: http://www.time.com/time/health/article/0,8599,1951968,00.html

EPIGENETICS: turning genes "on" and "off" is key e.g. Women: "the extra X" is "dormant"

What Did My Child Inherit? How Can That Knowledge Help Me?

Gene Basics, Epigenetics, Attachment

Sensory Processing Disorder - Sensory Over-responsivity

Impulsivity and Early Sexual Debut

Secondary Disabilities and Inherited Mental Health Issues

Alcoholism, Level of Response, Gene- Environment Interactions

The Pups of High Licking/Grooming Mums

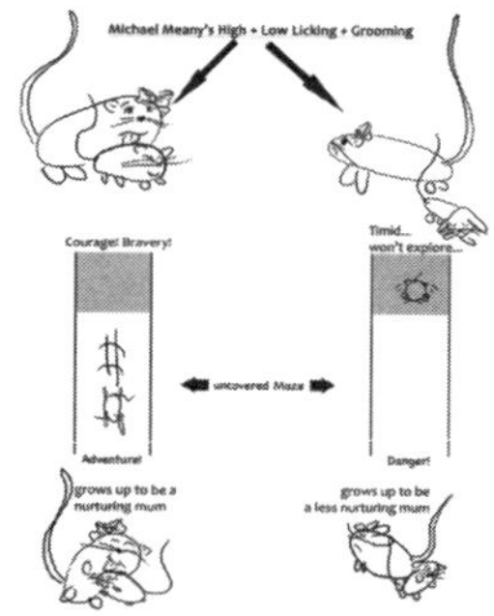

Higgins ES, Gorge MS. The Neuroscience of Clinical Psychiatry: The Pathophysiology of Behavior and Mental Illness. Philadelphia (USA): Lippincott, Williams and Wilkins; 2007, pg. 109

-less (pup) glucocorticoid release after stressed (restraint)

-less CRH messenger RNA in hippocampus (less stress reactivity in hippocampus)

-more glucocorticoid receptors in hypothalamus .. can turn stress down better

-increased resilience, less fear
SHOW GREATER WILLINGNESS TO EXPLORE NEW PLACES CURIOSITY (vs. guardedness)

Be vulnerable! explore + learn!

(CRF=CRH=Corticotropin Releasing Factor)

Hormonal Stress System: "HPA" Activation

Stress ⇒ Hypothalamus ⇒⇒ Pituitary ⇒⇒Adrenal (Cortex) ⇒⇒Body⇒⇒Cortisol Receptor
CRF or CRH ACTH Cortisol

Epigenetics, Altered Methylation *and Sperm*

Alcohol's effect on male gametes before conception are consistent with epigenetic effect

Haycock, 2009

Heavy alcohol consumption results in a decreased methylation of normally hypermethylated regions in *human sperm DNA*

Ouko, et al, 2009

Haycock PC, 2009. Fetal alcohol spectrum disorders: the epigenetic perspective. Biol Reprod. DOI 10.1095/ biorepod.108.074682

Ouko LA, Shantikumer K, Knezovide J, et al. 2009. Effects of alcohol consumption on CpG methylation in the differentially methylated regions of H19 and IG-DMR in males gametes-implications for fetal alcohol spectrum disorders. Alcoholism: Clinical and Experimental Research,DOI 10.111/j. 153020277.2009.00993.x

Attachment = (7) gene systems
Early = Reward Later =Obsession

VTA (ventral tegmental area) is a dopamine – rich area (1) which projects to Nucleus Accumbens

caudate (2)

Other Players

-Oxytocin + OTR (3) -in Nucleus Accumbens in an Estrogen (4) Progesterone (5) and Prolactin (6) Primed brain (in females)

-Vasopressin (7) and receptors in ventral pallidum (males)

Attachment can change epigenetic damage!

Higgins ES, George MS. The Neuroscience of Clinical Psychiatry: The Pathophysiology of Behavior and Mental Illness. Philadelphia (USA): Lippincott, Williams and Wilkins; 2007: pg.186

Sense of Self – Peter Fonagy

Sense of Self (as a person distinct from your mum)
Sense of Agency (you can "do things all by yourself")

Recognizing / dealing with emotions

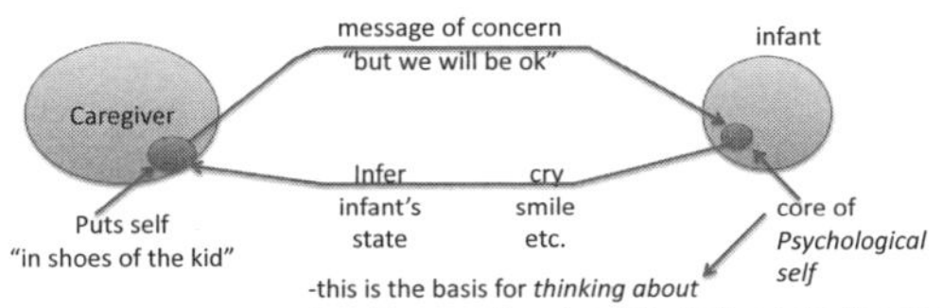

-this is the basis for *thinking about* thoughts or emotions (mentalization) vs. being "engulfed" by thoughts and emotions

-allows you to feel you are distinct from mom/dad/peers

Allen JG, Fonagy P, Bateman AW. 2009. Mentalizing in Clinical Practice. Washington,DC. American Psychiatric Publishing Inc.

Dr. Joel Paris' ideas re: really volatile people

-see suicidal ideas, self-harm and other crises as "a cry for help" and offer that help; be sure that attention to (albeit necessary) details at a time of crisis, for instance documenting the degree of suicidal intent, planning, access to means, etc., does not distract you from the critical work: which is attending to the "cry for help"

-the *foundation* of any work with volatile or distressed folks is the security of your *relationship with them*...maintaining that respectful relationship is a *primary goal* for without it "helpers" can do *nothing*

-(as a doctor) *NEVER "fire" a* patient (even if provoked by the patient not showing up to appointments, not taking meds as prescribed, or other "no-nos") because often the precipitant for another crisis (of self-harm or similar) is the patient's *perception of being abandoned by a social attachment.* Reasonable boundaries are great but the threat if they are broken must not be severing the relationship for the doctor-patient relationship *is the basis* on which any intervention is built

.....it is all about Attachment

Paris J Personality Disorders Over Time: Precursors, Course, and Outcome. Washington (USA) American Psychiatric Publishing Inc. 2003

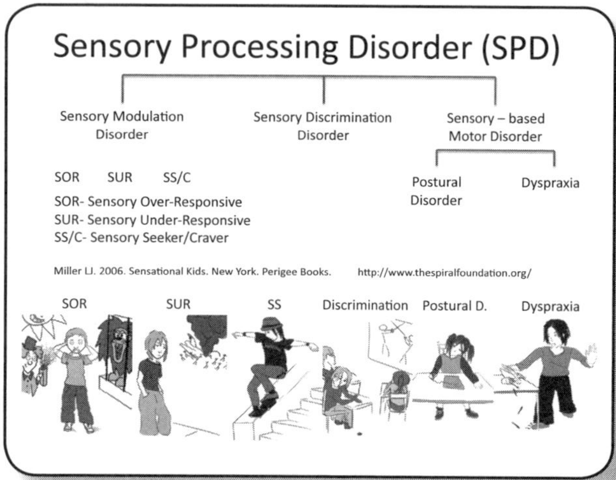
Sensory Processing Disorder (SPD)
Sensory Modulation Disorder
Sensory Discrimination Disorder
Sensory – based Motor Disorder
Postural Disorder
Dyspraxia
SOR SUR SS/C
SOR- Sensory Over-Responsive
SUR- Sensory Under-Responsive
SS/C- Sensory Seeker/Craver
Miller LJ. 2006. Sensational Kids. New York. Perigee Books.
http://www.thespiralfoundation.org/
SOR
SUR
SS
Discrimination
Postural D.
Dyspraxia

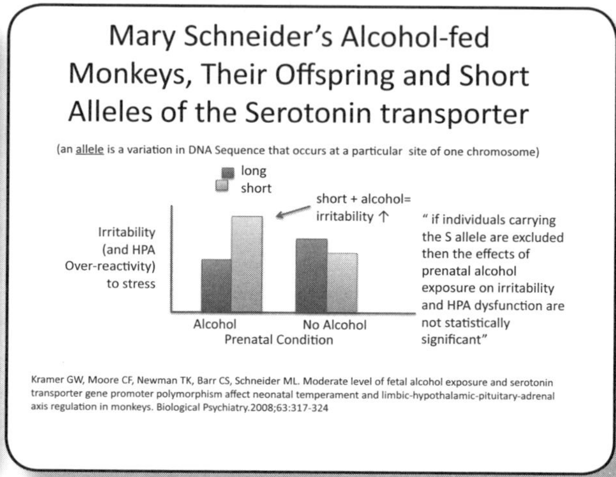
Mary Schneider's Alcohol-fed Monkeys, Their Offspring and Short Alleles of the Serotonin transporter
(an allele is a variation in DNA Sequence that occurs at a particular site of one chromosome)
long
short
short + alcohol= irritability ↑
Irritability (and HPA Over-reactivity) to stress
Alcohol
No Alcohol
Prenatal Condition
" if individuals carrying the S allele are excluded then the effects of prenatal alcohol exposure on irritability and HPA dysfunction are not statistically significant"
Kramer GW, Moore CF, Newman TK, Barr CS, Schneider ML. Moderate level of fetal alcohol exposure and serotonin transporter gene promoter polymorphism affect neonatal temperament and limbic-hypothalamic-pituitary-adrenal axis regulation in monkeys. Biological Psychiatry.2008;63:317-324

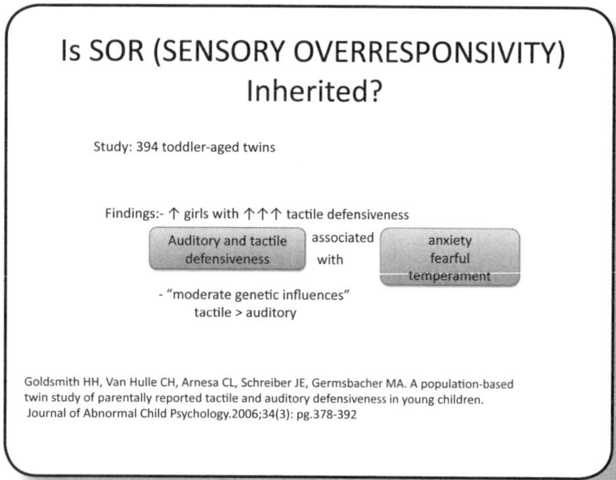
Is SOR (SENSORY OVERRESPONSIVITY) Inherited?
Study: 394 toddler-aged twins
Findings:- ↑ girls with ↑↑↑ tactile defensiveness
Auditory and tactile defensiveness
associated with
anxiety fearful temperament
- "moderate genetic influences"
tactile > auditory
Goldsmith HH, Van Hulle CH, Arnesa CL, Schreiber JE, Germsbacher MA. A population-based twin study of parentally reported tactile and auditory defensiveness in young children. Journal of Abnormal Child Psychology.2006;34(3): pg.378-392

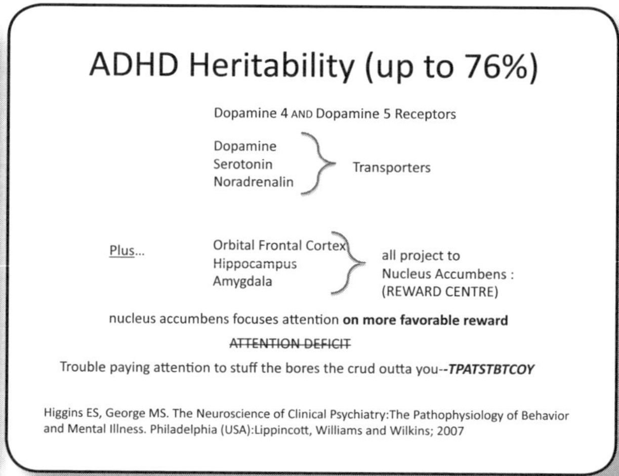
ADHD Heritability (up to 76%)
Dopamine 4 AND Dopamine 5 Receptors
Dopamine
Serotonin
Noradrenalin
Transporters
Plus...
Orbital Frontal Cortex
Hippocampus
Amygdala
all project to Nucleus Accumbens : (REWARD CENTRE)
nucleus accumbens focuses attention on more favorable reward
~~ATTENTION DEFICIT~~
Trouble paying attention to stuff the bores the crud outta you--TPATSTBTCOY
Higgins ES, George MS. The Neuroscience of Clinical Psychiatry:The Pathophysiology of Behavior and Mental Illness. Philadelphia (USA):Lippincott, Williams and Wilkins; 2007

Impulsivity May Relate To FASD

Sexual debut 16 or younger

-correlates to unintended pregnancy due to ↓ use of contraception

-immature cervix → ↑ Sexually Transmitted Disease,

↑ Pelvic Inflammatory Disease,

↑ Human Papillomavirus

-20-25% had been drinking

-if ↑ Conduct Disorder or Substance Use Disorders there is

↑ unprotected sex and

↑ sex in exchange for money or drugs

genetics influence disinhibitory traits: sensation seeking, impulsivity, non-conformity

Cavazos- Rehg PA, Spitznagl EL, Bucholz KK et al. Predictors of Sexual Debut at age 16 or younger [online]. Archives of Sexual Behavior ISSN. Oct 10, 2008: 1573-2800 10p

GABRA2

- ~~Different proteins~~ made by some Single Nucleotide Polymorphisms (SNPs)
- Changes how promoters and splicing variants work to change gene expression
- "Severe phenotype": alcohol *and drug* dependence, early age heavy drinking, larger binges, worse withdrawal, more Conduct Disorder (CD), Antisocial Personality Disorder (ASPD), Depression and "novelty seeking"
- **Kids from these families are at ↑ risk**

GABRA2: Odds Ratio of Alcoholism: 1.2, O.R. ~~Married:~~ 2.2!!

(Do you have one or two copies of the High Risk) GABRA2 Allele?

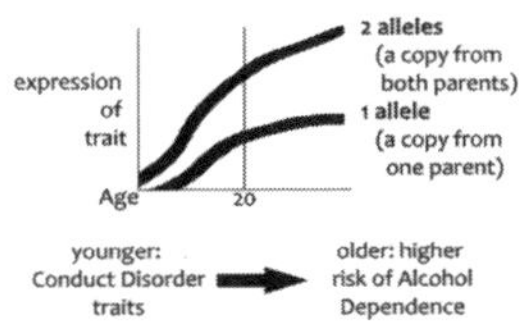

Edenberg H (2009)Symposium 70: Genetic Vulnerabilities for Drug Use and Co-morbid Mental Health Disorders: Genetics of Alcoholism and Related Endotypes (confrence presentation) Americain Psychiatric Assosiation Annual Meeting, San Fransisco

<u>Alcohol Dependence</u> Can Co-occur:

-Some genes increase risk of a cluster of behaviours called extreme "<u>externalizing</u> <u>disorders</u>"

(Conduct Disorder, Antisocial Personality Disorder, severe drug and alcohol dependencies)

<u>heritability of 80%</u>

-Alcohol Dependence also shares genetic risk with Nicotine dependence + caffeine use

Gelernter J, Kranzler HR. Genetics of alcohol dependence. Human Genetics.2009;126: 91-99

Variations in Nicotine Receptor Gene Cluster on Chromosome 15

CHRNA5
CHRNA3 } affect risk of
CHRNA4

developing dependence to
-Alcohol and
-Nicotine

Candidate Genes Associated with ↓Level of Response (LR)

GABRA alpha 6	COMT	5 HTT
GABRG2	DRD2 / ANKK1	ADORA
A5	DRD4	**NPY**
A1		
		ADH1B
KCNMA1	DGK2	ADH1C
CHRNA5	GNAS	CYPZE
	PK	

Schuckit MA. Adolf Meyer Award Lecture. How Alcoholism Develops: Identification of Genetic and Environmental Influences in a 25-year Longitudinal Study. American Psychiatric Association Meeting. 2009. San Francisco (Reference for this and the next 4 slides)

Stress Axis HPA Axis

an important mediator of the stress response
CRHR1 encodes the corticotropin releasing hormone receptor 1
2 SNPs: rs 242938
rs 1876831
associated with binge drinking in adolescents and adults with alcohol dependence

Gelernter J, Kranzler HR. Genetics of alcohol dependence. Human Genetics.2009;126: 91-99

40 Year Olds

all arrows (⟶) show statistically significant correlations

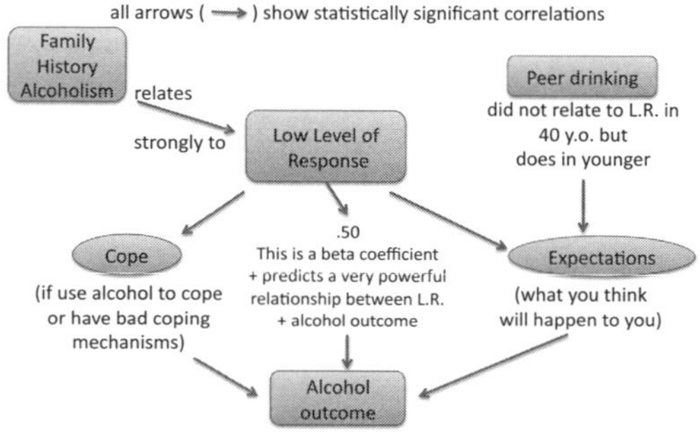

once the whole model is filled in how much of this outcome is predicted by by these factors? .49 (about ½)

Their Kids- 17 Years Old

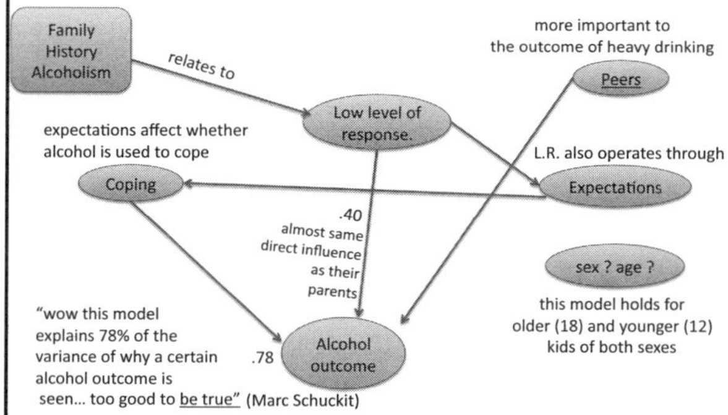

Could *Primary* Inheritance of Mental Health Problems relate to *Secondary* Disabilities

Trait of:	Heritability	Link to?
"Externalizing behaviors"	80%	trouble with law
Impulsivity	50-70%	school drop out
Emotional "dysregulation"	(slightly) less then 50%	anxiety disorder
Bipolar	Up to 70%	mental health, Drug use
Alcohol Dependence	50-60%	Substance Use Disorder
Nicotine Dependence	50-60%	Substance Use Disorder

Children with FASD are born with a considerable genetic burden which could emerge as "Secondary Disabilities". As with any inherited traits, our caregivers and professionals must.....BE RADICAL ----EXPLOIT YOUR MEASLEY 20-50% THAT YOU CAN INFLUENCE! "BOTTOM UP REBULILDING JOB" BRUCE PERRY, TRAUMA AND RELATIONSHIPS: DAVE ZIEGLER: RAISING CHILDREN WHO REFUSE TO BE RAISED, EDNA FOA: EFFECTIVE TREATMENT OF PTSD

Child KCNMA1 (TT OR TC), *Parent* Education + *Parent* Alcohol Use: Relationship to binge size in The *Child*

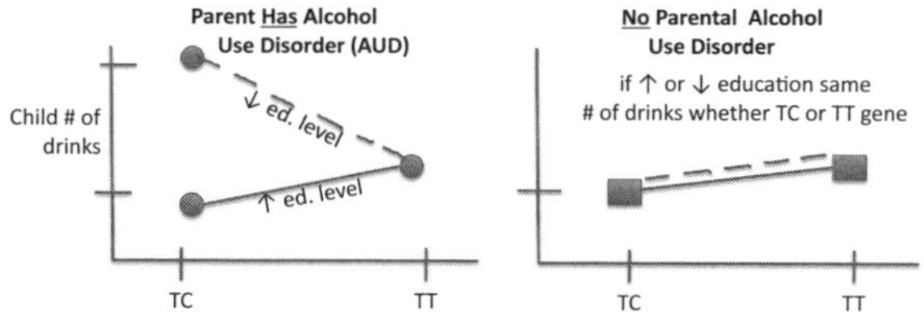

- IF YOU HAVE **TC** FORM OF KCNMA1 AND YOUR PARENTS HAVE **LOW EDUCATIONAL** LEVEL AND ARE **HEAVY DRINKERS** SEND YOUR FOLKS BACK TO SCHOOL!
- Low level of parent education influences AUD (in child) *if* parent has AUD themselves

Environmental Changes Influence *Expression* of a High Risk Gene

"Any one gene only explains **part** of the risk

AND anyhow, who wants to change a gene?"*

So *identify* genes that put people at High Risk and then make *robust changes* to environment to help

↓ expression of these High Risk genes

*Schuckit, Marc

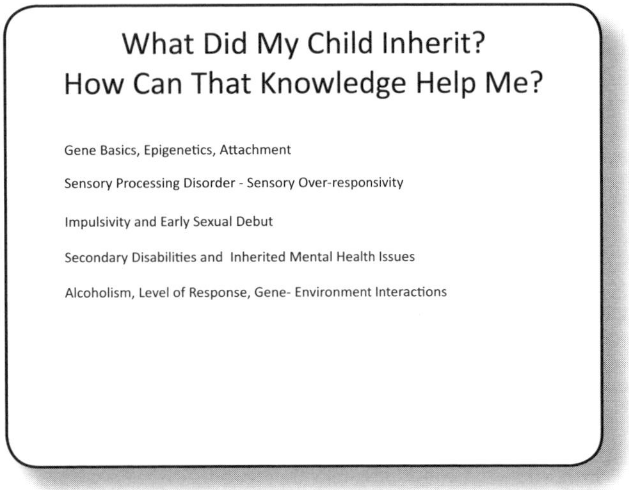
What Did My Child Inherit?
How Can That Knowledge Help Me?
Gene Basics, Epigenetics, Attachment
Sensory Processing Disorder - Sensory Over-responsivity
Impulsivity and Early Sexual Debut
Secondary Disabilities and Inherited Mental Health Issues
Alcoholism, Level of Response, Gene- Environment Interactions

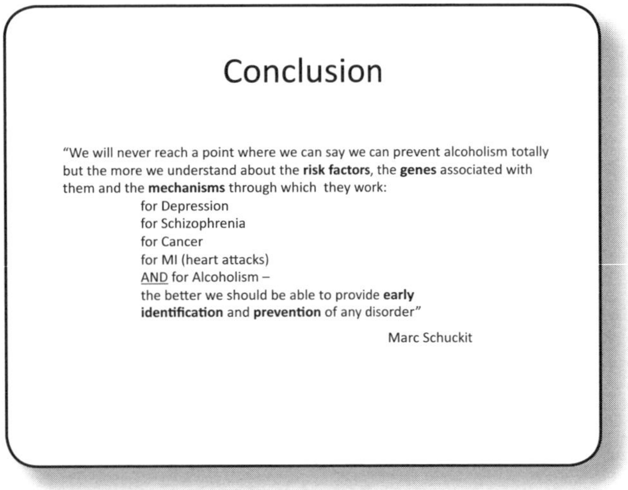
Conclusion
"We will never reach a point where we can say we can prevent alcoholism totally but the more we understand about the **risk factors**, the **genes** associated with them and the **mechanisms** through which they work:
for Depression
for Schizophrenia
for Cancer
for MI (heart attacks)
AND for Alcoholism –
the better we should be able to provide **early identification** and **prevention** of any disorder"
Marc Schuckit

Come To Your Senses

An Introduction to Sensory Processing Issues That Affect People Who Have FASD

Rod Densmore M.D. & Shannon Densmore O.T.

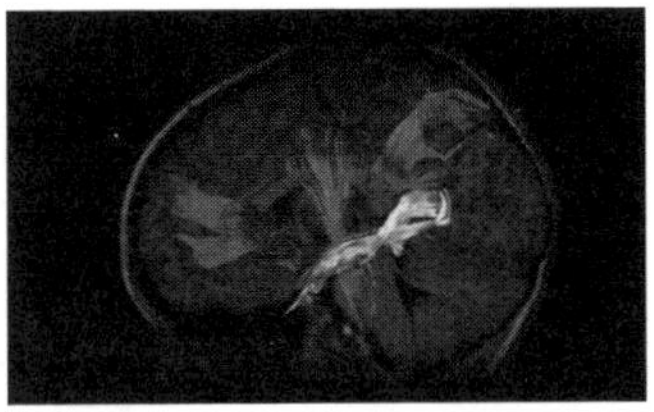

Thanks to Catherine Lebel and her research group at University of Alberta for permission to use this Diffusion Tensor MRI image

Perceptions Wakes Us Up!

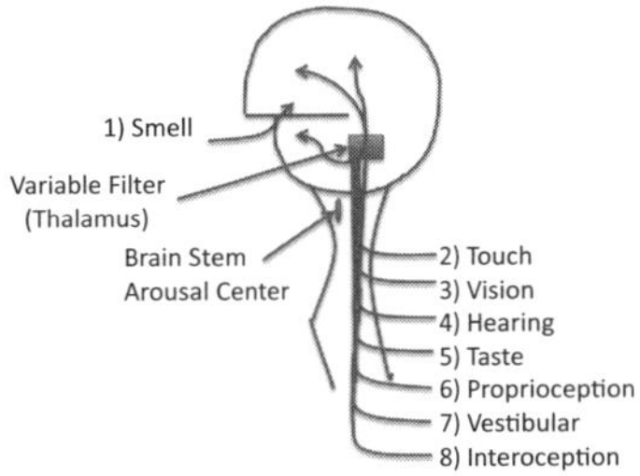

Senses

1- Smell (Olfactory)
2- Touch (Somatosensory)
3- Vision
4- Hearing (Auditory)
5- Taste (Gustatory)
6- Where joints + muscles are with respect to one another body (Proprioception)
7- Where body is with respect to gravity (Vestibular)
8- Perceptions from body organs e.g. bladder, bowel (Interoception)

"Internal" senses

consider also Immune System (XS "arousal" ?allergies) / Eye Contact

Energy/Arousal Level

Too "revved up" like Tigger

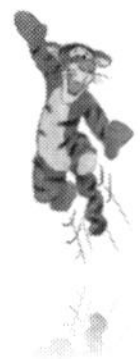

(What about "Just Right"?)

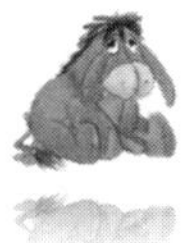

Too "sluggish" like Eeyore

Sensations are NOT "Silos" They "Talk to One Another"

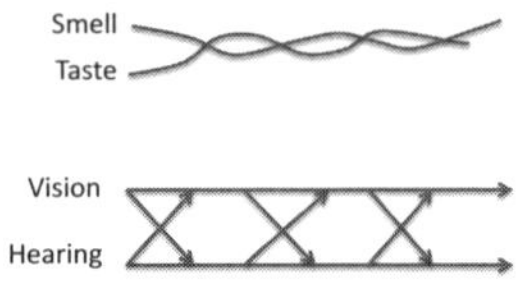

Foxe JJ. 2008. Sensory Processing Disorder and multisensory integration: Perspectives from Neuroscience. SPD Foundation 7[Th] International Symposium: Sensory Processing Disorder: Advanced Research and Innovative Practice. Boston, Mass. Nov 6, 2008

Sensory Processing Disorder (SPD)

- Sensory Modulation Disorder
  - SOR SUR SS/C
- Sensory Discrimination Disorder
- Sensory – based Motor Disorder
  - Postural Disorder
  - Dyspraxia

SOR- Sensory Over-Responsive
SUR- Sensory Under-Responsive
SS/C- Sensory Seeker/Craver

Miller LJ. 2006. Sensational Kids. New York. Perigee Books. http://www.thespiralfoundation.org/

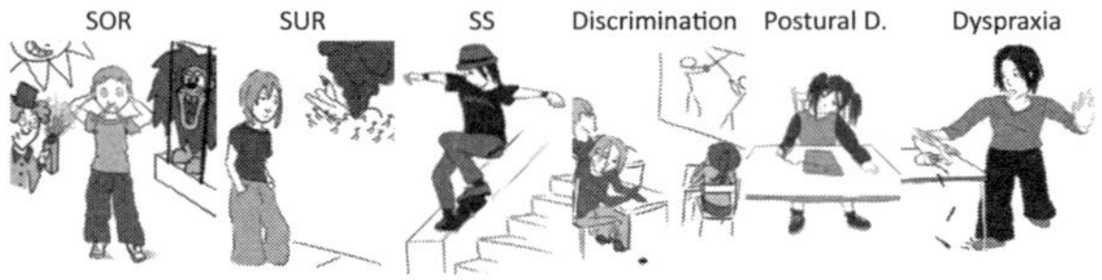

Perceptions/Sensory input can be:

-Too much (bombarding, overwhelming)

-Too little (hardly noticed)

-Muddled (unclear messages)

-Poorly Filtered (not sure what to pay attention to)

-We can crave/seek sensations

- "SENSORY PROCESSING IS THE ORGANIZATION OF SENSORY INPUT FOR USE" (Henry, D.)

Too Much = Sensory Over-responsivity

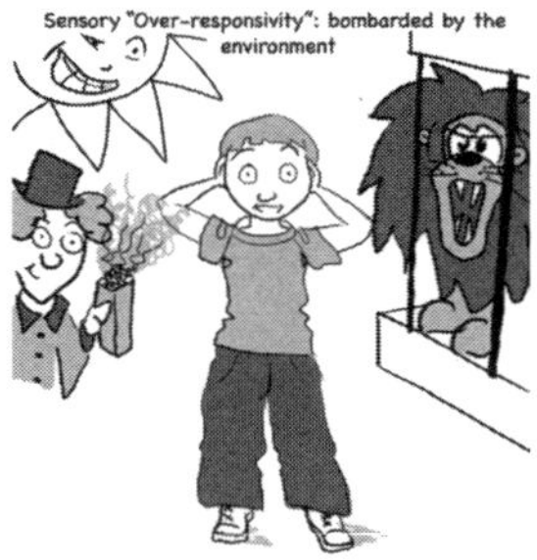

Too Little = Sensory Under-responsivity

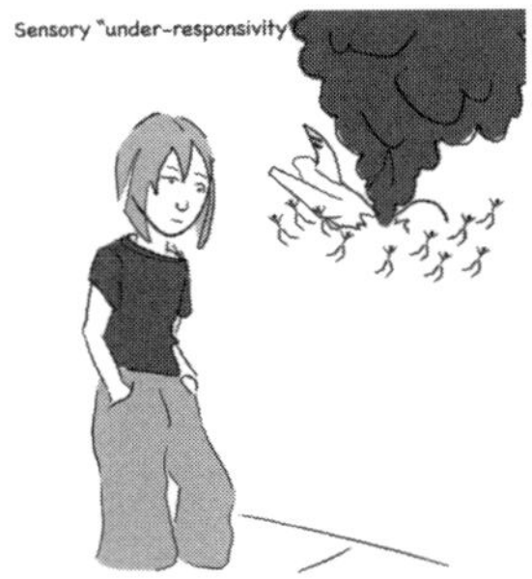

Muddled/Poorly Filtered = Sensory Discrimination

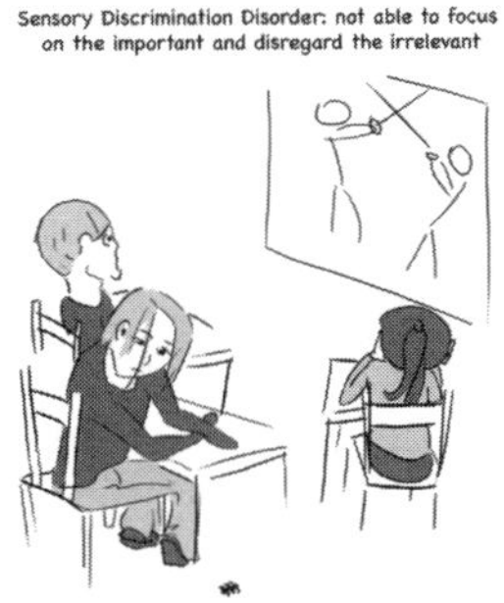

Sensory Seeking/Craving

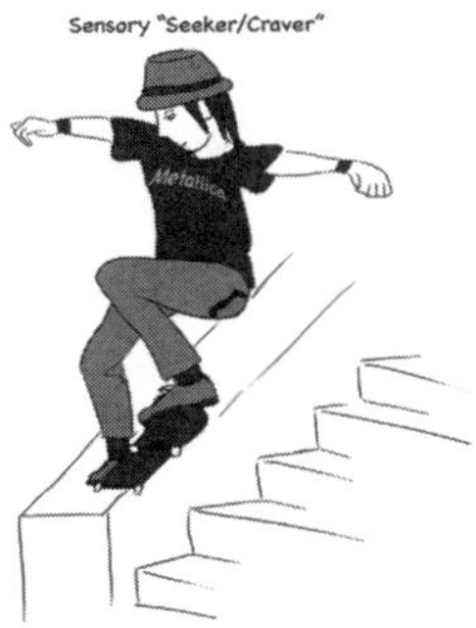

Praxis = Planning + Carrying Out a Muscle Movement

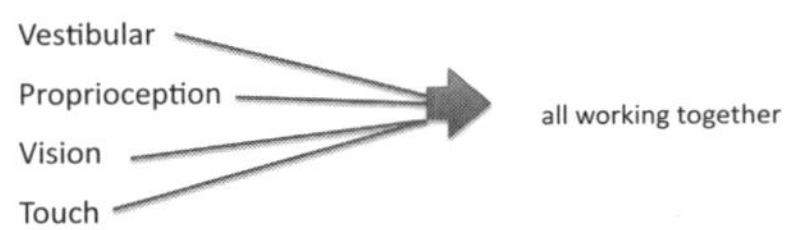

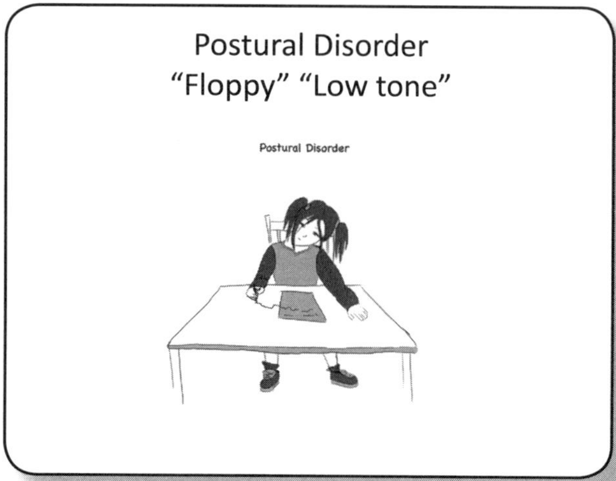
Postural Disorder
"Floppy" "Low tone"
Postural Disorder

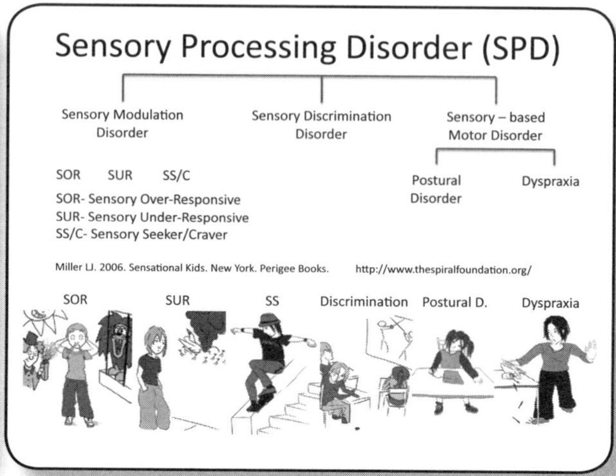
Sensory Processing Disorder (SPD)
Sensory Modulation Disorder
Sensory Discrimination Disorder
Sensory – based Motor Disorder
SOR SUR SS/C
SOR- Sensory Over-Responsive
SUR- Sensory Under-Responsive
SS/C- Sensory Seeker/Craver
Postural Disorder
Dyspraxia
Miller LJ. 2006. Sensational Kids. New York. Perigee Books.
http://www.thespiralfoundation.org/
SOR
SUR
SS
Discrimination
Postural D.
Dyspraxia

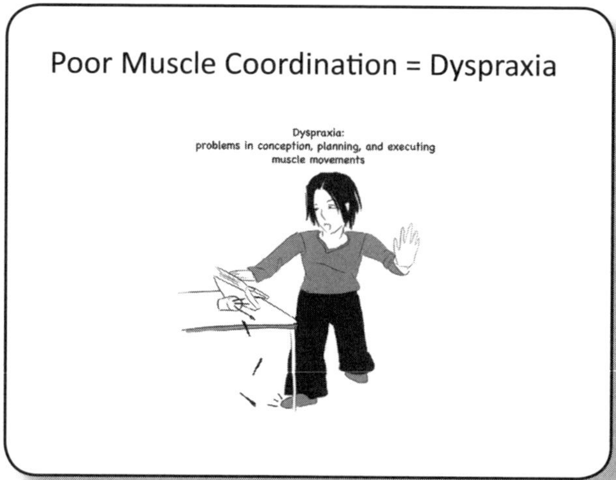
Poor Muscle Coordination = Dyspraxia
Dyspraxia:
problems in conception, planning, and executing muscle movements

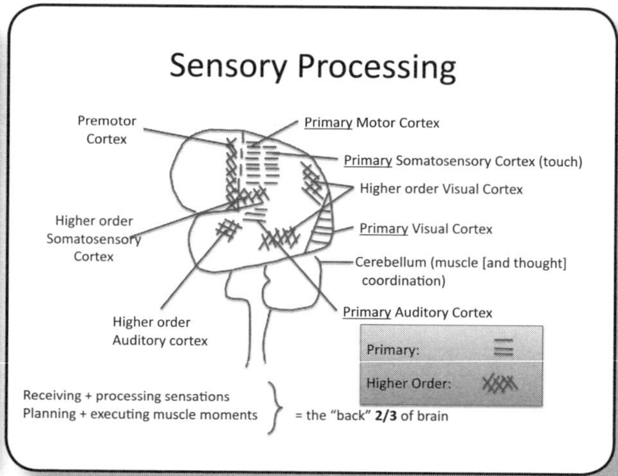
Sensory Processing
Premotor Cortex
Primary Motor Cortex
Primary Somatosensory Cortex (touch)
Higher order Visual Cortex
Higher order Somatosensory Cortex
Primary Visual Cortex
Cerebellum (muscle [and thought] coordination)
Primary Auditory Cortex
Higher order Auditory cortex
Primary:
Higher Order:
Receiving + processing sensations
Planning + executing muscle moments
= the "back" 2/3 of brain

Pathways that convey sensory information

P r o c e s s i n g s p e e d ⇓ ⇓

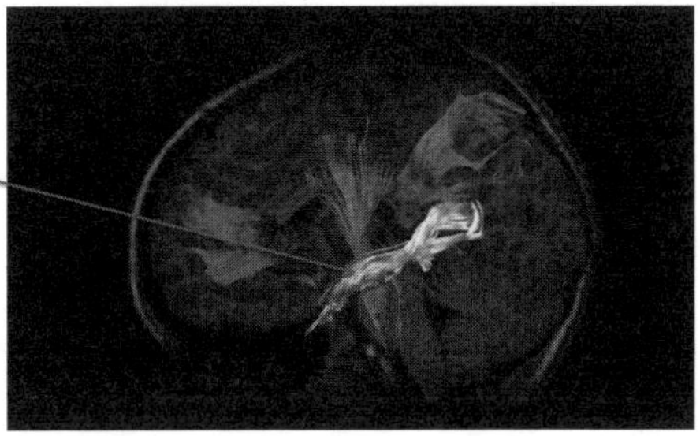

Acknowledgement: C. Lebel, U of A, Edmonton

ERP = Event Related Potentials

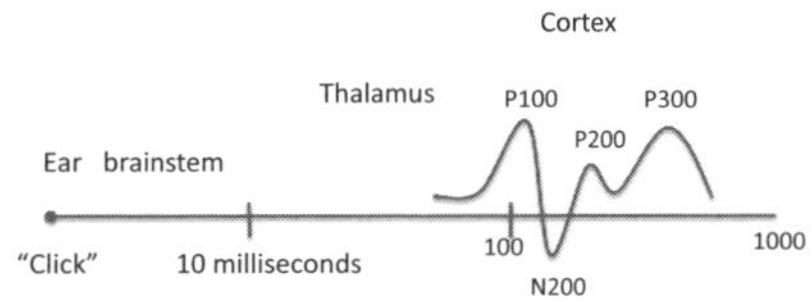

P= Positive N=Negative numbers are milliseconds after click
P100 mainly sensory
N100 sensory plus attention/ first awareness of
P200 influenced by attention
P300 cognitive = your brain evaluating the stimulus

"Visual" of Touch Discrimination problems caused by central processing deficits

SPD = A neurobehavioral disorder that interferes with a person's ability to regulate their behavioural responses to sensory input in a graded manner

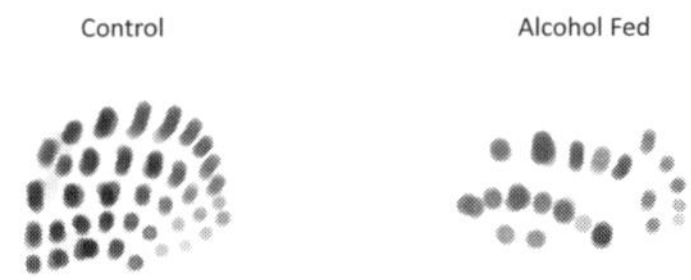

Adapted from: Powrozek TA, Zhou FC. 2005. Effects of prenatal alcohol exposure on the development of vibrissal somatosensory cortical barrel network. Brain Research Developmental Brain Research 155(2):135-146

Sensory Over Responsivity (SOR) Muddled Confusing Messages!

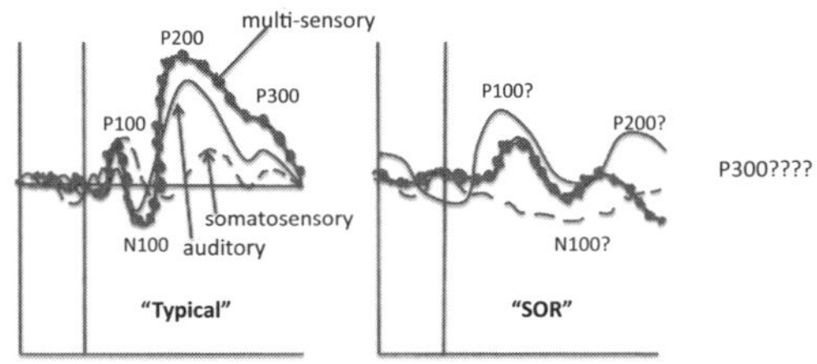

Based on: Brett-Green B, et al. Multi-sensory Integration in Children with S.P.D. Advanced Intensive Workshop on Diagnosis and Treatment of SPD Level One Aug 11-15, 2009. Sensory Processing Disorders Foundation, Denver Colorado

Outcome After Sensory Integration Treatment = *Neuroplasticity* (nerve cell growth + remodeling)

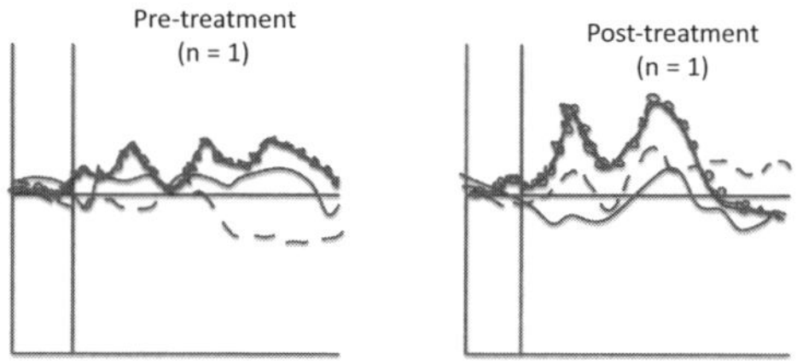

Based on: Brett-Green B, Miller LJ, Gavin WJ, Davies PL (2008) Multi-sensory Integration in Children: A Preliminary ERP Study. *Brain Research*. 1242: 283-290.

Neurosequential Model–Perry (www.childtrauma.org)

Frontal Cortex	**Insight/ reflective thinking**, Planning/ sequencing, Motor activity integration, **Modulation of Impulses,** Abstract thought, Morality/values/spirituality
Cortex	Speech articulation, Concrete thinking, Somato-Sensory integration, Time sense/delay gratification, Self-awareness, **Language (expressive and receptive)**
Limbic	Relational/sharing, **Attunement**, Affect/mood regulation, Play/pleasure, Short term memory/ learning, Threat response
Diencephalon/ Cerebellum	Co-ordination/balance, Sleep regulation, Appetite/ feeding/ satiety, Fine motor
Brainstem	Body Temp/ metabolism, Arousal/ self regulation, Attention/tracking, Blood pressure/ pulse rate, Extraocular movements, Breathing regulation

What "dose" of Multisensory Integration Therapy will "grow" brain connections for **Self-regulation**?

- Goal: have "top" (frontal cortex) regulate "lower" brain impulses/ urges....nice idea, but the connections between cortex and lower brain *must be there* if the child is to use them!
- If connections are not intact yet—(the brain develops from the bottom up)

how can we help it grow?

1) Sensory Integration Treatments 2) Bruce Perry

Body, Emotional, Cognitive Processing States **in response to threat** (Perry)

Devel. stage	15-30 +	8-15	3-8	1-3	0-1
Brain Area	Frontal Cortex	Cortex	Limbic	Midbrain/ cerebellum	Brainstem/ Autonomics
Thinking	Abstract	Concrete	"Emotional"	Reactive	Just Reflexes
Mental State	Calm	Alert	Alarm	Fear	Terror
Word Use	"New" ideas	Follow rules	Less words	Few words	No words
Threat Response					
Adaptive	Rest	Vigilance	Freeze	Flight	Fight
Hyperaroused	Rest	Vigilance	Resistance	Defiance	Aggression
Dissociative	Rest	Avoidance	Compliance	Dissociation	Fainting

Calm versus Alarm

Thinking	Abstract	Concrete	"Emotional"	Reactive	Just Reflexes
Mental State	Calm	Alert	Alarm	Fear	Terror
Word Use	"New" ideas	Follow rules	Less words	Few words	No words

Regular, Rhythmic, Age-appropriate Activities: see list in handout addendum

Patient D.L. 26, Single Mum

- FASD, diagnosed 2 years ago
- 8 yr. old son in care---wants full-time custody, social worker and psychologist thought unlikely because: quit gr. 9 (bored), lived mostly on the street, cocaine addiction age 16-24
- now is a hairdressing student
- Medications: Methylphenidate (Ritalin) not much help for attention, wt. loss, sleepless; Dexedrine: "made me feel weird--like outside myself"; Stratterra: some help for attention (not covered)

What dose of Regular, Rhythmic, Repetitive, Age-appropriate Activities will "Grow" circuits of self-regulation?

3-5 40-50 minute sessions per week

Perry BD. 2010. 9:00 a.m. – 12:00 p.m. Plenary: Introduction to the Neurosequential Model of Therapeutics: Application in Children Impacted by FASD 2010 Alberta FASD Conference: Promising Practices, Promising Futures. Feb 8, 2010, Calgary

Sensory Profile D.L. #1

- *Has* to smell everything
- *Bothered* by light touch, *distressed* by others touching her, *hates* cold water/ any kind of shower, "stiff" new clothes bother her
- *Does not* notice pain
- *Often* touching/twirling her hair, *loves* to sleep with **heavy blankets**, *bites* inside of cheek, *loves* to touch/has to touch everything
- Finger touch discrimination ⇓
- Words "jump around on the page"

Sensory Profile D.L. #2

- *Difficulty* concentrating if background noise
- Talks too loudly or too softly
- *Prefers* foods with strong tastes
- *Has* to fiddle/fidget, *restless* through a lecture, *loves* crunchy foods, *seeks out* crashing or "squishing" activities
- Car sick, throws up on carnival rides, very unsteady on a bus or subway
- *Tips* chair back on 2 legs, a thrill seeker—loves roller coaster
- *Over or under* sensitive to hunger sensations
- *Avoids* eye contact

Sensory Profile A.J. #1

(boy in grade 2, FASD, adopted as baby)

- Seems unaware of being touched
- Trouble keeping hands to self, *has* to touch
- Avoids eye contact
- Difficulty drawing, coloring, copying
- Reverses words
- Overly sensitive to loud noises
- Has trouble with 2-3 stage commands
- Hard to understand, mumbles
- Constantly in motion

Sensory Profile C.R.

(4 yr-old girl, *Mum* has FASD, she does not, "hard to look after"

- Likes weighted vest, heavy blanket, likes vibration toy, vibrating massager
- Holds hands over her ears, responds negatively to unexpected or loud noises
- *Very* loud, yells often, ignores people
- Distracted if background noise is present
- seeks all kinds of movement, never still
- Loves to spin on desk chair for extended periods, seeks twirling, merry-go-rounds, spinning
- Encopresis (involuntary stooling)

Sensory Profile A.J. #2

- Likes spinning/ whirling around
- Seems weaker than peers, tired esp. after school, confuses L. and Rt., difficulty learning new motor tasks, does not want to do sports (with others) but likes swimming and skating
- Difficulty drawing, coloring, copying
- Falls often
- Reverses words
- Hard to coordinate eyes to follow movement, keep place in reading, or copy from blackboard to desk--- "loses his lines" "hard to cooperate on eye tests"
- Avoids eye contact

Attention Issues?

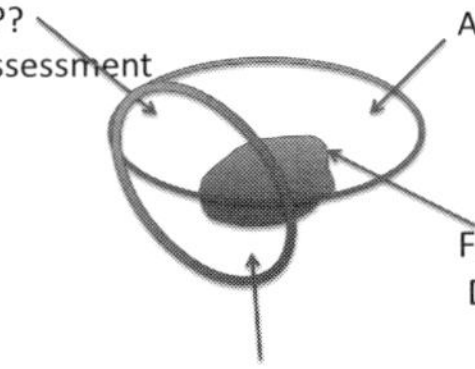

Also consider: Sleep Apnea, Concussion, Not Safe, Drugs or Alcohol

Why seek to understand SPD?

- Self esteem
- Reduced anxiety
- Better sleep, better self-regulation
- Success is more likely
- You, or your wife/husband/other kids have the same issues!
- "ADHD," "ODD," and Anxiety treatment without pills...at least if pills don't "work"
  PLEASE DO NOT FORGET TO ASK, "SPD??"

D.L. Sensory Profile - Sensory Profile Blank

Sense	Notes & Comments
Smell	Comments: Over ☐ Under ☐ Seek ☐
Touch	Comments: Over ☐ Under ☐ Seek ☐
Vision	Comments: Over ☐ Under ☐ Seek ☐
Hearing	Comments: Over ☐ Under ☐ Seek ☐
Taste	Comments: Over ☐ Under ☐ Seek ☐

D.L. Sensory Profile - Sensory Profile Blank

Sense	Notes & Comments
Proprioception	Comments: Over ☐ Under ☐ Seek ☐
Vestibular	Comments: Over ☐ Under ☐ Seek ☐
Interoception	Comments: Over ☐ Under ☐ Seek ☐
Eye Contact	Comments: Over ☐ Under ☐ Seek ☐

D.L. Sensory Profile

Sense	Over	Under	Seek	Discrimi-nation	Comments
Smell			✓		*Has* to smell everything
Touch	✓				Bothered by light touch, *distressed* by others touching her, *hates* cold water/
		✓	✓		*Often* touching/twirling her hair, *loves* to sleep with **heavy blankets**, *bites* inside of cheek,
				✓	Finger touch discrimination ↓
Vision				✓	Words "jump around on the page"
Hearing				✓	*Difficulty* concentrating if background noise
	✓	✓			Talks too loudly or too softly
Taste			✓		*Prefers* foods with strong tastes
Proprioception	✓				*Has* to fiddle/fidget, *restless*
Vestibular	✓				Car sick, throws up on rides,
			✓		*Tips* chair back on 2 legs, a thrill seeker - loves roller coaster
Interoception	✓	✓			*Over or under* sensitive to hunger
Eye Contact	✓				*Avoids* eye contact

Sensory Profile D.L. - Accommodations/ Strategies

Smell (D.L.)

Possible Accommodation Strategies	**Comment:**
» Pleasant fragrances - lavender calms, peppermint alerts	» *Has* to smell everything **(smell seeking)**

Touch (D.L.)

Possible Accommodation Stragegies	**Comment:**
» Light touch is *activating/* often *irritating* » She needs to be initiator of touch/hugs, etc. » Wash new clothes several times, use fabric softener, choose comfortable fabrics » Might be dissociation from abuse when she was a child - possibly will improve with treatment of PTSD symptoms » Heavy pressure might be both calming and alerting - at night a weighted blanket may help sleep, tight undergarments (body stockings) might help in the day	» *Bothered* by light touch, *distressed* by others touching her, *hates* cold water/ any kind of shower, *hates* cold water/any kind of shower, "stiff" new clothes bother her **(touch over-responsive)** » *Does not* notice pain **(touch under-responsive)** » *Often* touching/twirling her hair, (rhythmic) *loves* to sleep with **heavy blankets**, *bites* inside of cheek, *loves* to touch/has to touch everything **(touch seeking)** » Finger touch discrimination ↓ **(touch discrimination)**

Sensory Profile D.L. - Accommodations/ Strategies

Vision (D.L.)

Possible Accommodation Strategies

- http://www.insightlearning.ca will link you to Darren Sass, O.D. who is a Developmental Optometrist, other information: College of Optometrists in Vision Development (covd.org) and the Neuro-Optometric Rehabilitation Association (nora.cc)

Comment:

- Words "jump around on the page" **(visual discrimination or eye muscle coordination)**

Hearing (D.L.)

Possible Accommodation Strategies

- Try to obtain a hearing discrimination test - this is very different from the "pure tones in each ear in a sound-proof room" hearing test that is usually done - ask the audiologist specifically whether they check auditory discrimination and ask them to refer you to someone that does check this if they don't. Amplification devices can help discrimination issues.
- Auditory hypo-responsivity could respond to amplification.
- A "listening system" such as http://www.integratedlistening.com might be helpful for hypo or hyper-responsivity - lower tones calm and higher tones alert

Comment:

- *Difficulty* concentrating if background noise **(hearing discrimination)**
- Talks too loudly or too softly **(maybe auditory over or under-responsive)**

Sensory Profile D.L. - Accommodations/ Strategies

Taste (D.L.)

Possible Accommodation Strategies	Comment:
» Chewing cinnamon gum might help activate/ keep on task, learn some flavourful but simple recipes	» *Prefers* foods with strong tastes **(taste seeking)**

Proprioception (D.L.)

Possible Accommodation Strategies	Comment:
» Get some "fidgets" - little balls or other objects one can keep in the hands, sit on a "Movin'sit Cushion" so she can wiggle her lower body and not distract the class (available at: www.fdmt.ca)	» *Has* to fiddle/fidget, *restless* through a lecture, *loves* crunchy foods, *seeks out* crashing or "squishing" activities **(proprioceptive seeking)**

Vestibular (D.L.)

Possible Accommodation Strategies	Comment
» Not a great accommodation: "I take 2 or 3 gravol tablets so I can go on the roller coaster several times!"	» Car sick, throws up on carnival rides, very unsteady on a bus or subway **(vestibular over-responsive)**
» Hopefully these vestibular issues would respond to sensory processing disorder treatment sessions .	» *Tips* chair back on 2 legs, a thrill seeker - loves roller coaster **(vestibular seeker)**

Sensory Profile D.L. - Accommodations/ Strategies

Interiception (D.L.)

Possible Accommodation Strategies	Comment
» Hopefully these interoceptive issues might respond to multisensory integration sessions	» *Over or under* sensitive to hunger sensations

Eye Contact (D.L.)

Possible Accommodation Strategies	Comment
» Educate friends, instructors, counselors *not* to "force" eye contact	» *Avoids* eye contact **(eye contact over- responsive)**

C.R. Sensory Profile - Sensory Profile Blank

Sense	Notes & Comments
Smell	Comments: Over ☐ Under ☐ Seek ☐
Touch	Comments: Over ☐ Under ☐ Seek ☐
Vision	Comments: Over ☐ Under ☐ Seek ☐
Hearing	Comments: Over ☐ Under ☐ Seek ☐
Taste	Comments: Over ☐ Under ☐ Seek ☐

C.R. Sensory Profile - Sensory Profile Blank

Sense	Notes & Comments
Proprioception	Comments: Over ☐ Under ☐ Seek ☐
Vestibular	Comments: Over ☐ Under ☐ Seek ☐
Interoception	Comments: Over ☐ Under ☐ Seek ☐
Eye Contact	Comments: Over ☐ Under ☐ Seek ☐

C.R. Sensory Profile

Sense	Over	Under	Seek	Discrimi-nation	Comments
Touch			✓		Likes weighted vest, heavy blanket, likes vibration toy, vibrating massager
Hearing	✓				Holds hands over her ears, responds negatively to unexpected or loud noises
		✓			*Very* loud, yells often, ignores people
				✓	Distracted if background noise is present
Proprioception			✓		Seeks all kinds of movement, never still
Vestibular			✓		Loves to spin on desk chair for extended periods, seeks twirling, merry-go-rounds, spinning
Interoception		✓			Encopresis

Sensory Profile C.R. - Accommodations/ Strategies

Touch (C.R.)

Possible Accommodation Strategies

- Weighted blanket =10% body weight (in lbs) plus 1 pound as a starting point. Eg. 40lb child 4+1 = 5 lbs - first night she slept 10 hrs. - a record. [↑ serotonin], provide vibrating toys, massager - esp. ones that she can be in charge of.

Comment:

- Likes weighted vest, heavy blanket, likes vibration toy, vibrating massager **(touch seeking)**

Hearing (C.R.)

Possible Accommodation Strategies

- The more control she has over her environment the less surprises she will need to cope with - some "not-too-noisy" musical instruments (e.g. ukulele or harmonica, not drums!)
- Provide Mum with some headphones/ear protectors so she can function when her child is yelling - often the solution is getting the daughter something to eat but this was hard for mum when she could hardly function because of the extreme noise
- Turn off T.V. and radio, esp. during meals, reading time and getting to sleep time

Comment:

- Holds hands over her ears, responds negatively to unexpected or loud noises **(auditory hyper-responsivity)**
- *Very* loud, yells often, ignores people **(?possible auditory hypo-responsivity)**
- Distracted if background noise is present **(auditory discrimination issues)**

Sensory Profile C.R. - Accommodations/ Strategies

Proprioception (C.R.)

Possible Accommodation Strategies

» Playground prior to sleep or naps, "heavy work" activities "wheelbarrow walking",anything that involves lifting carrying pushing e.g. carry diaper bag, carrying in groceries, shovel snow with appropriate-sized shovel, push kid-sized grocery cart with bag of flour in it, bathtub: oversized pouring things e.g. 2 litre pop container or big watering can

Comment:

» seeks all kinds of movement, never still **(proprioception seeking)**

Vestibular (C.R.)

Possible Accommodation Strategies

» Sit in rocking chair or on "Therapy ball" - a therapy ball with handles on it and/or sitting the ball on a base that will keep it from rolling far is optimal, rolling over the large ball on tummy (legs held by mum) was also an enjoyable and helpful activity

Comment

» Loves to spin on desk chair for extended periods, seeks twirling, merry-go-rounds, spinning **(vestibular seeking)**

Sensory Profile C.R. - Accommodations/ Strategies

Interoception (C.R.)

Possible Accommodation Strategies

» Reduced awareness of body sensations can be influenced by impaired function of the insula. Mineral oil routines can help. Referral to Gastroenterology is wise - in BC: Dr Mark Kovacs, BC Children's Hospital

Comment

» Encopresis (involuntary stool) **(possible interoceptive hypo-responsivity)**

Results thus far (10 months):

» ↓ aggression

» ↓ time spent whirling, spinning

» ↑ social interaction with peers at daycare

» ↓ stress for Mum

» ↑ attention span--could sit at a table and make valentines

» ↑ now able to see her excellent fine motor skills and cognitive abilities....i.e. "unlocking her potential"

» ↓ need for supervision

» did still hit baby brother but was looking at O.T. and mum at the time...issue not gone but much more manageable

» mum less exasperated and has more energy and more positive and now is getting child into daycare on graduated entry basis

» Thus: family support, home programme for incorporating sensory principles into the family routines and dexedrine made a HUGE difference

A.J. Sensory Profile - Sensory Profile Blank

Sense	Notes & Comments
Smell	Comments: Over ☐ Under ☐ Seek ☐
Touch	Comments: Over ☐ Under ☐ Seek ☐
Vision	Comments: Over ☐ Under ☐ Seek ☐
Hearing	Comments: Over ☐ Under ☐ Seek ☐
Taste	Comments: Over ☐ Under ☐ Seek ☐

A.J. Sensory Profile - Sensory Profile Blank

Sense	Notes & Comments
Proprioception	Comments: Over ☐ Under ☐ Seek ☐
Vestibular	Comments: Over ☐ Under ☐ Seek ☐
Interoception	Comments: Over ☐ Under ☐ Seek ☐
Eye Contact	Comments: Over ☐ Under ☐ Seek ☐

A.J. Sensory Profile

Sense	Over	Under	Seek	Discrimination	Comments
Touch		✓			Seems unaware of being touched
				✓	Trouble keeping hands to self, *has* to touch
Vision	✓				Avoids eye contact
		✓		✓	Difficulty drawing, coloring, copying
		✓		✓	Reverses words
Hearing	✓				Overly sensitive to loud noises
		✓		✓	Has trouble with 2-3 stage commands
		✓		✓	Hard to understand, mumbles
Proprioception			✓		Constantly in motion
Vestibular			✓		Likes spinning/ whirling around

Comments re: Praxis is the coordinated planning and execution of (esp. new) muscle movements - depends on proprioception, and vestibular perceptions working together and movement correction by visual feedback

Symptoms of Praxis: Seems weaker than peers, tired esp. after school, confuses L. and Rt., difficulty learning new motor tasks, does not want to do sports (with others) but likes swimming and skating

» Difficulty drawing, coloring, copying
» Falls often
» Reverses words

Hard to coordinate eyes to follow movement, keep place in reading, or copy from blackboard to desk--- "loses his lines" "hard to cooperate on eye tests"

Sensory Profile A.J. - Accommodations/ Strategies

Touch (A.J.)

Possible Accommodation Strategies

» Random Showers: change the shower head setting and the temperatures a bit each time, brushing, bath shops sell Foot Rollers these feel weird at 1st then as you get used to them - feel good

Comment:

» Seems unaware of being touched **(touch under-responsivity)**

» Trouble keeping hands to self, *has* to touch **(touch seeking)**

Vision (A.J.)

Possible Accommodation Strategies

» Assessment by Devel. Optometrist, ball cap, sunglasses, do not force to look at you

» Practice eye activities, play games with flashlights, fibre optic lights, kaleidoscopes

» These are huge issues - needs O.T. assessment

Comment:

» Avoids eye contact **(visual sensitivity)**

» Difficulty drawing, coloring, copying **(sensory-based fine motor problem?)**

» Reverses words

Sensory Profile A.J. - Accommodations/ Strategies

Hearing (A.J.)

Possible Accommodation Strategies

- Chew gum to cover up background noises, headphones
- Help student plan out a task: "What materials do you need? What needs to be done first?"
- Sour candy, electric toothbrush- wake up mouth!

Comment:

- Overly sensitive to loud noises **(Auditory over-sensitivity)**
- Has trouble with 2-3 stage commands
- Hard to understand, mumbles **(Dyspraxia- verbal muscle planning?)**

Proprioception (A.J.)

Possible Accommodation Strategies

- Ball pit –whole body deep pressure input, lycra (exercise) wear

Comment:

- Bumps into things **(proprioception seeking)**

Vestibular (A.J.)

Possible Accommodation Strategies

- Swimming, rock climbing, trampoline, doing cartwheels, sliding down circular slide, weighted back pack

Comment

- Likes spinning/ whirling around Always in motion **(vestibular seeking)**

Sensory Profile A.J. - Accommodations/ Strategies

Praxis (A.J.)

Possible Accommodation Strategies

» Develop a functional level of arousal throughout the school day by providing organizing sensory inputs such as:

» Rt/Lt confusion: practice shaking hands

» Don't force into team sports

» Draw in sand or shaving cream for tactile input

» Use cardboard with cutout for reading

» Sit near front of class to reduce distance to board

Comment

» Seems weaker than peers, tired esp. after school, confuses L. and Rt., difficulty learning new motor tasks, does not want to do sports (with others) but likes swimming and skating

» Difficulty drawing, coloring, copying

» Falls often

» Reverses words

» Hard to coordinate eyes to follow movement, keep place in reading, or copy from whiteboard to desk--- "loses his lines"

Age Appropriate, Rhythmic, Repetitive, Fun Activities/ Warm, nurturing "Together time" to help Self-regulation

» **Babies:** Mothers: cuddles, higher pitched, sing/song "motherese," snuggle time face to face, rocking, stories. Fathers: bouncing, "airplanes," snugglie-walking facing outwards, songs, music, stories

» **Toddlers:** swings, music, dance

» **School aged:** music (but not 5 new songs each week), dance, martial arts, walking, interactive metronome

» **Teens:** above,"The Wild Devine" http://www.wilddivine.com/ Yoga, Tai chi, drumming, strumming guitar

Parent Resources for Sensory Issues SHANNON'S FAVOURITES/ ROD'S FAVOURITES

Assessment and Treatment Facilities:

1. Children's Therapy and Family Resource Centre
   250-371-4100
   website:
   www.kamloopschildrenstherapy.org
2. Gail Johnson, private O.T., Kamloops
   250-434-6762
   email: mindinmotion.OT@shaw.ca
3. Leanne Godwin, private O.T., Vernon
   250-542-3089
   email: info@meridianrehab.ca
4. Shuswap Children's Association, Salmon Arm
   Shannon's Favorite
   250-833-0164
   website:
   http://www.shuswapchildrensassociation.ca/ ...Shannon's Therapy Room!
5. **Developmental Optometrists: Darren Sass O.D.,**
   Rod's Favorite
   604-455-0477 (Langley)
   website: www.insightlearning.ca
   Brent Neufeld O.D. (Calgary) email: drneufeld@canada.com
   Brenton Loose O.D. (Prince George) email: bloose20-20@telus.net
6. **Sensory Questionnaire, website: http://www.sensory-processing-disorder.com/sensory-processing-disorder-checklist.html**
   Rod's Favorite

Books/Websites/Resources:

1. FASD Relationships Website: www.fasdrelationships.ca FASD 101 Fetal Alcohol Spectrum Disorder for a General Audience, Interview with Myles Himmelreich--achieving success.
2. Sensory Processing Disorder Canada website: www.spdcanada.org
3. Dr. Bruce Perry's organization: ChildTraumaAcademy website: http://www.childtrauma.org/
4. Dr. Lucy Miller's organization: SPD Foundation: www.spdnetwork.org
5. *Shannon's Favorite Rod's Favorite* **Dr. Jane Koomar's organization:** www.otawatertown.com, www.thespiralfoundation.org/
6. Diane Henry's organization: website: www.henryot.com
7. Sensory Integration Global Network website: http://www.siglobalnetwork.org/
8. Mary Sue Williams, Sherry Schellenberger's Therapy Works Inc. "How Does Your Engine Run?" programme website: www.alertprogram.com
9. Developmental Optometry websites: http://www.oepf.org/, http://covd.org/, http://www.nora.cc/
10. Williams MS, Schellenberger S. 2001. Take Five! staying alert at home and school. Albuquerque, New Mexico: Therapy Works Inc.
11. Reebye P, Stalker A. 2008. Understanding Regulation Disorders of Sensory Processing in Children: Management strategies for parents and professionals, London (U.K.): Jessica Kingsley Press.
12. *Rod's Favorite* **Miller LJ. 2006. Sensational Kids: Hope and Help for Children with Sensory Processing Disorder. New York: Penguin Books**
13. Henry DA, Kane-Wienland M, Swindeman. 2007. Tools for Tots: Sensory strategies for toddlers and preschoolers. Glendale,Arizona: Henry O.T. Services Inc.
14. Mucklow N. 2009. The Sensory Team Handbook: A hands-on tool to help young people make sense of their senses and take charge of their sensory processing. Kingston,Ontario: Michael Grass House

15. Wilson LF. 2009. Squirmy Wormy: how i learned to help myself. Arlington,Texas: Future Horizons Inc.

16. Yack E, Aquilla P, Sutton S. 2002. Building Bridges Through Sensory Integration: Therapy for children with autism and other pervasive developmental disorders. Arlington Texas: Future Horizons Inc.Kranowitz CS. 2004. The Goodenoughs Get in Sync. Las Vegas: Sensory Resources

Equipment

1. Innovaid (Diane Luzny-weighted blankets and vests) 780-467-7627 website: www.innovaid.ca

Shannon's Favorite

2. Hugz4me The Sensory Place (fidget toys, etc.) website: www.hugz4me.com
3. FDMT Educational materials and sensory toys 866-465-0559 website: www.fdmt.ca
4. Stickids Muscles, Motion 'n Touch software (Meryle Lehn) website: http://stickids.com/index.html
5. Kid's Companion Chewelry (oral-motor tools) 902-762-0186 website: www.chewelry.ca/
6. School Specialties Canada: Sensory Solutions (main supplier in Canada for large sensory equipment) 866-519-2816 website: schoolspecialtyonline.net

NEUROBIOLOGY OF FASD For a General Audience

Rod Densmore, M.D., Parent of a young adult who has FAS

IDEAS

History – Screams (when forced to "Sit still") Sensory Overload/Integration
– trial: lower light, quieter, able to "get up," able to "move"

Toxic – judgmental V.P.
– poorly informed ADHD=Distracted ***if not engaged***
– does not know what she does not know
– primitive "fair" all equal…not all get what needed

Burned out isolated mother
no "place of rest" or validation
decreased support for her daughter,
decreased feelings about her

WHY ARE WE HERE: B.B.

B.B. 14 ♀ loves to read, creative

Grade 8 (West Vancouver) **hates** school, wants to quit, can't sit still, "vibrates," "forgets" homework, prefers low lights, no music, soft clothes

Mom – anxious, tense
– yelling match with Doctors
– worried re Ritalin – no help anyways

"Vice principal" – What do you mean "Doctor"

She is: (manipulative) – no problems playing all day in the gym
(lazy) – won't hand in homework

IF YOU DON'T LAUGH, YOU WILL CRY

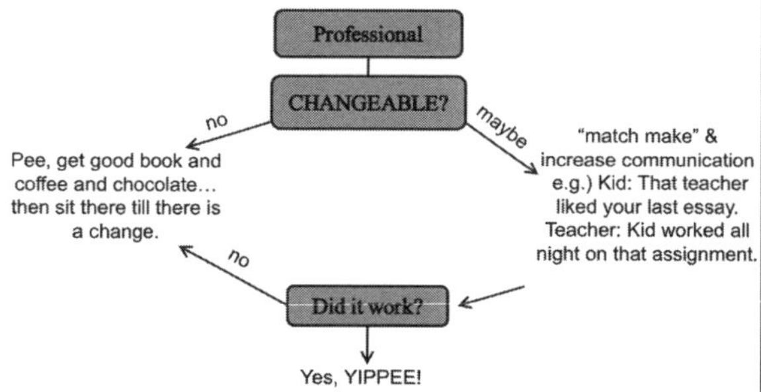

FINALLY…SOME USEFUL ACRONYMS

"NURMU"

Noncompliant
Uncooperative
Resistant
Manipulative
Unmotivated

(Dubovsky, Dan)

+

"PTHD"

PMS
Tired
Hungry
Depleted

(Rod)

Righteous Indignation

① Curious – where's that from?
② Can we hang on to the relationship
(Neufeld, Gordon)

A
T
T
A
C
K

NURMU <u>Never</u> before Rule out and Treat:
*ADHD
*Sensory Processing
*Learning Disabilities
*Attachment

DSM-5 (2013)

Importance of Relationships

"a place of rest" - Gordon Neufeld, *Hold On To Your Kids* DVD Series

BEACH SRH (ed.) 2006. *Relational Process and DSM-V.* p 21

"Social Relationships form the *foundation* of human society… however glaringly little research exists on the biological mechanisms underlying the formation and maintenance of social relationships."

BRAIN MECHANISMS AFFECTED BY FASD

<u>TODAY</u>

- Attention
- Executive Function
- Memory/Learning
- Music
- Speech and language
- Depression
- PTSD

<u>ALSO</u>

- Stress
- Reward Centre/Addictions
- Abuse/Trauma/Attachment
- Sleep problems
- Other gifts: art, drama, humour, exuberance, good with old/young/ animals
- Sensory issues
- Affililiative/ interpersonal/ social attachment systems

SOCIAL *RECOGNITION*

Social Recognition	Where	If a Problem
Is it a face?	Fusiform Gyrus	Not sure who
Is it happy/mean?	Superior Temporal Gyrus and Sulcus	Safe to approach?
Go or stay?	Amygdala and Prefrontal Cortex (PFC)	Like to approach?

E.g. Williams Syndrome all above brain areas do not work well
➔ Slow PFC takes a while to process information---
"hyper social, indiscriminate"

Sensory Problems

For example ***vision***: for example reading the whiteboard

1) Retina problems, double vision
2) Tracking / focus/accommodation →Developmental Optometrist
3) Fuzzy borders
4) Slow pathway from vision center (occipital lobe) to where you figure out the *meaning* of the word (temporal lobe)
5) Impaired ability to ANTICIPATE what you should see in future (catch a ball / safely cross the street)

A BASIC CIRCUIT

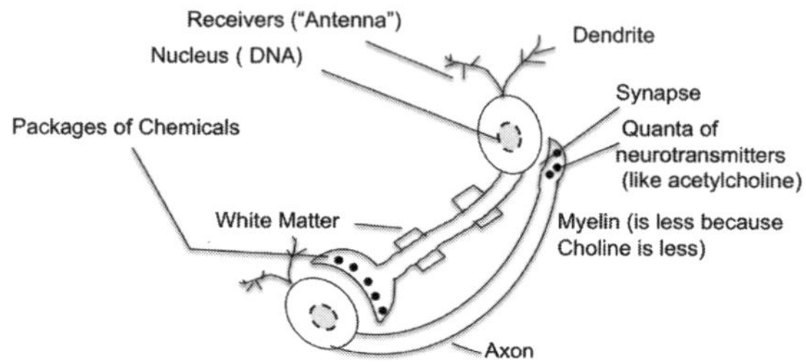

100 Billion Neurons (in Cortex) (More in Cerebellum!)
5000 Trillion Synapses

<u>Some</u> Areas Affected by Prenatal Alcohol Exposure (on MRI, MRS)

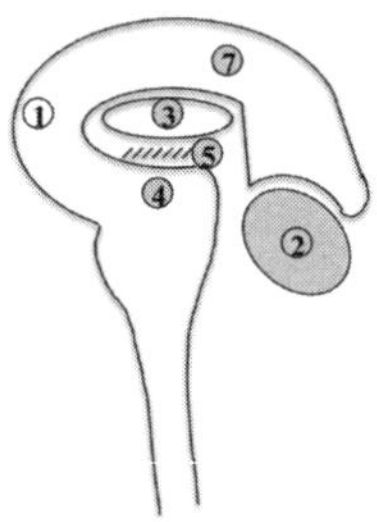

1- Frontal Lobes – executive function
2- Cerebellum Vermis (middle)
- coordination of muscles and attention and learning procedures
3- Corpus Callosum – R/L coordination
4- Caudate – executive function, memory
5- Hippocampus – calming, memory
6- Decreased white matter – processing speed
7- Parietal Lobe – spatial location, movement
8- Temporal Lobe (outside **5**) – memory
9- Decreased Choline leads to decreased I.Q.

SPEECH and LANGUAGE

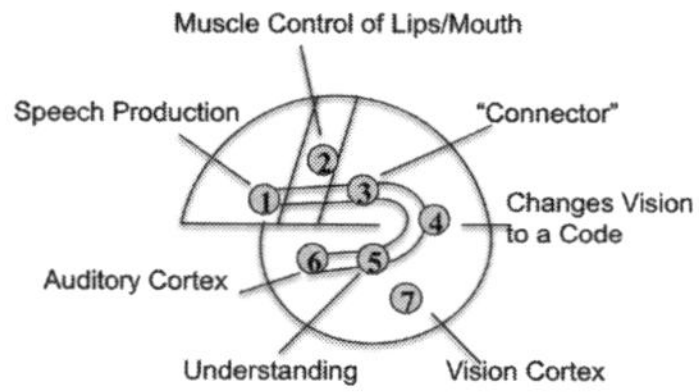

① Broca's
② Motor cortex
③ Arcuate Fasciculus
④ Angular Gyrus
⑤ Wernicke's

(1) Broca's
(Steven Hawkins)

- *Articulate* speech decreased
- Understands ⇨ heard
  ⇨ Read
- Content is ok… except:
  - ⇨ verbs
  - ⇨ connecting words (e.g.) "by" *

(5) Wernicke's
(least favourite politician)

- Fluent *
- Poor comprehension *
- "relentlessly steady and rapid word flow" *
- Could read words but not act on them does not seem to understand meaning (or act on the input)*

* Often seen in those who have FASD

WHY ARE YOU GETTING UP?
Corpus Callosum and "Lying"

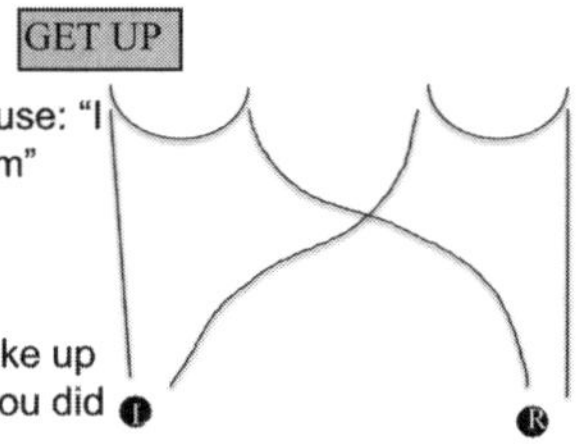

Makes up a coherent excuse: "I have to go to the bathroom"

"Cognitive backfill"

Cognitive – do it, then make up a reason to explain why you did it!

Source: *The Accidental Mind,* David Linden, 2007, p. 228

TO REPEAT A SPOKEN WORD

Repeat Spoken Word

- (6) Ear leads to auditory cortex
- (5) Wernicke – now understood as word
- (3) connector
- (1) words converted to a code for muscle movement of speech
- (2) message to motor cortex to move lips and tongue

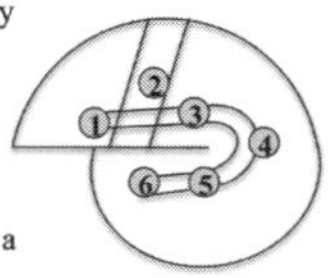

Also

- Areas next to (1) and (5)*
- Caudate *
- Thalamus
- Cerebellum *
- The (R) side too! (C.C.*)
- (C.C. = 200 million axons)

3 C's COGGINS, COHESION, COHERENT

- Coggins T. 1998. "Analysing narrative productions…" Clinical Linguistics & Phonetics12(3): 221-236
- *Frog, Where are you* - (Mercer Meyers, 1969)

What Happens ⇦ COHESION ⇨ What's Up

What Do They Do ⇩ ⇩ What Do They Want to Do

Get the "gist" * = Frog went missing – escaped.

Kids with FAS	Peer/age controls
0/2	8-10/12

COHERENCE

	Informative/ Able to Infer	Vague	Irrelevant or Inaccurate	No Response
FAS	19%	71%	8%	2%
Control	48%	48%	4%	0%

"READING" SOCIAL SITUATIONS

Ramachandran VS, Oberman L. 2007. Broken Mirrors, A Theory of Autism. Scientific American Reports. pp. 20-29.

If see a hand moving…	we fire neurons in the same area as if we moved it.
If see a person crying…	we fire neurons in same area as if we were crying.

READING – STEP #1 – VISION and HEARING (otitis media)

Kerstin Strömland

- Globe size decreases
- Visual acuity decreases / refraction errors
- Strabismus (esp. inward) squint
- Optic nerve (retina) ⇨Increased Blood vessels
  - ↳ Decreased Neurons

INITIAL LEARNING OF WORDS is the fruit of attachment -(Neufeld, G.)

Initially keep Mom & Dad close by:	**What if we are/have:**
Touch/Feeling	Tactile defensive *
Taste (Breast milk)	Oral & taste problems *
Sight	Acuity & conjugate gaze problems *
Smell	
Hearing	Earaches/Eustachian tube problems

Remember increase or decrease of sensations* can complicate "attunement"
IF above goes well ➤ learn words by imitation (starting 25 weeks)

Attunement = "Dance" of getting "in synch"
"A PLACE OF REST"

"MOTHERESE" = "PRE-WORD" ***Synchronous*** Comunication

Baby looks up, bright eyes

Mom or Dad talk "motherese" playful, friendly, high pitched.

Gurgles, coos

More "motherese"

Ends with Mom and Baby matching (happy) states

Babe and Mom in a synchronized "dance" (close attention, match emotional tone … result = ahh!)

FASD

- bombarded by sensations
- slow processing = hard to "get in synch"
- too agitated to settle
- distracted ++

No ahh No snuggle

Mom's feeling of competence decreased

To do: decrease over stimulation, support mom +++

INATTENTION

Kodituwakku, P: "significantly lower on a test of language comprehension"

Slow info processing leads to decreased comprehension

Gets distracted – off on a tangent. ← decreased persistence relates to inattention

ADHD → Inattention
ADHD → Hyperactivity/impulsivity

"ADHD is the most likely disguise for FASD" – (O'Malley, K.)

CONSIDER THESE ISSUES – MEDICAL WORK UP

(ADHD or Depression or Anxiety)

- TSH
- Ferritin/iron
- Vit D 2000 units
- Omega 3 2000 mg+
- Epilepsy? – EEG
- Sensory processing
- Disrupted sleep/ obstructive sleep apnea

If "usual" meds do not work: THINK ATYPICAL SEIZURES OR HEAD INJURY AND TREAT IT ANYWAYS. (Lamotrigen, Valproic acid, etc.)

IMPULSIVITY

WHAT DRIVES IT?-(Hollander, E.)

Compulsivity
Anxiety
SSRI

Inattention
Hyperactivity
Dexedrine

Craving
Addiction
Naltrexone

Unstable mood
Mood stabilizer
-Topiramate
- Lithium
- Valproate

Genetics – Paris, J. ~ 70 % Penetrance

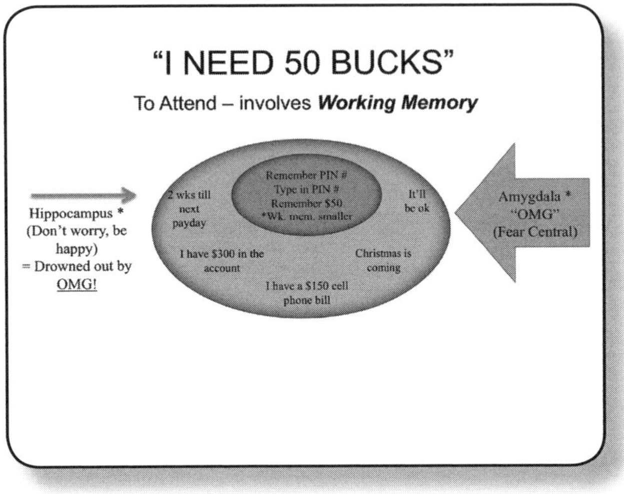
"I NEED 50 BUCKS"
To Attend – involves Working Memory
Hippocampus *
(Don't worry, be happy)
= Drowned out by OMG!
Remember PIN #
Type in PIN #
Remember $50
*Wk. mem. smaller
2 wks till next payday
It'll be ok
I have $300 in the account
Christmas is coming
I have a $150 cell phone bill
Amygdala *
"OMG"
(Fear Central)

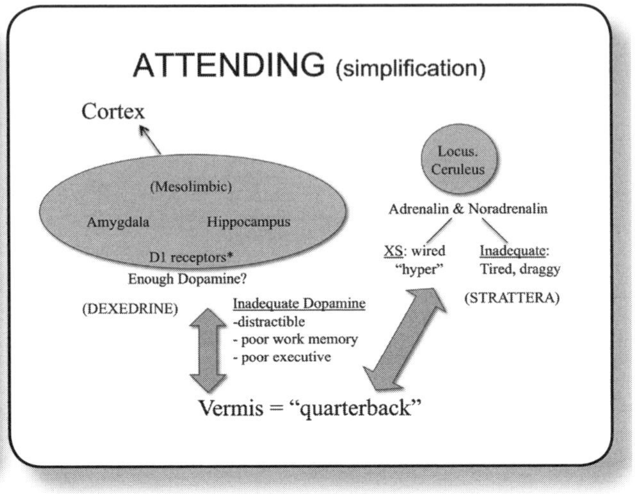
ATTENDING (simplification)
Cortex
(Mesolimbic)
Amygdala
Hippocampus
D1 receptors*
Enough Dopamine?
(DEXEDRINE)
Inadequate Dopamine
-distractible
- poor work memory
- poor executive
Locus. Ceruleus
Adrenalin & Noradrenalin
XS: wired "hyper"
Inadequate: Tired, draggy
(STRATTERA)
Vermis = "quarterback"

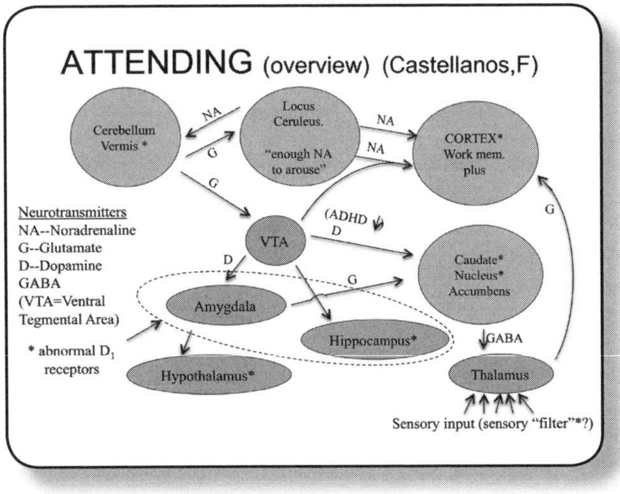
ATTENDING (overview) (Castellanos,F)
Cerebellum Vermis *
Locus Ceruleus.
"enough NA to arouse"
CORTEX* Work mem. plus
NA
G
VTA
(ADHD
D
Caudate* Nucleus* Accumbens
Amygdala
Hippocampus*
Hypothalamus*
Thalamus
GABA
Neurotransmitters
NA--Noradrenaline
G--Glutamate
D--Dopamine
GABA
(VTA=Ventral Tegmental Area)
* abnormal D1 receptors
Sensory input (sensory "filter"*?)

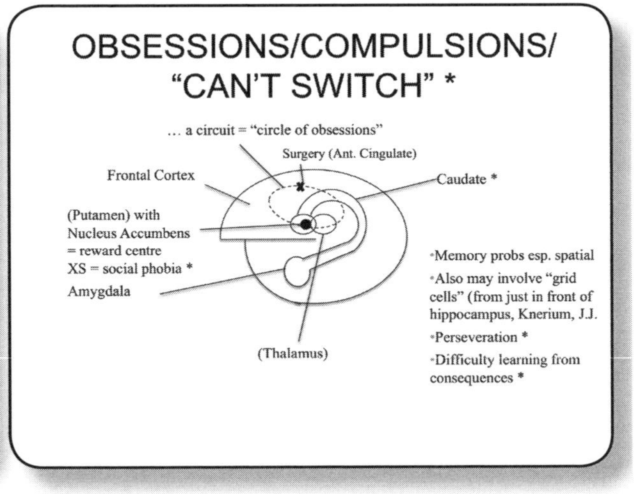
OBSESSIONS/COMPULSIONS/ "CAN'T SWITCH" *
… a circuit = "circle of obsessions"
Surgery (Ant. Cingulate)
Frontal Cortex
Caudate *
(Putamen) with
Nucleus Accumbens
= reward centre
XS = social phobia *
Amygdala
(Thalamus)
•Memory probs esp. spatial
•Also may involve "grid cells" (from just in front of hippocampus, Knerium, J.J.
•Perseveration *
•Difficulty learning from consequences *

"ADHD IS THE MOST LIKELY DISGUISE FOR FASD…"-(O'Malley, K.)

"<u>Standard</u>" <u>ADHD</u>

- Focus and Sustain worse
- Imbalance of Fronto-Nigro-Striatal Dopamine Pathway (where Ritalin works)

<u>ADHD *of FASD*</u>

- **Encode** and **shifting attention** worse
- More of a problem of abnormal D_1 Receptors in mesolimbic area (where dexedrine works)

MEMORY – STARTS WITH A MESSAGE BETWEEN NEURONS

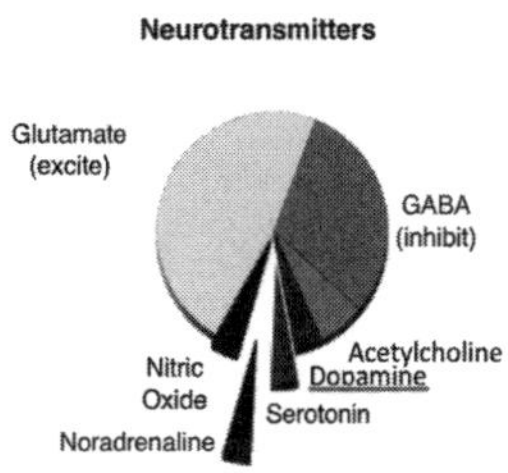

- Amino acids – Glutamate and GABA
- Catecholamines – Dopamine and Noradrenalin
- Histamine
- Acetylcholine (from caudate* and putamen) together with Dopamine (from substantia Nigra) control muscles
- Neuropeptides – Oxytocin and Vasopressin and CRF
- Gases Nitric Oxide

31

The ADHD *of FASD* (continued)

- Often has earlier onset –infant may meet criteria for "Regulatory Disorder" esp. "hard to warm up (emotionally) or difficult to settle"… leads to problems getting "in synch" with parents (attunement)
- More side effects esp. to Ritalin (esp. generic)
- "Ritalin" should not be used in Native American Children with FASD because of lack of effectiveness and more side effects esp. growth suppression
- More Psychiatric diagnoses Depression, Anxiety, and explosiveness
- Complex learning disorders are more common (especially math and higher order language)

Mgt: sensory integration, language therapy, special schooling, non-verbal play therapy, meds, parent education, and supportive family therapy.

MEMORY – LONG TERM POTENTIATION – (Higgins, E.S.)

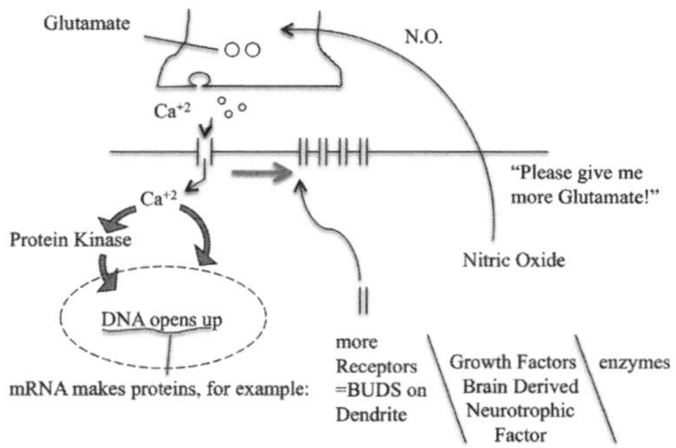

Memory – Learning : 3 Issues

Declarative
Facts
Episodes
(1)**Hippocampus**
↓New Cells
↓BDNF

Procedural
Academic Skills
how to write, spell, punctuate, form letters, sound out words
(2) **Cerebellar circuits**

Rules / Routines are compensatory strategies to overcome procedural problems

BUT OVERLOAD (3) **WORKING MEMORY (Frontal Lobe)**

33

MUSIC #2

"meme" – an idea spread mind to mind

Hip Hop 1) Kid is moving "in synch"
2) Now kid will get message

e.g. Kayne West John Stevens (Legend)

Also: Playing instrument Singing \ Is a complex task \ It changes your nerves!

An increase in signals from Auditory Cortex (increases verbal skills?)

An increase in signals from Somatosensory Cortex (increases muscle coordination?)

"hear the note" = (R) side Wernicke's workout!

MUSIC/HUMOUR LEADS TO INFLUENCE - (Goleman, D.)

- When we play/sing together our **Right Hemisphere** activity "gets in synch" with next player
- Synchronize in thought, in movement, in brain waves
- Likely "mirror neurons"
- Also…

"little cements a social interaction as well as a great laugh together… laughter may be the shortest distance between two brains"

Pissed Off Ready to Blow → (Why Try) → Foosball! → (Leads to) → laugh silly → (Leads to) → Social Bond and Influence

DEPRESSION IN PREGNANCY-
Effect on Baby

- Stress/Depression/Alcohol in Mom leads to increase in cortisol (stress reactivity) ***in kids***
- Mechanism: sensitivity of Hypothalamus-Pituitary-Adrenal Axis to stress is increased
- More neglect/less nurturing care leads to: "lower early a.m. cortisol and 'flatter' circadian rhythm" … sleep problems *
- **1st:** Baby attunes to Mum… by being "in synch" with Mum, **then…**small babies can calm down (not by themselves)
- Parental WARMTH is the dimension most predictive for child to avoid mental health and substance use problems (Kender, K.S.)

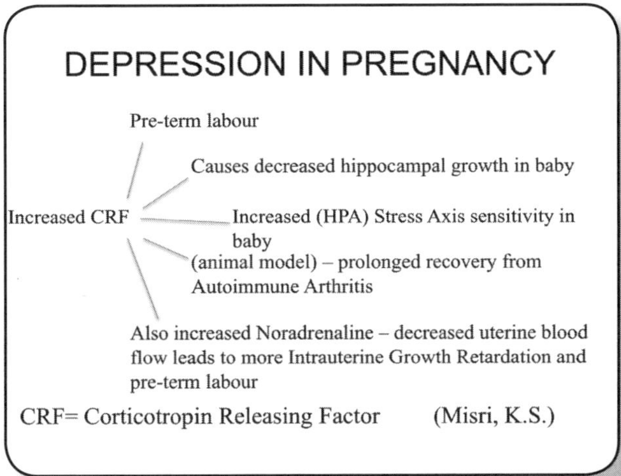

DEPRESSION (Am Psychiatric 2007 meeting)

"less than 50% of Depressed are detected in Primary Health Care settings … and few are offered evidence-based care"

Depression is a: common, disabling, chronic ***medical*** illness

U.S. 2006:	$83.1 Billion
Depression changes the *Relative Risk*:	1.5 Fatal Heart Attack
	1.7 Stroke
	1.7 Type II Diabetes
also…BDNF	*Decreased* in Prefrontal cortex and Hippocampus
	Increased in Nucleus Accumbens Reward Centre

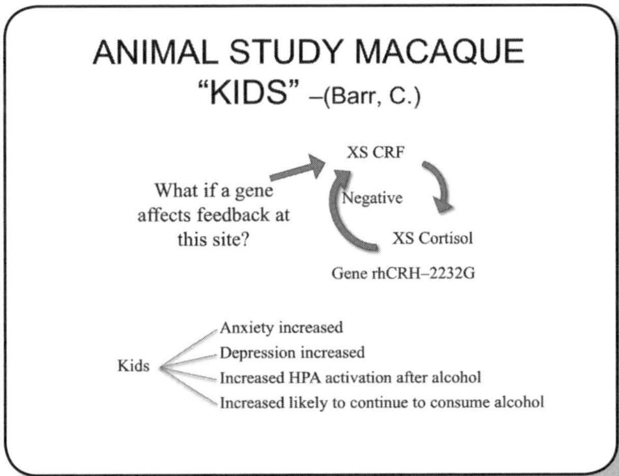

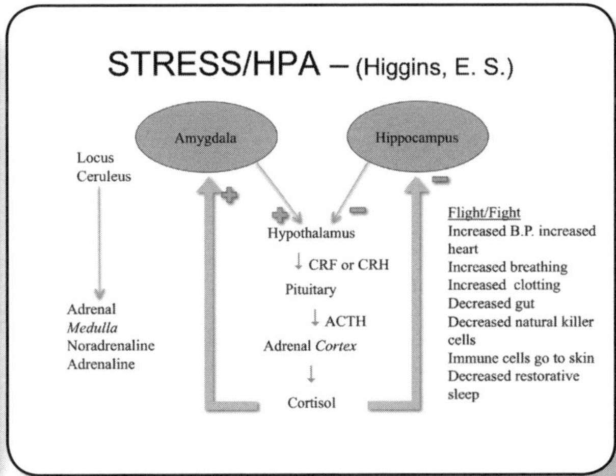

GETTING THE BALANCE RIGHT

"BURNED OUT"
Low Cortisol
Dysthymia
Hypothyroid
Autoimmune increased
Chronic Fatigue

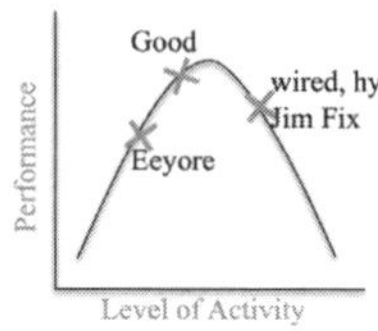

"STILL ON OVERDRIVE"
Hi "everything"
Melancholia
Hyperthyroid
Heart attack

Great Resources: *The Relaxation Response*, H. Benson
or: Benson Henry Institute for Mind Body Medicine:
http://www.mgh.harvard.edu/bhi/

STIGMA, SHAMING,SHUNNING

… a primal threat to the core of self.

Our most basic need = acceptance and belonging

The worst trauma involves an intension to personally harm i.e. the trauma was purposely inflicted

- An experiment: hostility/shaming/rejection … "reliably triggers the HPA Axis to produce some of the highest levels (of stress hormones) of any laboratory stress simulation ever recorded. RESULT=LEARNED HELPLESSNESS

(Goleman, D. p. 231)

PTSD

1) Re-experiencing (e.g.) Flashbacks (Hippocampus)
2) Avoidant/Numbing symptoms (e.g.) less able to talk about traumatic memories (decreased PFC-Broca's)
   also decreased ability to extinguish fear (medial and ventral PFC)
3) Hyperarousal via Hyperactive Amygdala

Tells Loc.Ceruleus to make XS Adrenaline Noradrenaline

Tells Hypothalamus to make CRF and Cortisol

Stress Soup:

Adrenaline	increase
Noradrenalin	increase
CRF	increase
Cortisol	increase or decrease (later)

LESS PTSD

- Just an accident
- Nothing personal
- Some sense of effectiveness
- Asian, white
- Moderate income
- Higher education/I.Q. (over 115: 1/5 PTSD vs. those less than 100)
- Isolated trauma
- Married/male/younger
- Lots of social connections
- No anxiety symptoms

MORE PTSD

- Intentionally harmed
- Personal attack
- Unable to change situation
- African American
- Low or very high
- Less able to "work around" the trauma
- Previous or chronic trauma
- More Cortisol, CRF etc
- Smaller hippocampus due to decreased BDNF
- "Kindling" of Amygdala

(Mancini, A. D.)

GOOD NEWS – Toxic memories can be "FLUID" ON RETRIEVAL

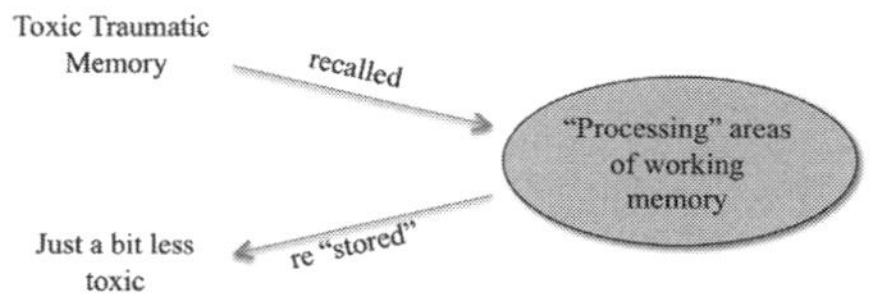

Key = If <u>SAFE</u> … if therapist can help you be "at rest"
(Higgins, p. 199)

ELLEN LIVES IN STRESS CITY – SO DOES HER CAREGIVER

Approach:

- Unhurried, safe, a place of rest … always "collect" a smile/nod before "directing," slow conversation, written instructions

(Visit #5)

- **Went with her** to RCMP (had sister who verified evidence)
- Kids always present, tried to help them
- See Mum as having great love for them and interest in them, tried to help get $ and respite for caregiver
- PTSD – medications, supportive counseling, try to help, decrease the stress – regular appointments same time each week/ reminders
- Health – cancer screen, birth control, vaccines Hep B, A, meningitis, flu
- Assessment leads to social worker dialogue

Wish List:

- Supported housing/job (good in sign language)
- "Intrusive support" for $, food, and relationships

WHY ARE WE HERE: Ellen

Ellen –35— probably has FASD

- When Ellen was 2 yrs old: family apprehended by police – parents drunk driving – 3 kids went to foster care
- Grew up Nanimo foster care
  - Sexual abuse X years by foster father, foster mother beat her, teachers x3 did not believe her.
- 2 kids, Dad not around, welfare, lives in Vancouver
- Lives with lady from church – "tense" (burned-out caregiver)
- 2 kids (9 & 13); doing well, but 13-year old is the "boss of Mum"
- Kids are at small Christian School
- Poor dental state, had cleft lip repair, superficial, nervous, **breast cancer**
- Had quit cigarettes
- Never drank

REFERENCES

Kodituwakku P, Coriale G Fiorentino D, et al. 2006. Neurobehavioral Characteristics of Children with FASD. Alcoholism: Clinical and Experimental Research 30(9): 1558-1559

Hollander E. 2007. "Impulsivity – What Drives It," Syllabus and Proceedings Summary American Psychiatric Association Meeting 2007, accessed Sept, 2007 at http://www.psych.org/

Paris J. Personality Disorders over Time: Pre-cursors, Course and Outcome. 2003. Washington, DC: American Psychiatric Publishing

O'Malley K. 2007. ADHD and Fetal Alcohol Spectrum Disorders (FASD). New York: Nova Science Publishing.

Castellanos FX, Swanson J. 2002. Biological underpinnings of ADHD. In. Sandberg S. (Editor) Hyperactivity and Attention Disorders of Childhood 2nd Ed. Cambridge,UK: Cambridge University Press. p 349

Knerium JJ. 2007. The Matrix in Your Head. Scientific American Mind, June/July 2007, pp. 42-49

Barr CS. 2003. Serotonin Transporter Gene Variation is Associated with Alcohol Sensitivity in Rhesus Macaques Exposed to Early-Life Stress. Alcoholism: Clinical and Experimental Research 27(5): p 812

REFERENCES

Neufeld G, Maté G. 2004. Hold on to Your Kids! Why parents matter more than peers. Toronto: Vintage Canada.

Higgins ES, George MS.2007. The Neuroscience of Clinical Psychiatry. Philadelphia: Lippincott, Williams, and Wilkins: Philadelphia p. 58

Goleman D. 2006. Social Intelligence: The New Science of Human Relationships. New York: Bantam Books pp. 45-46

Kender KS, Prescott CA. 2006. Genes Environment and Psychopathology: Understanding the causes of Psychiatric and Substance Use Disorders. New York: Guilford Press

MISRI KS. 2006. Pregnancy Blues. New York: Delacorte Press.

Mancini AD, Bonanno GA. 2006. Resilience in the Face of Potential Trauma. Journal of Clinical Psychology62 (8): 971-985

NEUROBIOLOGY OF ATTACHMENT

Rod Densmore, M.D., Adoptive Dad

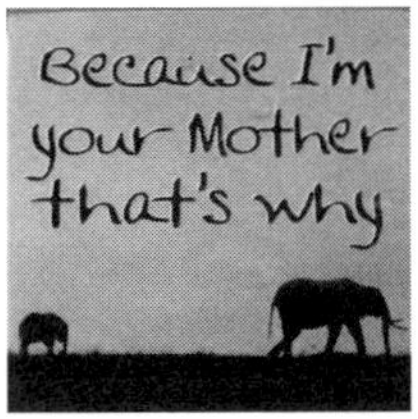

It should be like this

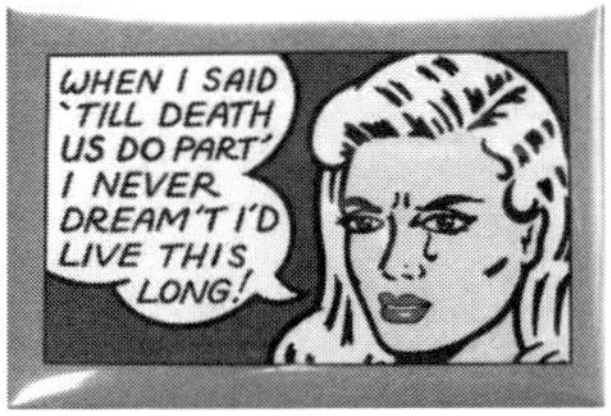

Not like this! (disclaimer ≠ my wife!)

ROOTS OF ATTACHMENT

- 1. To be with (touch, feel, see, hear and taste)
- 2. To imitate (act, look, sound and dress like)
- 3. To " Please," to be loyal to
- 4. To honor, to be important to
- 5. To love, give our heart to
- 6. To keep secrets of, be confidante of.
- *allows* curiosity, learning, interdependence

Neufeld, G DVD series : *Power to Parent* available at gordonneufeld.com

ATTACHMENT

- Contact, closeness, a sense of belonging
- "A place of rest"
- Its our #1 need (even more than food and shelter for it is how we *access* food and shelter).

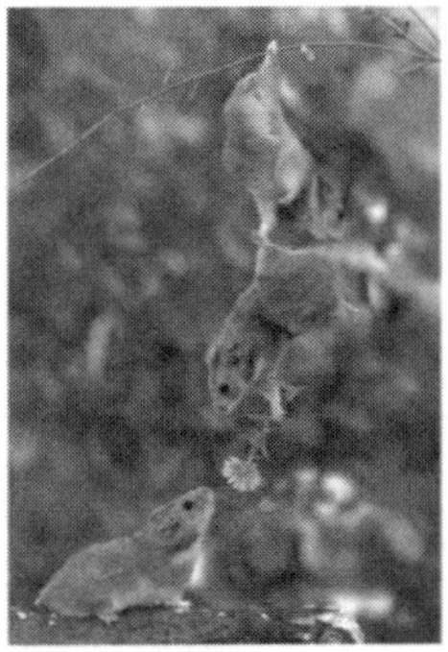

Attachment

cry → pick up empathetically "ride mum down" → **ahhh... relax** → curiosity exploration → tired, hungry, dirty → cry

Get close = Get Love

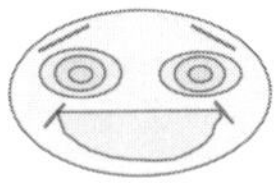

Abuse

cry

swat (never 100%)
yell

much ↓ relaxing, hyper-
vigilant = always on alert

wary even
whether to cry
or approach

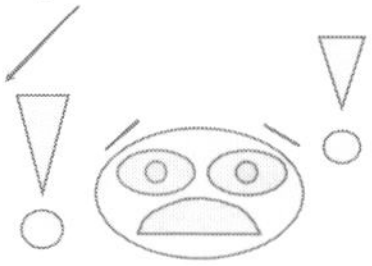

Get close= Get hurt
so- don't *depend*, do it all yourself, don't be vulnerable

Attachment is ~~Important~~ CENTRAL to development

- It is *biological*
- Involves 2 "players" (at least)
- Is *basis* for *relationship....*
- Which is the basis for *sense of self* (vs. not self)
- Which allows one to see others' points of view (theory of mind)

Neglect

cry

ignored

why bother

numb out
don't cry

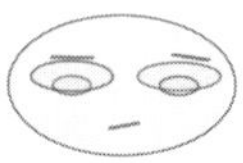

Get close= Nothing happens
Give up after initial struggle-- maybe attach to something else- dog, rocking etc...

FASD

- 1. Involves damage to some attachment structures BUT ALSO
- 2. An *increased* need for being able to depend on *stable, ongoing, nurturing* attachments to competent adults that care...
- Building attachments= Hard work but not hopeless .... caregivers get DEPLETED

"Stable nurturing home"**(good attachments)**: 3-4X ⇩ Secondary Disabilities
Streissguth AP, et al. 2004. Risk factors for adverse life outcomes in Fetal Alcohol Syndrome and Fetal Alcohol Effects. Developmental and Behavioral Pediatrics. 25(4): 228-238

This session: Attachment Busters and ideas to ⇩ them

How Depleted Do Caregivers Get?

Caregiver Strain Questionnaire Robinson B. 1983. Journal of Gerontol38: 344-348
(yes or no)... a score of 7 or over suggests enough stress to cause health problems

Disturbs sleep disturbed	Other demands on my time
Causes Inconvenience	Forces Emotional Adjustments
Is a Physical Strain	Involves coping with behaviours which are upsetting
Restricts free time	Forces Work Adjustments
Requires Family to Adjust	Causes Financial Strain
Forces changes in Personal Plans	Can Overwhelm You

n=35 average score 10.5/12 Whitecrow..."insensitive"...Rod:...maybe a tool for us to improve on /for counselors or clinicians to use with a client

Adaptive Function: Our Kids' (FASD) and Ours (Overwhelmed)

Adapt= ability to "get it", "apply it" and "modify it"

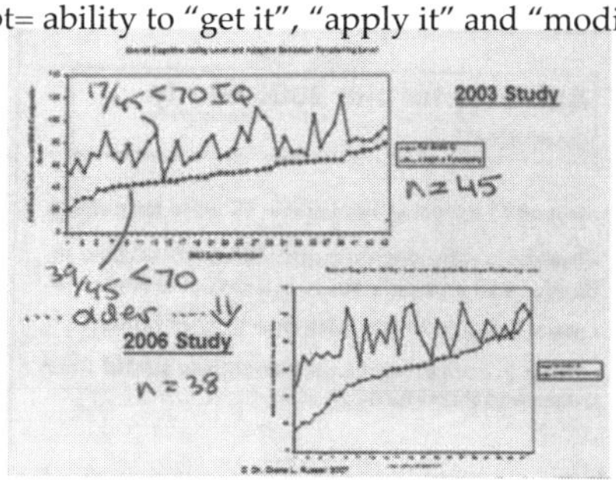

Russell D. 2007. 2nd Intl. Conf. on FASD Syllabus. Vancouver. UBC p.54

Role of Caregiver in FASD

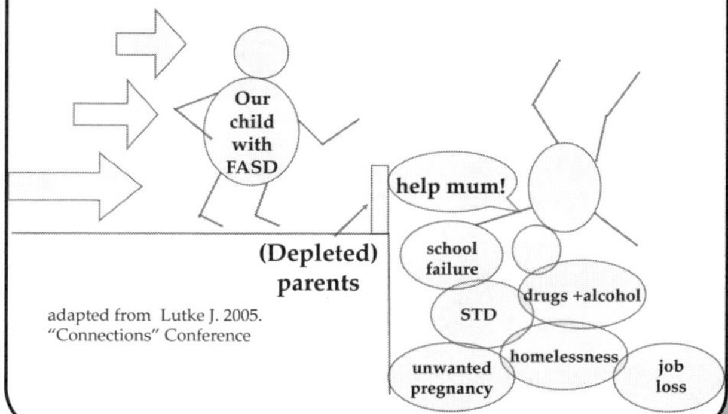

adapted from Lutke J. 2005.
"Connections" Conference

Who Is the "Slow Learner"

If caregivers expect:	To result in:
"Tough love"	"Compliance"
"Consequences"	"Cooperation"
Raised voice	"I get it"
Repeated demands	Bonding, understanding

1. **You assume your child can hold (in working memory):**
   a) the impulse to swipe the "cool" ipod
   b) and the idea: "BUT" I will get into trouble

2. **You assume the child is not "guarded" or "closed off"** to your influence (i.e not saying "I don't care, Whatever", etc.)

in FASD --**1.** and **2.** are unlikely.....so "back off" and rebuild the relationship if you meet resistance

REDUCTIONISTIC VS DEVELOPMENTAL

what is the "bottom line?" "what needs to grow so a child *wants* to cooperate?"

- The fruit of years of depending on and connection to caregivers = *wish* to cooperate, look out for, be obedient to, and to please
- Yeah - "the truth of the matter" is he must pay attention, respect authority, honor elders, etc....
- *No.....* "success will be *through* attachments" Gordon Neufeld

KEYS: attitude towards kid, "you can depend on me"
not "lording it over" → grudging "compliance"
→ sabotages relationships
"Collect" first get their eye, a smile, a nod — Then give directions or a correction

John Gottman: (http://www.gottman.com/) "soft start up"

COST OF "DARN KID NEEDS TO GROW UP, LEARN HIS LESSON, ETC."

Child	You
- ⇧distant, disconnected, negative, guarded, defensive, defended - ⇩likely to do what you want	-Try to "force compliance" by coercion...utter defeat, lash out at spouse, dog, other kids, you feel incompetent (to the core)

-when relationship needs are not met by caring adults the child may try peers, drugs, alcohol

Cost= where is the kid at 3 a.m.? and secondary disabilities ⇧
because
relationship is the *only* "conduit" / access point to influence

Adapted quote: To the extent a child is not mature they *depend* on their relationship with adults who care for them to "shoehorn" them into adulthood. Neufeld G. DVD course: *Making Sense Out of Adolescence*

"NO TIME FOR THAT PSYCHOLOGIST STUFF", NOT "REALISTIC"

- -To you, it is self evident you *are entitled to be angry* and the *child must change ...*
- consider mbmi.org : *Post MI patients*

Anger	Cost	Maybe smarter
cut off by driver on freeway	sticky platelets, ↑B.P. + pulse rate, ↑clot proteins,↓clot dissolving, changes in artery lining **= *another* heart attack !**	that guy is stupid - maybe for a reason

... COST of self-evident entitlement (to be angry) is TOO HIGH!!!

REQUIREMENTS TO BENEFIT FROM "TOUGH LOVE"

Brain required

-Be *undefended* ** enough "to care" i.e. not overwhelmed by amygdala* overresponse or XS sympathetic nervous system tone*
-Big enough working memory* (to hold "lesson" on line)
-Enough R⇔ L communication through corpus callosum* to "work on creative solutions"

Thinking required

-*See* error of their ways/repent
-*See* better alternative
-*Choose* better alternative
-Set aside immediate wants
-Choose what's best in the long term
-Be *vulnerable* enough to see error of their ways and "need to change"

*For FASD? , For **any** kid if upset??..For me??
** Gordon Neufeld

AN ATTACK IS A "RELATIONSHIP BUSTER" SO HOW DO CAREGIVERS RESPOND??

Attacks, Meltdowns, "Incidents", Aggression

5 Issues	**Ideas**
1) Cornered? →	Don't coerce / corner
2) Surprised (by a transition) →	Plan transition / use routines or habits
3) Overstimulated →	Understand and plan for sensory processing pattern
4) "Out of the blue" violence you must consider →	Temporal lobe (or other Traumatic Brain Injury) / epilepsy Consider: mood stabilizers like carbamazepine, lamotrigine, gabapentin
5) The perception of being abandoned by a social attachment →	So-far-as-possible "Bridge" any transitions or separations (G Neufeld)

TO REDUCE FRUSTRATION

A) ***Can*** something *external* be changed?

Yes

- Well, then help change it

No

-Say, "No" firmly *but be sympathetic*
e.g. hostile (scared) patient: "I *wish* it were possible to do this anaesthetic and *guarantee* no side effects "
e.g. 4yr. old: "I *wish* you could have a cookie before dinner but that is not allowed in the Daddy Book" ("Agent of futility and angel of mercy") G.Neufeld

ATTACKS, AGGRESSION...A DEEPER UNDERSTANDING

G. Neufeld: "Expressions of *Foul Frustration*"

-See it as something not working for the child, something frustrating him/her

-If you had ⇩ *words for feelings* (alexithymia), felt always *put down*, "a failure" (despite trying) *you'd be frustrated too*

-If we see attack as a ***frustration gone afoul...***

-Primes our wish to help ⇩ frustration in the child

TO REDUCE FRUSTRATION – WHEN THE EXTERNAL SITUATION *CANNOT* BE CHANGED

B) So...if some *external* frustration cannot be changed the child may need to change *himself* i.e. *adapt*?

-Try to encourage sadness about what does not work... touch it gently... the energy changes G.Neufeld

e.g.
(Very ill) dad cried when son came over ⇨ "We will cry with you *first* before son visits" ⇨ ***Tears shed,*** then energy changed ⇨ Move on to build memories

Remember Diane Russell?.. in FASD: ***Adaptability*** impacted even more than I.Q....could this be related to perseveration, compulsions? (the "compulsion circuit" involves caudate*, cingulate, prefrontal cortex*, nucleus accumbens, thalamus*)

HORMONES AND ATTACHMENT

Mummy Rats
(hormonally primed)

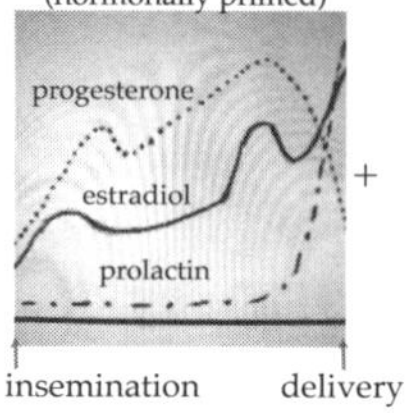

\+ **oxytocin** (not just milk let down and uterus contraction) = *more* attraction to pups and *less* fear so ⇧defense vs intruders

Oxytocin - in pre-optic area (anterior hypothalamus) in a hormonally-primed mum = Attachment

(graph adapted from Higgins ES, et al. 2007. The Neuroscience of Clinical Psychiatry. Philadelphia. Lippincott. p. 178)

TILL DEATH DO US PART VS THE HOLLYWOOD SWINGER

Prairie Vole	**Meadow Vole**
Enduring partner for life	Promiscuous, ↓attachments
Dad helps rear the young	Abandon young in 2 weeks!!!

amount of oxytocin and vasopressin in the brain is similar...but....

OTR' + V1aR ⇧ in reward centre

OTR' and V1aR ⇩ in reward centre

(OTR'= oxytocin receptor)
(V1aR= vasopressin receptor)

so...maybe we have her figured out now??

"Oh why can't i have more OTR's in my Nucleus Accumbens????"

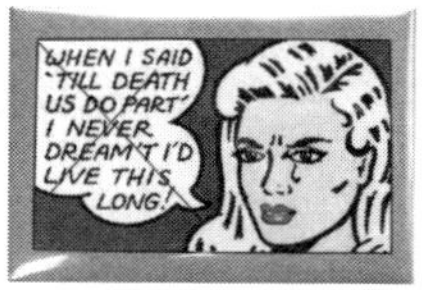

HAVING PUPS (AND BABIES) IS REWARDING

Players:
- -Hippocampus
- -Amygdala
- -Orbitofrontal (Bottom) Prefrontal Cortex
- -Ventral Tegmental Area

-All work though *Nucleus Accumbens* and ⇧ dopamine there in response to exposure to infants

-One mechanism of alcoholism is ***reduced sensitivity* of reward system** so joy of more *subtle* rewards (babies, chocolate, sex) may be less... i.e. need "BIG HIT" of alcohol, cocaine, etc.) to stimulate the nucleus accumbens...could this be one reason why chronic substance abuse might result in ⇩ attachment ...

-So parents need more supports as natural positive feedback/ joy of motherhood is not as rewarding

A Hurtin' Country Song if we are silly we will increase salience in the amygdala and improve retention eh??

to the tune of "Stand by Yer Man"

VTA=Ventral tegmental area NA=Nucleus Accumbens
OTR'=Oxytocin Receptor V1aR=Vasopressin Receptor

He: Give me more V1aR's in my littl' VTA (and NA),
She: Give me more OTR's in my VTA too big boy,
He: Make her Dopamine receptors in her VTA light
up fer *me*,
Not fer that smooth talkin' city-slicker of a
meadow vole varmint that's bin snoopin' 'round,
She: Make me depend on that Budweisser to excite
my mu recepters less ....so I can....
STAND BY MY MAN!!

Canadian Licking and Grooming Rats (Michael Meaney's Gp @ McGill) ...or... We do stink don't we?

Pups handled- have improved resilience to stress *when adults*!...

Q: handling = great for stress?

A: Nope!

Licking and grooming (to get the stink off) is great for stress

Higgins, et al. p.109

Stress can ⇩ our resilience and ⇩ our ability to attach

Depressed Humans

If treat mums who are depressed:

their children have ↓ depression, ↓ anxiety, and ↓ behavior disorders

Why?

probably related to reducing the methylation of the part of DNA *which codes for protein* BDNF

(Higgins p.183)

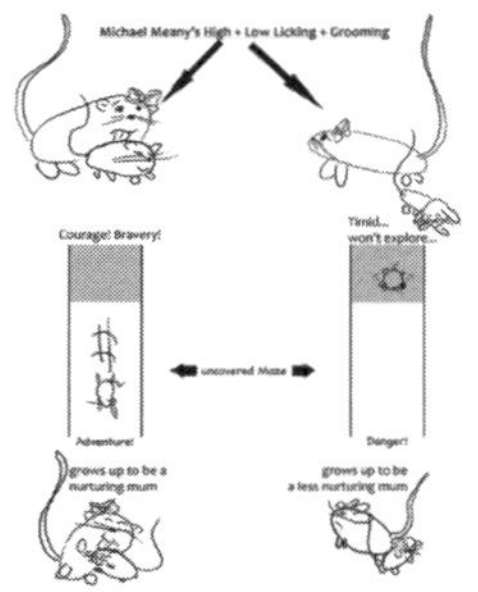

Higgins ES, Gorge MS. The Neuroscience of Clinical Psychiatry: The Pathophysiology of Behavior and Mental Illness. Philadelphia (USA): Lippincott, Williams and Wilkins; 2007, pg. 109

-less (pup) glucocorticoid release after stressed (restraint)

-less CRH messenger RNA in hippocampus (less stress reactivity in hippocampus)

-more glucocorticoid receptors in hypothalamus .. can turn stress down better

-increased resilience, less fear SHOW GREATER WILLINGNESS TO EXPLORE NEW PLACES CURIOSITY (vs. guardedness)

Be vulnerable! explore + learn!
(CRF=CRH=Corticotropin Releasing Factor)

Hormonal Stress System: "HPA" Activation
Stress ⇒ Hypothalamus ⇒⇒ Pituitary ⇒⇒ Adrenal (Cortex) ⇒⇒
CRF or CRH ACTH Cortisol

Chronic Defeat...and Solutions!

↑ methylation of DNA...so ↓ BDNF can be made

-Antidepressant
-Lithium
-exercise
-(probably) psychotherapy

→ *acetylation* of histone- doesn't "bump methyl off" the DNA.... but does let mRNA "in" so BDNF can be made (lets the suitor in the back door)

DEPRESSION (IN PART)

1) Localized ↓ in BDNF activity in Nucleus Accumbens - result = needs more to "register" or "appreciate" a reward...hopelessness can ↑

2) not enough BDNF in hippocampus and prefrontal cortex → less able to "calm down"

(Higgins p.236)

SO LETS APPLY THIS

<u>Joanne (24)</u>
- *-her* mum drank +++
- *-she* did not drink with her pregnancy =Jason
- -"derailed" by loud noise
- -has not hit him
- -calls her mum 15x/d.

<u>Jason (3)</u>
- -touch sensitive
- -texture sensitive
- -fussy eater (coordination of swallow ↓, food preference++)
- -*screams* when hungry..
- - ↓knowledge when *full*
- -"regulatory disorder"

Issues: What are the genetics of Joanne's eggs soaked in alcohol in utero?, birth father

Joanne- headphones during meal prep

Jason-O.T.- calms with heavy pressure

-Dietician- thicker foods more satisfying

COULD THIS BE RELATED TO SOME BIRTH MUMS?

If alcohol dependent---women who tried but were *unable to remain abstinent* after treatment vs those that could remain abstinent had:

1) about 50% lower BDNF
   a) ↓P.F.C.-calming
   b) ↓hippocampus- memory and calming

2) acoustic startle

<u>Fit?</u> <u>child with FASD</u> fussy eater "colic" poor sleeper + if <u>birth mum or any parent</u> has "acoustic startle" =

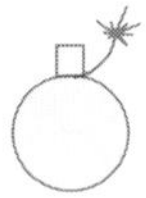

<u>Idea</u> approachable non-judgmental support +++ e.g.)France prenatal videos for higher risk mums

SO LETS APPLY THIS #2

<u>Francine (38)</u>
- -unhappy childhood
- -dyslexia, put downs,very religious- message ="Austin is the one"
- -very touch and noise sensitive
- -asked for help from MCF 6 times
- -in distress---hit him......
- mortified/suicidal

<u>Austin (9)</u>
- -adopted Honduras
- -"viral infection", ↑ fever, ↓weight gain
- -hyper++, rough, loud
- -will NOT "purr" (G. Neufeld)

<u>Issues</u>- Infertility (PTSD), <u>core</u> violation of sense of self, sensory sensitivities= care of Austin at times, overwhelming

<u>Plan</u>- Recognize HIGH RISK, RESPITE, ACCESS TO HELP

<u>Please</u>- no one miss the next Francine!

ALEXITHYMIA- "NO WORDS FOR EMOTIONS"

Measure: -Toronto Alexithymia Scale (TAS-20)
-High = Over 60

Key: at the *core* of our *ability* to be social* → are these skills:

- -process experience into emotions
- -attend to/ regulate emotions
- -find words/ ways to communicate emotions to and from others

Ref.: O'Malley, K (ed.) *AHDH and Fetal Alcohol Spectrum Disorders.* Nova Biomedical, New York. 2007 p.229

*esp important to "automatic/quick" social reciprocity...problems mean "getting" social cues will take longer Ref: Goleman,D. 2006.*Social Intelligence-the new science of human relationships.*Bantam, New York.

MIRROR NEURONS

"we effortlessly gain a feel for what goes on in the mind of other people ... this social intuition may rest on brain mechanisms I call *shared circuits* ... these translate the *actions, sensations* and *emotions* of others into our own."

parietal + premotor cortex

somatosensory+ insular cortex

Lesion? - ↓understand emotions of others
- ↓experience certain emotions yourself

Keysers, C. May, 2007. *American Psychiatric Assoc. Annual meeting Syllabus and Proceedings Summary* p.144

FASD AND ALEXITHYMIA

If Alexithymia

↓Blood flow from in Ⓡ Frontal (where *comprehend facial + vocal expression)*

↓Blood flow in Ⓡ parietal (where *process emotions)*

O'Malley p.230

FASD -PFC, parietal, corpus callosum, processing speed, ??? mirror neurons

ABUSIVE + NEGLECTFUL ENVIRONMENTS

"provide limited opportunities for children to learn how to efficiently cope with and express painful emotions"

childhood trauma →
- high TAS-20
- affect/mood dysregulation
- self injury

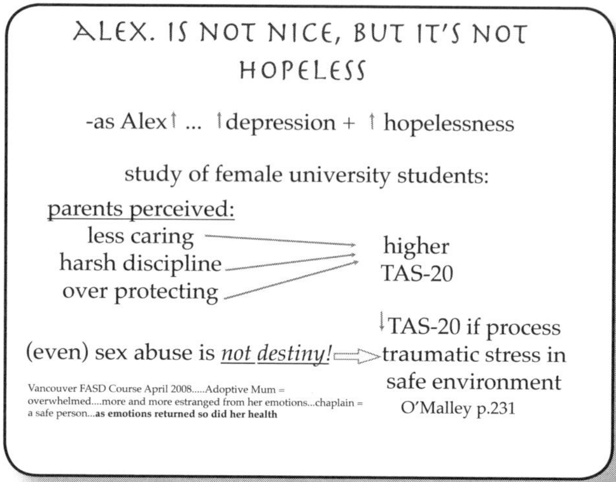
Alex. is not nice, but it's not hopeless
-as Alex↑ ... ↑depression + ↑ hopelessness
study of female university students:
parents perceived:
less caring
harsh discipline
over protecting
higher TAS-20
↓TAS-20 if process traumatic stress in safe environment
(even) sex abuse is *not destiny!*
O'Malley p.231
Vancouver FASD Course April 2008.....Adoptive Mum = overwhelmed....more and more estranged from her emotions...chaplain = a safe person...**as emotions returned so did her health**

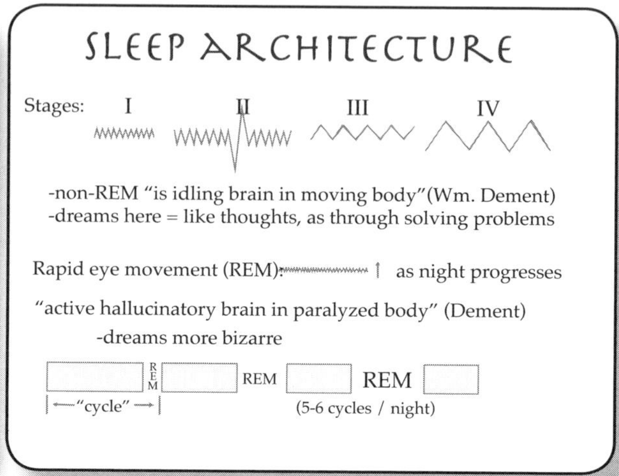
Sleep Architecture
Stages: I II III IV
-non-REM "is idling brain in moving body"(Wm. Dement)
-dreams here = like thoughts, as through solving problems
Rapid eye movement (REM): ↑ as night progresses
"active hallucinatory brain in paralyzed body" (Dement)
-dreams more bizarre
REM
REM
REM
"cycle"
(5-6 cycles / night)

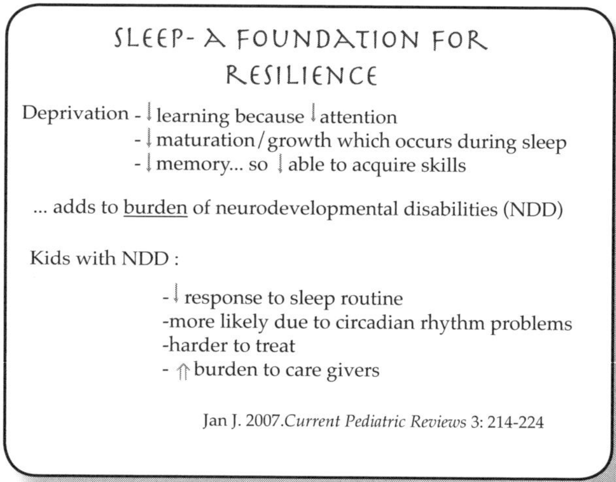
Sleep- a foundation for resilience
Deprivation - ↓learning because ↓attention
- ↓maturation/growth which occurs during sleep
- ↓memory... so ↓able to acquire skills
... adds to burden of neurodevelopmental disabilities (NDD)
Kids with NDD :
-↓response to sleep routine
-more likely due to circadian rhythm problems
-harder to treat
- ⇑burden to care givers
Jan J. 2007.*Current Pediatric Reviews* 3: 214-224

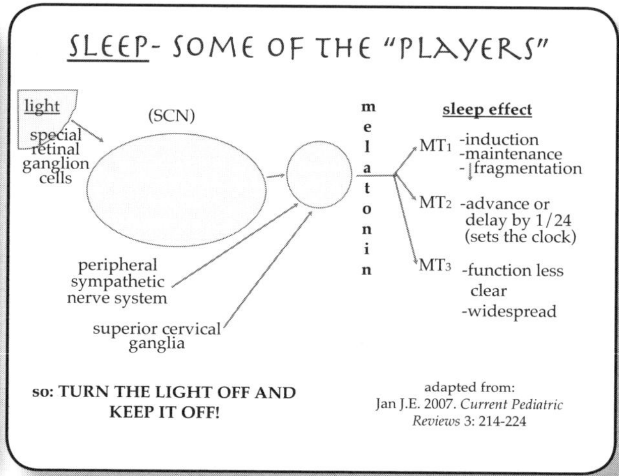
Sleep- some of the "players"
light
special retinal ganglion cells
(SCN)
peripheral sympathetic nerve system
superior cervical ganglia
melatonin
sleep effect
MT1 -induction -maintenance -↓fragmentation
MT2 -advance or delay by 1/24 (sets the clock)
MT3 -function less clear -widespread
so: TURN THE LIGHT OFF AND KEEP IT OFF!
adapted from: Jan J.E. 2007. *Current Pediatric Reviews* 3: 214-224

MELATONIN- OTHER ACTIVITIES

- pre + postnatal eye +brain development
- neurogenesis
- growth
- free radical scavenger
- antioxidant
- helps reflux, epilepsy, osteoporosis, B.P., sarcoid, septic shock, cancer, radiation therapy

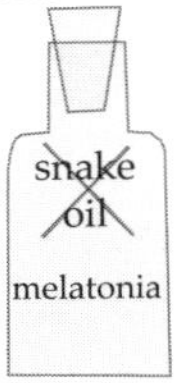

BAD COMBINATION FOR ATTACHMENT

Baby with FASD

- inconsolable crying, restlessness
- possible damage to pineal ✧
- ↓priming of melatonin receptors
- ↓able to recognize *cues* for sleep e.g.) it's 9p.m., teeth /story / sleep *sequence*

Birth mum **Adoptive** **Foster**

- acoustic startle
- infertility
- not like other kids
- advice does not work
- ↓ sleep leads to
- ↓ coping

✧Jan JE. personal communication 2008

CIRCADIAN RHYTHM SLEEP DISORDERS

=misalignment of internal clock (SCN) with the social norm
-most common e.g.) "delayed" sleep phase syndrome" =wake up to early +irregular sleep - wake pattern

Low melatonin — head injuries / alcohol-induced brain damage

if **Birth Mum** has alcohol dependence and/or head injuries she may make less melatonin

Fetus - receives all its melatonin from mum - this primes his/her MT1, MT2, MT3 receptors

Baby - no melatonin produced till 2-3 months when pineal "comes on line"

IF WANT TO TRY MELATONIN

U.K.=Drug Store vs. Canada/U.S.= Health Food Store
"Beware source variation of active ingredients" Kieran O'Malley

maybe in the future: extended release melatonin or

Agomelatine: +(agonist) melatonin receptors and -(antagonist) at serotonin 2C receptors
Bourin,M. et.al. 2004 Antidepressant-like activity of S20098 (agomelatine) in the forced swimming test in rodents:involvement of melatonin and serotonin receptors. *Journal of Psychiatry and Neuroscience* 29(2):126-133

melatonin: may need highish dose but always start low

toddlers: 1-2 mg.
older kids: 2-4 mg. (10 mg. not unheard of in devel. delay)

Attachment in FASD Further Reading

For M.D.'s, O.T's, S.L.P.'s, Psychologists, etc... scientific reports (often with jargon ++)

-on **importance of caregiver bond to outcomes** for children with special needs... and how professionals can work with families to enhance these bonds:

Almbery B. et al. 2000. The Interplay of Institution and Family Caregiving: relations between patient hassles, nursing home hassles and caregiver burnout. *International Journal of Geriatric Psychiatry* 15 : 931-939 (some aspects of Alzheimer caregiver- patient interactions may be very relevant for pediatric caregiver - child interactions)

Hastings RP. 2002. Parental stress and behavior problems of children with developmental disability. *Journal of Intellectual and Developmental Disability* 27(3): 149-160

Kumpfer KL, Fowler MA. 2007. Parenting skills and family support programs for drug-abusing mothers. *Seminars in Fetal and Neonatal Medicine* 12: 134-142

Sadler LS, et al. Promising outcomes in teen mothers enrolled in a school-based parent support program and child care center. *Journal of School Health* 77(3): 121-130

Kaslow NJ, et al. 2006. *Relational Processes and DSM-V -neuroscience, assessment, prevention, intervention.* Washington,DC: American Psychiatric Publishing Inc.

Attachment in FASD Further Reading (continued)

-on a model for **professional - family interrelationships**:

Cooley WC. 2004. Redefining primary care for children with special health care needs : The primary care medical home. *Current Opinions in Pediatrics* 16: 689-692

-on a current, practical application of neurobiology to behaviors:

O'Malley, K.D. (editor) 2007. *ADHD and Fetal Alcohol Spectrum Disorders.* New York: Nova Science.

Higgins ES, George MS. 2007. *The Neuroscience of Clinical Psychiatry - the pathophysiology of behavior and mental illness.* Philadelphia: Lippincott, Williams and Wilkins. (esp. chapter 14 "social attachment " is lucid and insightful... a small, precise, well illustrated book)

Niccols A. 2007. Fetal Alcohol Syndrome and the developing socio-emotional brain. *Brain and Cognition* 65: 135-142

Attachment in FASD Further Readings (continued)

-on how such concepts can be relevant **even when families are/have been "dysfunctional"**(mine has been!) and **even when** (like me) **initial outcomes are poor:**

Ziegler D. 2000. *Raising Children Who Refuse to be Raised - parenting skills and therapy interventions for the most difficult children.* Phoenix: Acacia Press.

Vermeiren R, et al. (editors) 2006. Juvenile Justice. *Child and adolescent psychiatric clinics of North America* 15(2) (The entire volume looks at professional - family - child interactions)

Rich P. 2006. *Attachment and Sexual Offending - understanding and applying attachment theory to the treatment of juvenile sexual offenders.* Chichester, UK: John Wiley.

-on approach to **defensive, often hostile and resistant** (often for good cause - because they are **stigmatized**) clients involved in drug abuse:

Bellack AS, et al. 2007. *Behavioral treatment for Substance Abuse in people with serious and persistent mental illness - a handbook for mental health professionals.* New York: Routledge. I have a dream..it would be for all care providers to use this model/ approach…it is elegant.

Attachment in FASD Further Reading (continued)

For parents, caregivers, the jargon-averse!
-on **practical interventions**:

Let's Talk FASD - parent driven strategies in caring for children with FASD. 2005. VON Canada, Public Health Agency of Canada FASD National Strategic Projects Fund. This can be downloaded from www.von.ca/fasd

Ziegler D. 2000. *Raising children who refuse to be raised* - see above - scientifically very accurate yet "accessible" to a general audience

-on **burnout- prevention/recovery**:

Domar AD, Dreher H. 2000. *Self Nurture - learning to care for yourself as effectively as you care for everyone else.* New York: Viking.

Benson Henry Institute for Mind Body Medicine:
http://www.mgh.harvard.edu/bhi/

Attachment in FASD Further Readings (continued)

on ways of **preserving/re-establishing attachments in the midst of behavioural difficulties:**

Neufeld G. 2010. 8 session DVD series: *Power to Parent-The Vital Connection.* In my opinion, this is the most practical application of Attachment Theory to the question of ,"What do I do now for/with this (behaviourally-challenged) child?"...Disclaimer: I am one of about 80 who have taken Dr. Neufeld's training to facilitate these DVD courses...the idea is that participants don't just listen but get a chance to really work with the concepts and apply them to their kids' issues. The facilitator training was about 100 hours with Dr. Neufeld and his interns.
I prepared a toolkit on FASD-specific brain differences and their relevance to *The Vital Connection* DVD course *Power to Parent* for the FASD Relationships book.

Neufeld G, Mate' G. 2005. *Hold on to your kids-why parents need to matter more than peers.* Toronto: Vintage Canada.
This book is great at *explaining* concepts of attachment but I think the facilitated DVD course is the best way to *understand* and learn *how to apply* these concepts--it is "hands-on" teaching.
DVD, book, and facilitator-led course information is at www.gordonneufeld.com

Attachment in FASD Further Reading (continued)

For educators, counselors:

Ylvisaker M, Jacobs HE, Feeney T. 2003. Positive support for people who experience behavioral and cognitive disability after brain injury - a review. *Journal of Head Trauma Rehabilitation* 18(1): 7-32
Mark Ylvisaker has a most elegant, simple, relevant model for how to work effectively with disabled kids and their families. This article gives an introduction to his ideas.

a quote: "Kids with traumatic brain injuries and FASD both have damaged executive function---they need a **"roll up your sleeves/get in there" collaborative "coaching"** approach working, as much as possible, **within the areas of the child's interests** is optimal. The *topics* to work on are those of **everyday life**---getting your books to school, getting up in time to make it to work, getting your project done, getting to school, working through conflicts from the playground, etc."

Ylvisaker M. 2003. Personal communication.

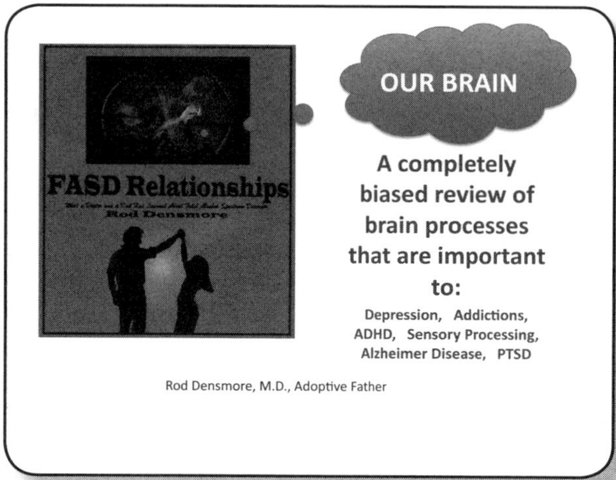
FASD Relationships
Rod Densmore
OUR BRAIN
A completely biased review of brain processes that are important to:
Depression, Addictions, ADHD, Sensory Processing, Alzheimer Disease, PTSD
Rod Densmore, M.D., Adoptive Father

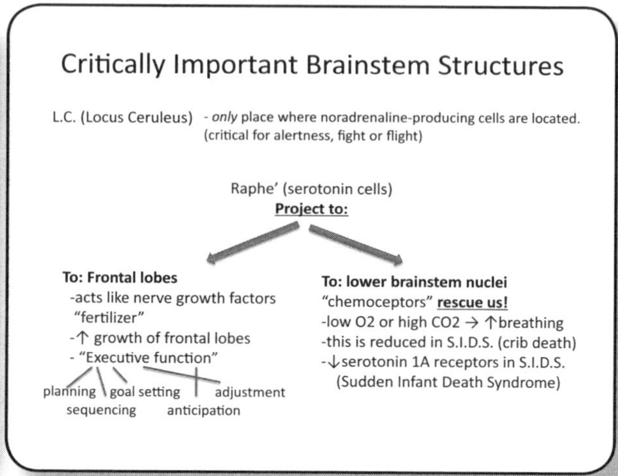
Critically Important Brainstem Structures
L.C. (Locus Ceruleus) - only place where noradrenaline-producing cells are located. (critical for alertness, fight or flight)
Raphe' (serotonin cells)
Project to:
To: Frontal lobes
-acts like nerve growth factors
"fertilizer"
-↑ growth of frontal lobes
- "Executive function"
planning
goal setting
adjustment
sequencing
anticipation
To: lower brainstem nuclei
"chemoceptors" rescue us!
-low O2 or high CO2 → ↑breathing
-this is reduced in S.I.D.S. (crib death)
-↓serotonin 1A receptors in S.I.D.S.
(Sudden Infant Death Syndrome)

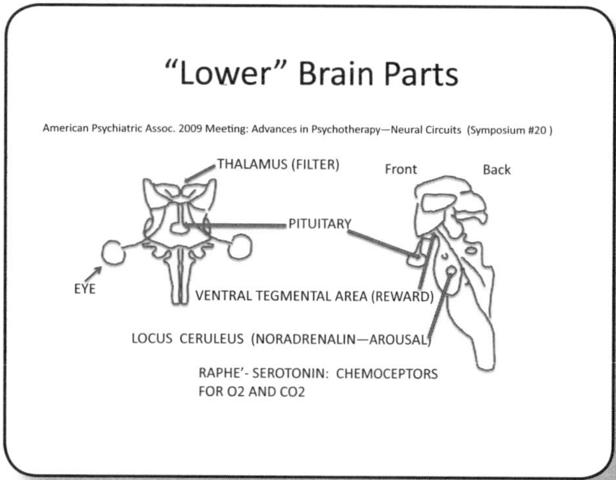
"Lower" Brain Parts
American Psychiatric Assoc. 2009 Meeting: Advances in Psychotherapy—Neural Circuits (Symposium #20)
THALAMUS (FILTER)
Front
Back
PITUITARY
EYE
VENTRAL TEGMENTAL AREA (REWARD)
LOCUS CERULEUS (NORADRENALIN—AROUSAL)
RAPHE'- SEROTONIN: CHEMOCEPTORS FOR O2 AND CO2

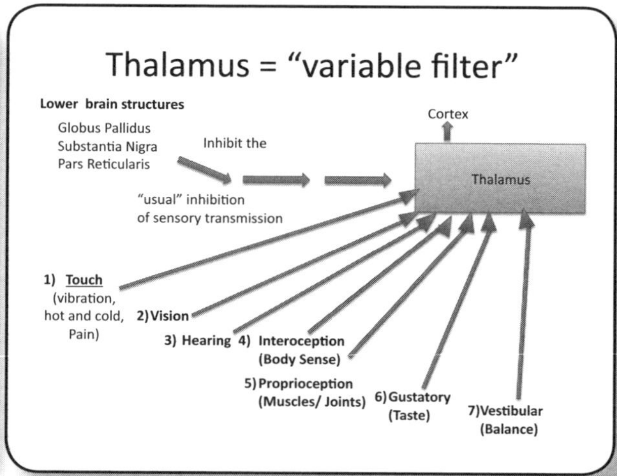
Thalamus = "variable filter"
Lower brain structures
Globus Pallidus
Substantia Nigra
Pars Reticularis
Inhibit the
"usual" inhibition of sensory transmission
Cortex
Thalamus
1) Touch (vibration, hot and cold, Pain)
2) Vision
3) Hearing
4) Interoception (Body Sense)
5) Proprioception (Muscles/ Joints)
6) Gustatory (Taste)
7) Vestibular (Balance)

Basal Ganglia = "The Striatum"

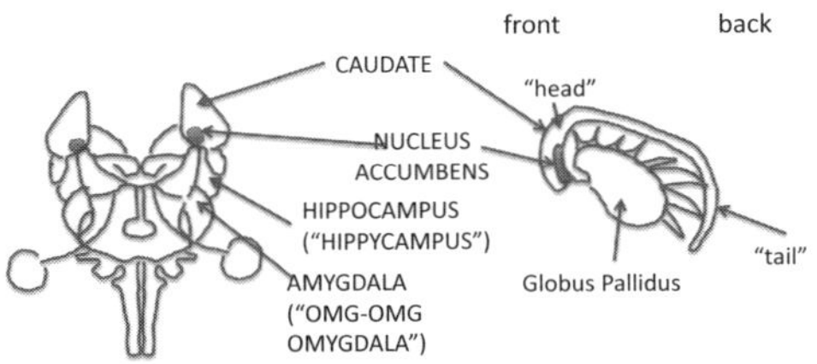

OMG OMYGDALA= "FEAR CENTRAL"
HIPPY= DON'T WORRY, BE HAPPY CAMPUS= NEW LEARNING

40-60% of *level of response* to alcohol is due to heritable factors

If ↓ ***sensitivity*** to alcohol → more alcohol is required to achieve effect

Kids- savor the Gewurztraminer
- debate the "peatiness" of single malt

-want to *get drunk*

EARLY: If ↓ Sensitive
needs more to "get high"
→ leads to higher intake
can't just sneak it out of liquor cabinet
→ get into peer groups were "norm" is 4-8 not 1-2

LATER: Causes of reinstatement of heavy drinking

1) Stress
2) Social cues
3) Small "priming" doses of alcohol
4) Withdrawal avoidance

Reward System

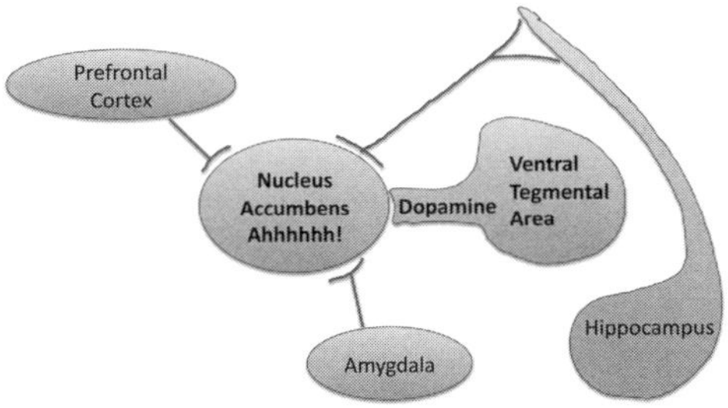

Why Do I Return To Heavy Drinking?

-smell beer
-imagine taste on a hot day
-see "ice cold Kokanee"
-see friends who you drunk with

- Ondansetron*
- Naltrexone*

1) "cues" excites:
- Orbital and Dorsolateral Prefrontal Cortex
-Ventral striatum
-Nucleus Accumbens / Ventral Tegmental Area
-Insula
=the brain's pattern for CRAVING

2) Stress
-causes ↓ activation of medial Prefrontal Cortex
-small dose of Aripiprazole* reverses this *not funded by phamacare

Myric H (2009) Advances in Substance Abuse: Pharmacologic Treatment of Alcoholism. American Psychiatric Association Meeting May 16-21/09 San Francisco

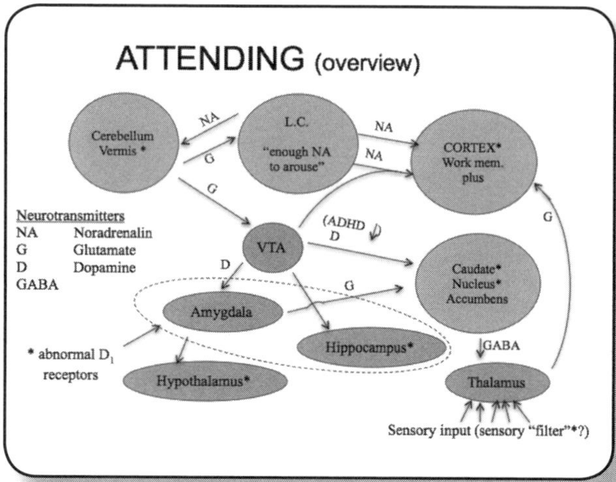
ATTENDING (overview)
Cerebellum Vermis *
L.C.
"enough NA to arouse"
CORTEX* Work mem. plus
NA
G
VTA
(ADHD D
D
Caudate* Nucleus* Accumbens
Amygdala
Hippocampus*
Hypothalamus*
Thalamus
GABA
Neurotransmitters
NA Noradrenalin
G Glutamate
D Dopamine
GABA
* abnormal D1 receptors
Sensory input (sensory "filter"*?)

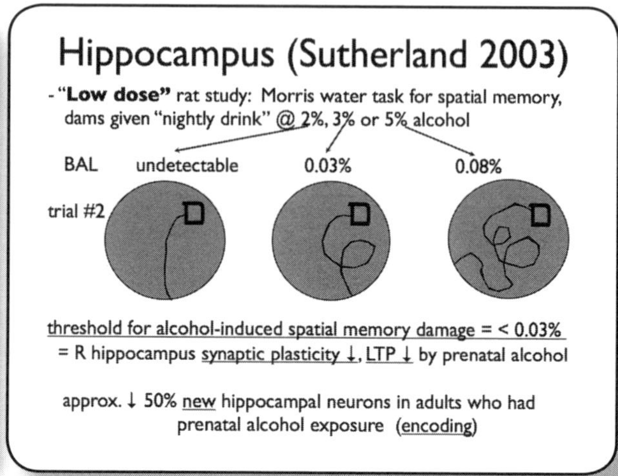
Hippocampus (Sutherland 2003)
- "Low dose" rat study: Morris water task for spatial memory, dams given "nightly drink" @ 2%, 3% or 5% alcohol
BAL undetectable 0.03% 0.08%
trial #2
threshold for alcohol-induced spatial memory damage = < 0.03%
= R hippocampus synaptic plasticity ↓, LTP ↓ by prenatal alcohol
approx. ↓ 50% new hippocampal neurons in adults who had prenatal alcohol exposure (encoding)

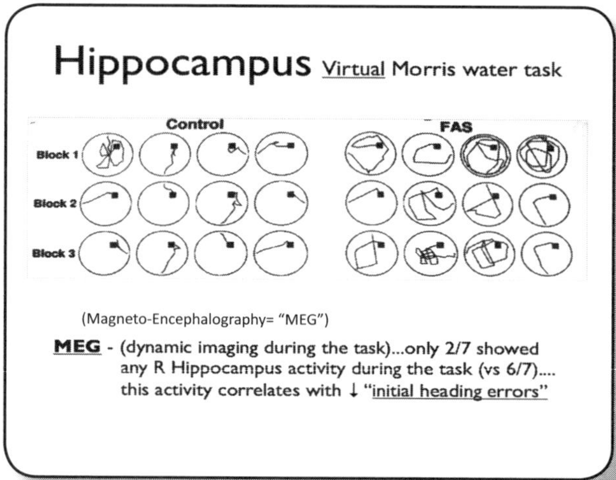
Hippocampus Virtual Morris water task
Control
FAS
Block 1
Block 2
Block 3
(Magneto-Encephalography= "MEG")
MEG - (dynamic imaging during the task)...only 2/7 showed any R Hippocampus activity during the task (vs 6/7).... this activity correlates with ↓ "initial heading errors"

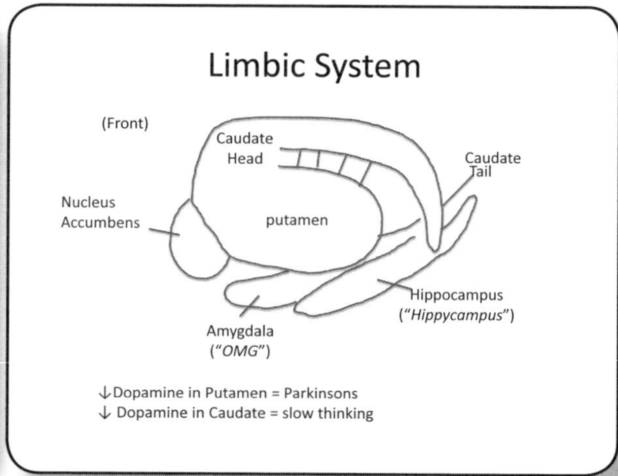
Limbic System
(Front)
Caudate Head
Caudate Tail
Nucleus Accumbens
putamen
Hippocampus ("Hippycampus")
Amygdala ("OMG")
↓Dopamine in Putamen = Parkinsons
↓ Dopamine in Caudate = slow thinking

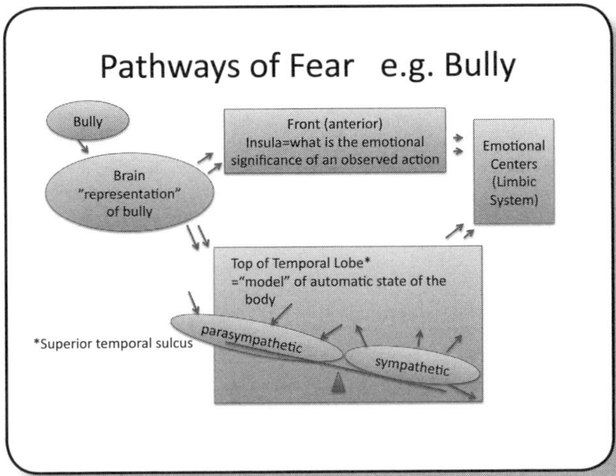
Pathways of Fear e.g. Bully
Bully
Brain "representation" of bully
Front (anterior) Insula=what is the emotional significance of an observed action
Emotional Centers (Limbic System)
Top of Temporal Lobe* ="model" of automatic state of the body
parasympathetic
sympathetic
*Superior temporal sulcus

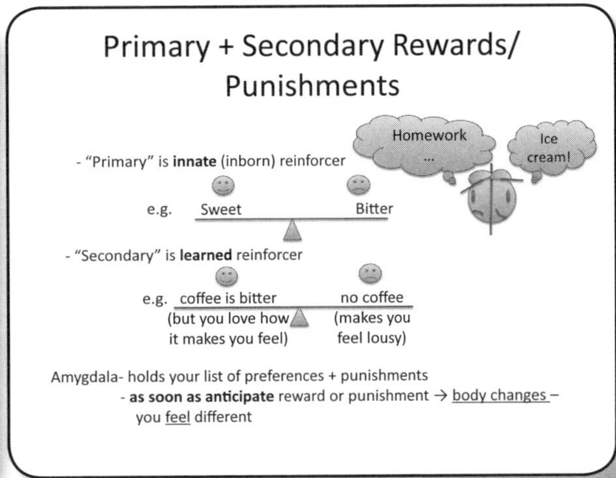
Primary + Secondary Rewards/ Punishments
Homework ...
Ice cream!
- "Primary" is innate (inborn) reinforcer
e.g. Sweet
Bitter
- "Secondary" is learned reinforcer
e.g. coffee is bitter (but you love how it makes you feel)
no coffee (makes you feel lousy)
Amygdala- holds your list of preferences + punishments
- as soon as anticipate reward or punishment → body changes – you feel different

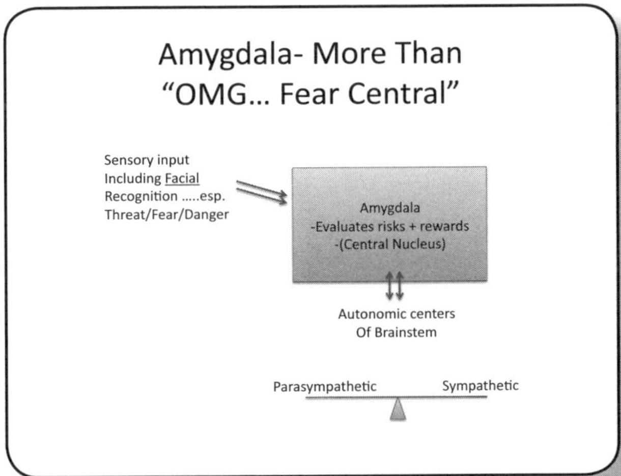
Amygdala- More Than "OMG... Fear Central"
Sensory input Including Facial Recognition .....esp. Threat/Fear/Danger
Amygdala -Evaluates risks + rewards -(Central Nucleus)
Autonomic centers Of Brainstem
Parasympathetic
Sympathetic

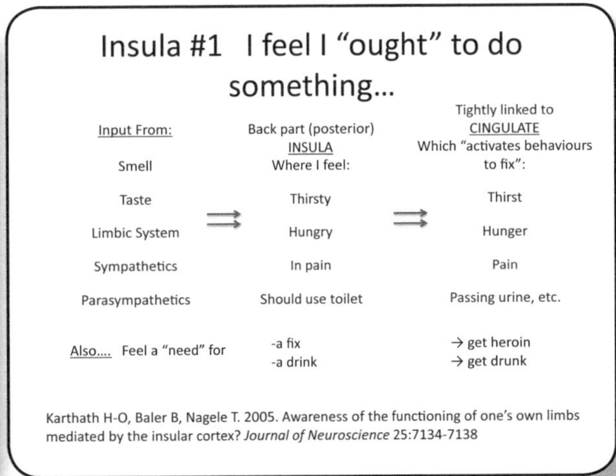
Insula #1 I feel I "ought" to do something...
Input From:
Smell
Taste
Limbic System
Sympathetics
Parasympathetics
Back part (posterior) INSULA Where I feel:
Thirsty
Hungry
In pain
Should use toilet
Tightly linked to CINGULATE Which "activates behaviours to fix":
Thirst
Hunger
Pain
Passing urine, etc.
Also.... Feel a "need" for
-a fix
-a drink
→ get heroin
→ get drunk
Karthath H-O, Baler B, Nagele T. 2005. Awareness of the functioning of one's own limbs mediated by the insular cortex? Journal of Neuroscience 25:7134-7138

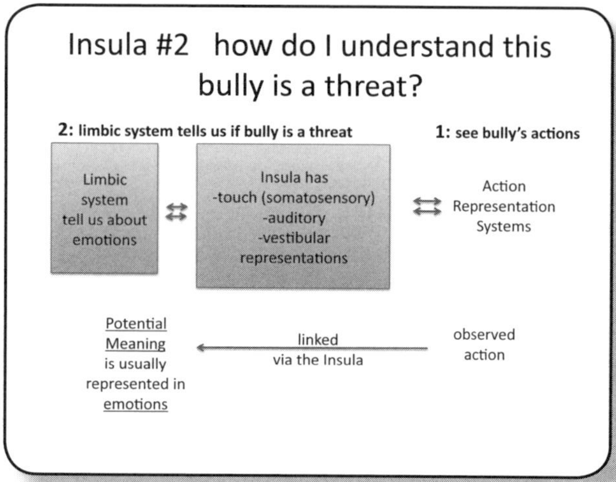
Insula #2 how do I understand this bully is a threat?
2: limbic system tells us if bully is a threat
1: see bully's actions
Limbic system tell us about emotions
Insula has -touch (somatosensory) -auditory -vestibular representations
Action Representation Systems
Potential Meaning is usually represented in emotions
linked via the Insula
observed action

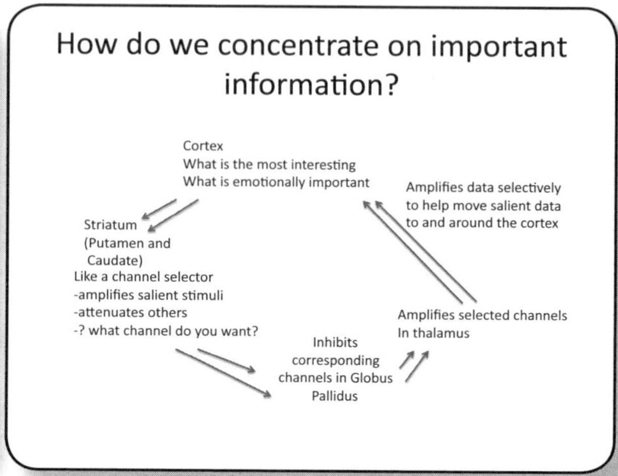
How do we concentrate on important information?
Cortex
What is the most interesting
What is emotionally important
Amplifies data selectively to help move salient data to and around the cortex
Striatum (Putamen and Caudate)
Like a channel selector
-amplifies salient stimuli
-attenuates others
-? what channel do you want?
Amplifies selected channels In thalamus
Inhibits corresponding channels in Globus Pallidus

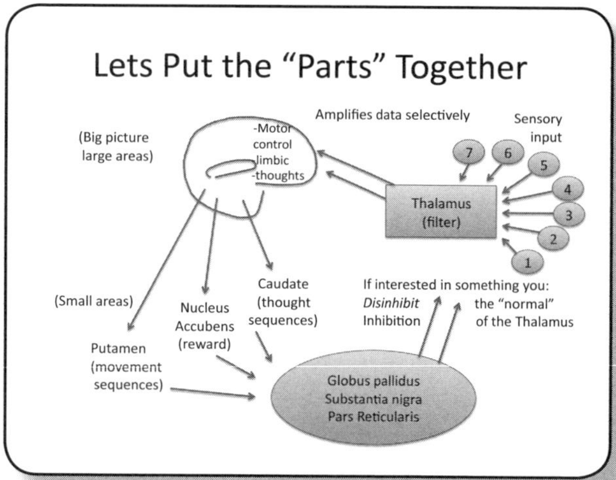
Lets Put the "Parts" Together
(Big picture large areas)
-Motor control
-limbic
-thoughts
Amplifies data selectively
Sensory input
7
6
5
4
3
2
1
Thalamus (filter)
(Small areas)
Putamen (movement sequences)
Nucleus Accubens (reward)
Caudate (thought sequences)
If interested in something you:
Disinhibit Inhibition
the "normal" of the Thalamus
Globus pallidus
Substantia nigra
Pars Reticularis

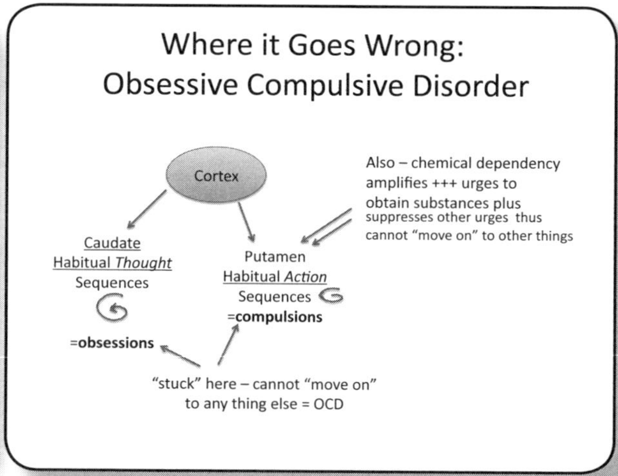
Where it Goes Wrong: Obsessive Compulsive Disorder
Cortex
Also – chemical dependency amplifies +++ urges to obtain substances plus suppresses other urges thus cannot "move on" to other things
Caudate
Habitual Thought
Sequences
=obsessions
Putamen
Habitual Action
Sequences
=compulsions
"stuck" here – cannot "move on" to any thing else = OCD

Depression #1 (functional MRI) Talk Therapy (CBT) vs. Meds (SNRI)

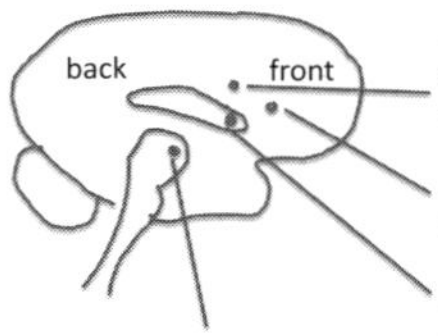

↓Activity in Orbitofrontal Cortex with CBT and SNRI (highly involved with amygdala) mediates emotional responses (over emotional)

↓activity in Dorsolateral Frontal Cortex With CBT + SNRI (area of sadness + self-blame)

↑activity in Anterior Cingulate* with CBT (emotional "clutch")

↓ activity Thalamus* with CBT (better filter)

*Improvements correlate to success of treatment

Kennedy A (2007) Am. J. Psychology 164: 778-788

Depression #3

Symptoms	Possible mechanism	Why
-Sleeping disturbance	HPA (stress system) (fight or flight) overactivity	Excess stress hormones, XS corticotropin releasing hormone = depressed feelings, ↓restorative (slow- wave) sleep
-Restless Cannot relax	HPA overactivity	XS Adrenalin = imbalance of sympathetic vs. parasympathetic
-Anhedonia (loss of enjoyment)	Dysfunction in reward center ↑ cells in Nucleus Accumbens	Needs bigger "hit" to stimulate reward center
-Poor problem solving	Less Anterior Cingulate activity	Organizing thoughts
	Less Corpus Callosum activity	This links the 2 sides of the brain---allows "lateral" thinking i.e. really creative problem solving

Depression #2

Symptoms	Possible Mechanism	Why
- Feels "picked on" ashamed guilty	Overactive Rt. Dorsolateral Prefrontal Cortex	This is an area of processing self-referential emotional stimuli (self blame)
- "Oversensitive" irritable	Overactive Orbitofrontal Cortex	Area of emotion processing
-↓ Concentration "cannot learn"	Reduction in Hippocampus function ↓ cells ↓neurogenisis	Area of encoding of memories

Chronic defeat and its solutions

Methylation of DNA Histones is ↑ the the point where access of RNA to the part
of DNA which codes for BDNF (Brain-derived Neurotrophic Factor—a protien that acts like "brain cell fertilizer") is blocked

Lithium
Exercise
Antidepressants
ECT

} Can "acetylate" these methylated histones which causes an "opening up" of tightly bound DNA so RNA can access to DNA (then RNA is able to make BDNF)

Neurobiology of Attachment

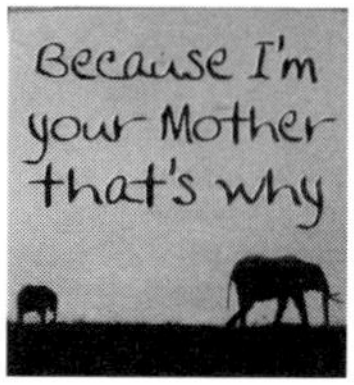

It should be like this

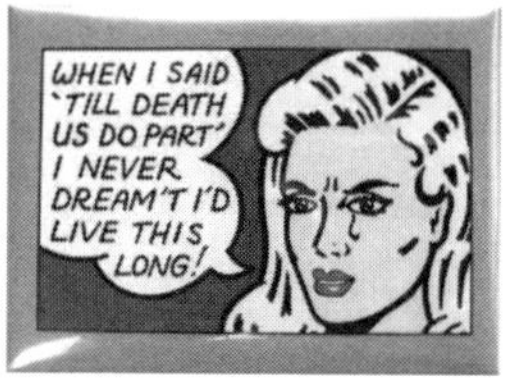

Not like this

Attachment

cry → pick up empathy "ride mum down" → ah... relax → curiosity exploration → tired, hungry, dirty → cry

Get close = Get Love

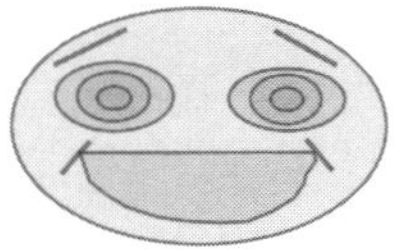

Attachment

- Contact, closeness, a sense of belonging
- Its our number one need (even more than food and shelter for it is how we *access* food and shelter).

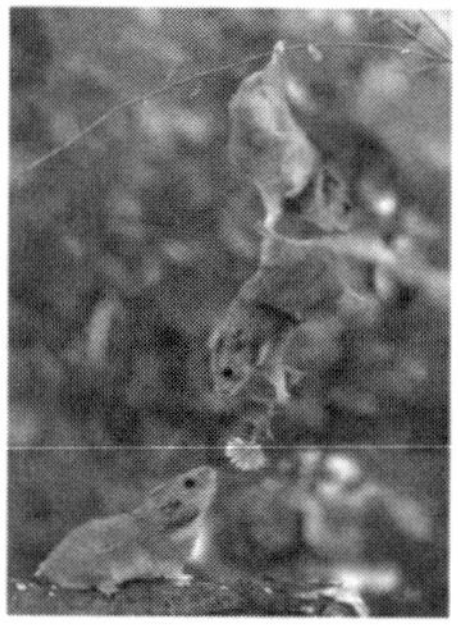

Abuse

cry → swat (never 100%) yell → no relaxing hyper-vigilant = always on alert → even wary re whether to cry or approach → cry

Get close= Get hurt
so- don't *depend*, do it all yourself, don't be vulnerable

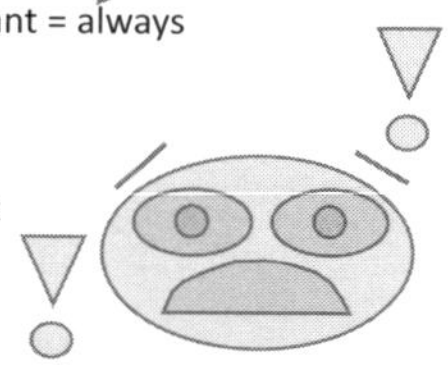

Neglect

cry

numb out
don't cry

ignored

why bother

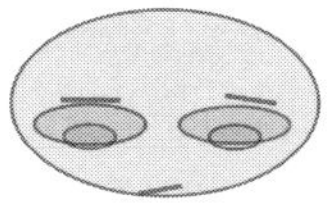

Get close= Nothing happens
Give up after initial struggle-- maybe attached to something else- dog, rocking etc...

Canadian Licking and Grooming Rats (Michael Meaney, et al. @ McGill)...or... We Do Stink Don't We?

Pups handled- have improved resilience to stress when adults!

Q: handling = great for stress?

A: Nope!

Licking and grooming (to get the stink off) is great for stress

Attachment is Important CENTRAL to development

- It is *biological*
- Involves 2 "players" (at least)
- Is *basis* for *relationship*
- Which is the basis for *sense of self* (vs. not self)
- Which allows one to see others' points of view (theory of mind)

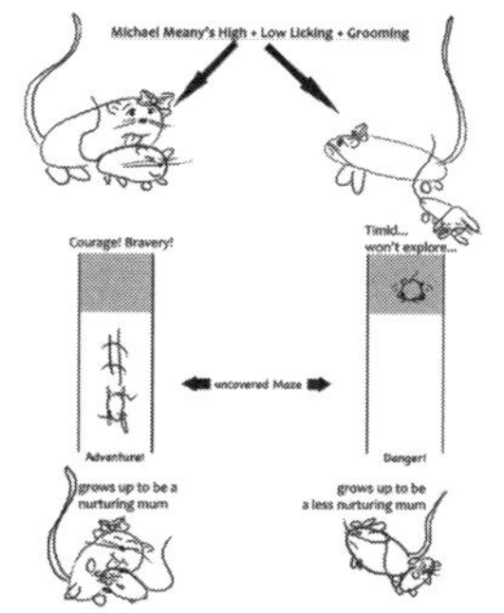

Higgins ES, George MS. The Neuroscience of Clinical Psychiatry: The Pathophysiology of Behavior and Mental Illness. Philadelphia (USA): Lippincott, Williams and Wilkins; 2007, pg. 109

The Pups of High Licking/Grooming Mums

-less (pup) glucocorticoid release after stressed (restraint)

-less CRH messenger RNA in hippocampus (less stress reactivity in hippocampus)

-more glucocorticoid receptors in hypothalamus .. can turn stress down better

-increased resilience, less fear
SHOW GREATER WILLINGNESS TO EXPLORE NEW PLACES CURIOSITY (vs. guardedness)

Be vulnerable! explore + learn!

(CRF=CRH=Corticotropin Releasing Factor)

Hormonal Stress System: "<u>HPA" Activation</u>
Stress ⇒ <u>H</u>ypothalamus ⇒⇒ <u>P</u>ituitary ⇒⇒<u>A</u>drenal (Cortex) ⇒⇒
CRF or CRH — ACTH — Cortisol

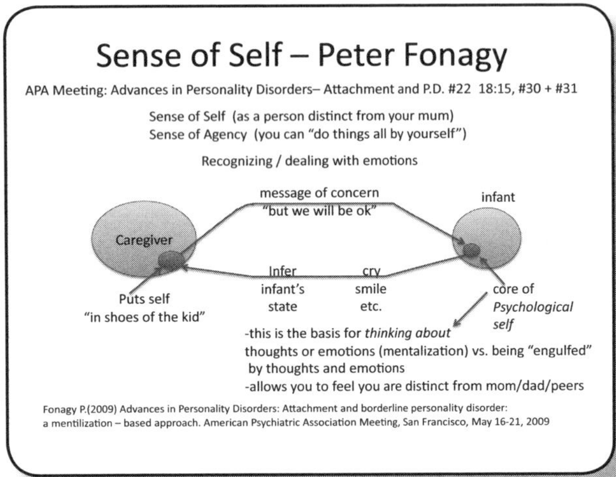
Sense of Self – Peter Fonagy
APA Meeting: Advances in Personality Disorders– Attachment and P.D. #22 18:15, #30 + #31
Sense of Self (as a person distinct from your mum)
Sense of Agency (you can "do things all by yourself")
Recognizing / dealing with emotions
message of concern
"but we will be ok"
infant
Caregiver
Infer
infant's
state
cry
smile
etc.
Puts self
"in shoes of the kid"
core of
Psychological
self
-this is the basis for thinking about thoughts or emotions (mentalization) vs. being "engulfed" by thoughts and emotions
-allows you to feel you are distinct from mom/dad/peers
Fonagy P.(2009) Advances in Personality Disorders: Attachment and borderline personality disorder: a mentilization – based approach. American Psychiatric Association Meeting, San Francisco, May 16-21, 2009

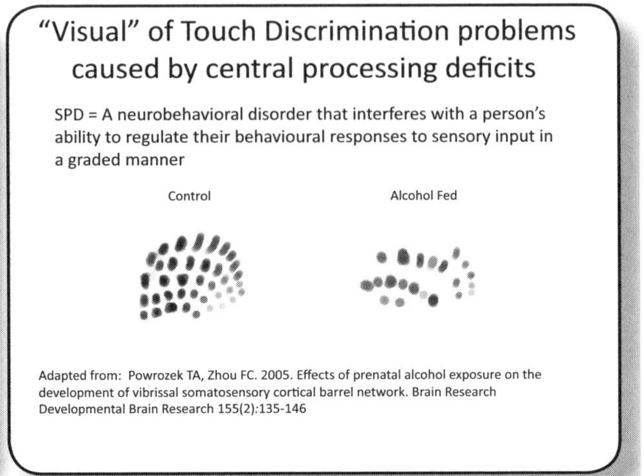
"Visual" of Touch Discrimination problems caused by central processing deficits
SPD = A neurobehavioral disorder that interferes with a person's ability to regulate their behavioural responses to sensory input in a graded manner
Control
Alcohol Fed
Adapted from: Powrozek TA, Zhou FC. 2005. Effects of prenatal alcohol exposure on the development of vibrissal somatosensory cortical barrel network. Brain Research Developmental Brain Research 155(2):135-146

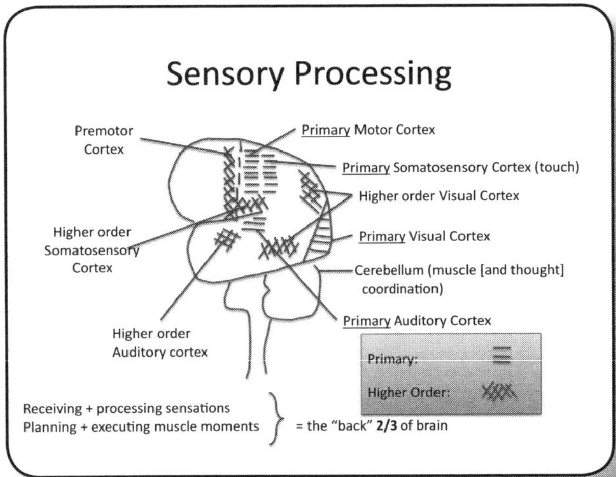
Sensory Processing
Premotor Cortex
Primary Motor Cortex
Primary Somatosensory Cortex (touch)
Higher order Visual Cortex
Higher order Somatosensory Cortex
Primary Visual Cortex
Cerebellum (muscle [and thought] coordination)
Primary Auditory Cortex
Higher order Auditory cortex
Primary:
Higher Order:
Receiving + processing sensations
Planning + executing muscle moments
= the "back" 2/3 of brain

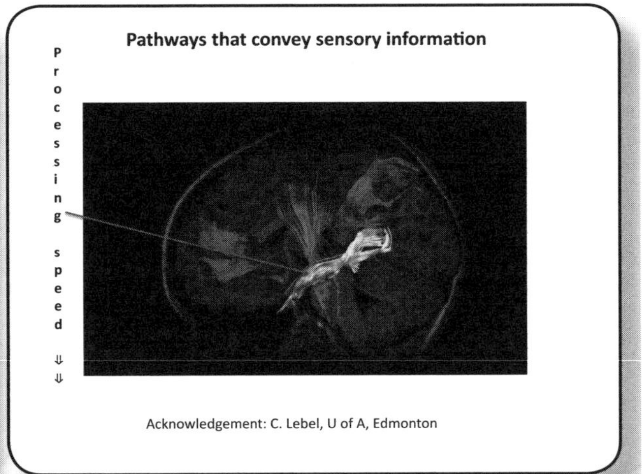
Pathways that convey sensory information
Processing speed
Acknowledgement: C. Lebel, U of A, Edmonton

Sensory Processing Disorders: What Do We See?

- Reacts negatively to loud unexpected sound
- Avoid tastes which most kids like
- Distressed by hair brushing, cutting nails
- Emotional, reactive, edgy, fearful, anxious
- Always climbing, bashing into things or people!
- Always rocking/ spinning
- "Eeyore" – sluggish
- Clumsy

Sensory Over Responsivity (SOR) Muddled Confusing Messages!

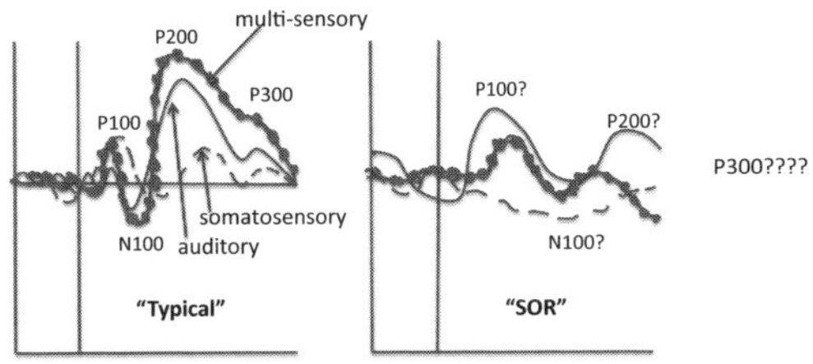

Based on: Brett-Green B, et al. Multi-sensory Integration in Children with S.P.D. Advanced Intensive Workshop on Diagnosis and Treatment of SPD Level One Aug 11-15, 2009. Sensory Processing Disorders Foundation, Denver Colorado

ERP = Event Related Potentials

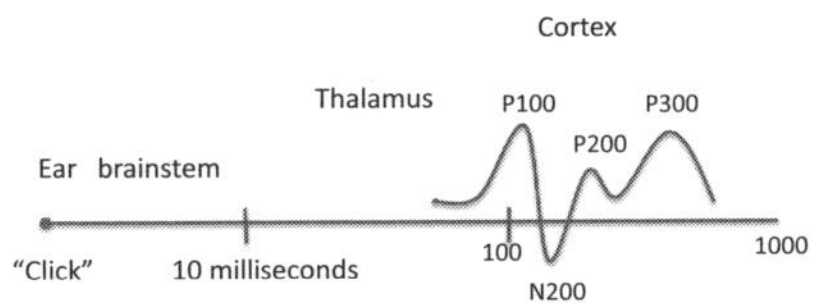

P100 mainly sensory
N100 sensory plus attention/ first awareness of
P200 influenced by attention
P300 cognitive = your brain evaluating the stimulus

Outcome After Sensory Integration Treatment = *Neuroplasticity* (nerve cell growth + remodelling)

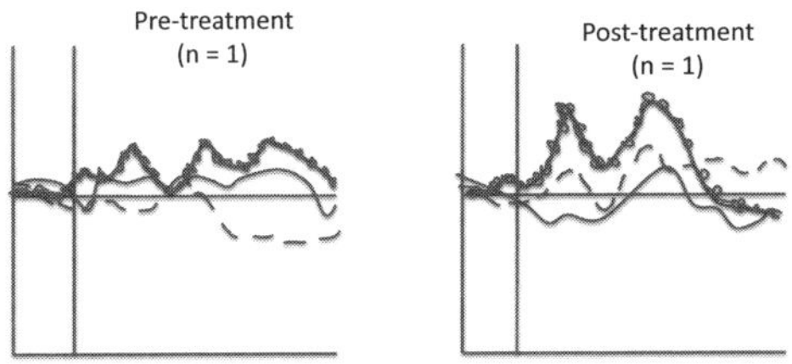

Based on: Brett-Green B, Miller LJ, Gavin WJ, Davies PL (2008) Multi-sensory Integration in Children: A Preliminary ERP Study. *Brain Research*. 1242: 283-290.

Attention Issues?

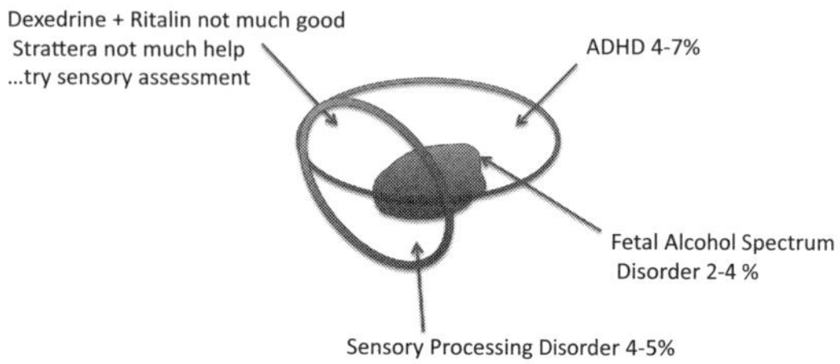

Also: Obstructive Sleep Apnea, Concussion, Not Safe, Drugs or Alcohol

PTSD

Re-experiencing
- -can't get trauma out of mind
- -nightmares
- -flashbacks (common)

Hypervigilance
- -constantly on the watch
- -"jumpy"
- -startles

Numbing or Avoiding
- -avoids going out on their own
- -unable to feel sad or happy
- -avoids certain activities

(specific to PTSD and if worse predicts harder to treat)

PTSD= Post Traumatic Stress Disorder

A1		A2				
Witness or experience threatened or actual death, serious injury or threat to physical integrity of self or others	⇉	Initial Response: Fear helplessness horror	⇉	Acute Stress Disorder (up to 30 days)	⇉	**PTSD** (Over 30 days)

40-90%
Women>Men

Resiliency

- -Internal locus of control (external = "it's all his/her fault" → helplessness)
- -Long- standing optimism
- -Having a sense of humour
- -Having a religious affiliation
- -Higher Socio-economic situation

Pandya A. (2009) PTSD and Disaster Psychiatry. American Psychiatric Association Annual Meeting. San Francisco. May 16-21, 2009

Prevention/Early Intervention

e.g. 1) Refugees from storm

-Disaster response center/camp feels like a "fishbowl" →privacy, at times, is needed

-But also—tendency to isolate

-If ↓ control have ↓ power

-Develop disaster camp into "village" with village council → promote sense of self- efficacy

e.g. 2) Rape Victim

-Beta blockers (propranolol), Alpha blockers (prazocin) may help ↓ flashbacks, nightmares and *consolidation* (and assist in *extinction*) of traumatic memories

-ventilate *if* it does not inflame

-"exposure therapy" like listening to a tape of a narrative of the trauma while doing relaxation exercises such as progressive muscle relaxation

In PTSD The Brain Acts *Like You Are In A Dangerous Situation ALL THE TIME*

Hyperarousal

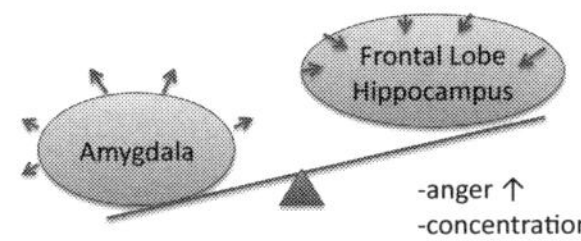

-anger ↑
-concentration↓

1) **Amygdala** -hyperresponsiveness to stimuli that are reminders of trauma

2) **Frontal Lobe** (esp. medial part) -volume loss
-↑PTSD...... ↓activation of F.L.
-anger dyscontrol, failure of extinction of memory = medical PFC is "taken off line" "you can't put the clutch in to put the brakes on"

3) **Hippocampus** -volume loss↓, neurons↓, function↓, ↓activation on functional MRI
-overgeneralization of threat i.e. "safe" not discerned from "dangerous"
-largest # of the stem cells to make new neurons CAI area

Successful treatment: PTSD *or Substance Abuse* = growth of new neurons on imagining studies

PBD: Key Points *required* for recovery

-recovery is NOT passive

-*learning* that old fears do not fit new situations

-goal = Frontal lobe + hippocampus can "talk" amygdala out of excessive "wind-up"

In PTSD The Brain Acts Like You Are In A Dangerous Situation ALL THE TIME (continued)

4) Anterior Cingulate Cortex... ↓activation in PTSD
this area lets you **put the clutch in so you can put the brakes on!!**

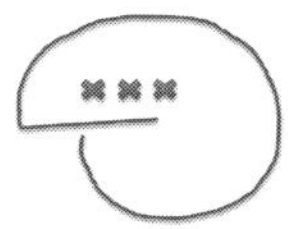

-interrupts emotional stimuli
-allows for processing your response
=THE CLUTCH
-moves in or out to govern whether you engage:

Sympathetic nervous system
= the accelerator
-↑ in PTSD

Parasympathetic nervous
System =the brakes
↓in PTSD

"Speechless Terror"

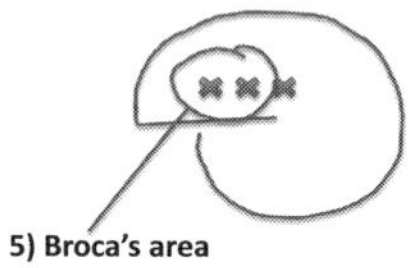

-suppressing of Broca's speech area during traumatic re-experiencing

-If you say or write a narrative of the trauma

(In a safe setting) it allows re-encoding of the memories in a less terrifying format

Threat Response System

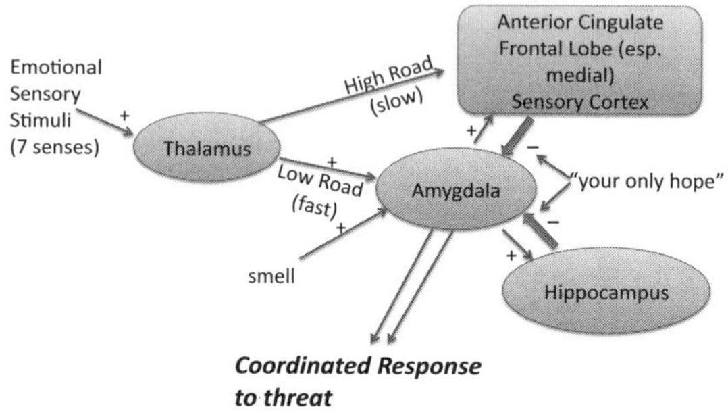

Problem: Memory Is Not In Area You Can Treat Easily

-subcortical memories mostly somatosensory (ie touch)

-**most trauma memories are held here**

Cortical memories are mostly Verbal + symbolic

-but we try to use this area (words and symbols) to extinguish traumatic memories

"your only hope is your cortex when you have PTSD... you've GOT to get it re-engaged"

Kosten T (2009) Neurobiologic determinants of the Comorbidity of PTSD and Substance Abuse. In: Symposium 35: PTSD and Alcoholism, emphasis on returning veterans. American Psychiatry Association Annual Meeting, San Francisco. May 16-21, 2009

If "Your Only Hope" Is <u>Learning</u> (Not All Is A Threat) Then How Can We ↑ Learning?

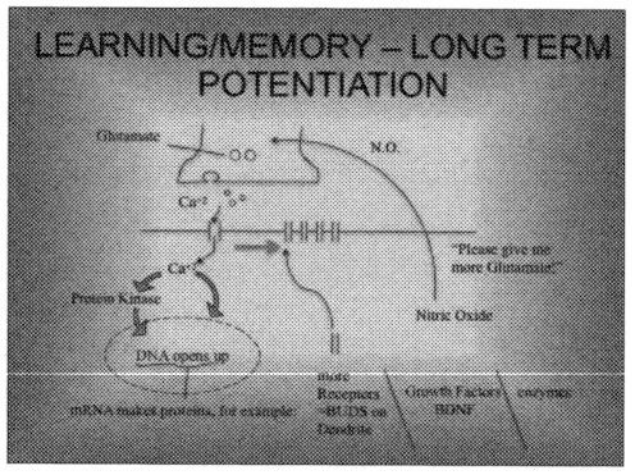

-Learning is also called "long term potentiation"

-Depends on 1) NMDA+ AMPA glutamate receptors

2) calcium, "a second messenger"

3) Kinases

4) Protein Synthesis

Dementia

-Alzheimer Disease 60-70%
-Vascular Dementia 5-10%
-"reversible" up to 19%

Meds- painkillers, psychotropics, steroids, gravol
Metabolic- ↓Na, ↑Ca, ↓Liver, ↓Kidney, ↓B12, ↓Thyroid
Depression- up to 9%
Alcohol abuse/ dependence 2%
Normal pressure Hydrocephaus 3%

Apostolova LF, Cummings JL. Neuropsychiatric aspects of Alzheimer Disease and other dementing illnesses in: *The American Psychiatric Publishing Textbook of Neuropsychiatry and Behavioral Neurosciences Ed 5th Edition.* Yudofsky SC, Hales RE editors (2008) American Psychiatric Publishing, New York. Pages 935-967

↑ Altzhiemer Disease if:

↑ Amyloid precursor proteins (e.g.) Down Syndrome

↑ *ratio* of **beta** and **gamma/ alpha** secretase

This will ↑ A-beta 42 protein production

which activates capsases

which cleave tau protein

which ↑ NFT

Shadlen M-F, et al. (May 2009) Dementia Syndromes, UpToDate version 17.2 DVD medical reference

Alzheimer Disease

1) Amyloid –beta protein **deposits** between neurons

Amyloid Precursor proteins *

Cleaved by beta-secretases* and gamma secretases
(normally cleared by "alpha-secretases")

"A-beta 42" Protein
-sets up plaques between neurons

*Curcumin (curry)
* Cholesterol ↓ agents

+++Inflamation excitotoxicity ↑ cell death

2) "**Neurofibrillary Tangles**" (NFT) within neurons

-NFT are an excessively phosphorylated form of the microtubule – associated protein **"TAU"**
-↑ NFT + ↑ Cognitive decline

*Blocked by
-memantidine
-Li
-valproate

3) **Loss of neurons** esp. hippocampus

Risk Factors in Dementia/ Solutions

↑ cholesterol	simvastatin, lovastatin
diabetes (low insulin)	weight loss*, avoiding high blood sugar
inactivity	exercise*
social isolation	social connection*
not challenging self cognitively	learning new things*
low educational level	adult learning*
inflammation	antioxidants: -omega 3, fish; ~~vit E~~ (controversial); -vit C ?; -maybe simvastatin, etc.
traumatic brain injury	helmets esp. if carry Apo E episolon 4 allele
depression	screen + treat it*
solvent exposure	youth programs!
pessimism	↓ stress + ↑ positive emotional states and people

***DANCE!**

Schadler M-F, et al. (May 2009) Risk Factors For Dementia, UpToDate version 17.2 DVD medical reference

Future

-now: **Vit E** = alpha tocopherol – what about *natural source Vit E* = mixture of 4 tocopherols and 4 tocotrienols. - drweil.com

-↑ **inflammatory markers**: -fibrinogen (but not C. Reactive Protein)
? Monitor? -interleukin -6
-intracellular adhesion molecule -1
above appear to predict ↑ cognitive deadline

-↑ **antioxidants** –see drweil.com
tumeric, deeply colored fruits + veggies: blueberries, blackberries, raspberries, yams, sweet potatoes, green tea

- at present - ↑ vegetables ↓ Alzheimer Disease symptoms
- Mediterranean diet = ↑ fruits + veggies, whole grains, beans, nuts, seeds, olive oil low to moderate fish, poultry, and dairy + low intake of red meats

-studies soon will be reported- to <u>slow progression</u> of Alzheimer Disease: -vitamin E
-selegiline

Omega 3's

EPA- eicosapentaenoic acid
DHA- docosahexaenoic acid
-lower triglyceride levels
-antinflammatory
-antiarrhythmic
-immune enhancing
-nerve cell stabilizing
-↓ clot formation

EPA	**DHA**
Tends to be stimulating	Tends to be sedating

It seems a dose of 3 grams/day of EPA + DHA is effective for ADHD
Amen DF. 2008. Magnificent Mind at Any Age. New York (NY): Harmony Books; p. 83

"We have XS omega 6 + 9 in our diets already"
Do not take supplemental omega 6 + 9
Weil A. (2002) personal communication

Genetics and FASD
For Health Professionals

Dr. Rod Densmore

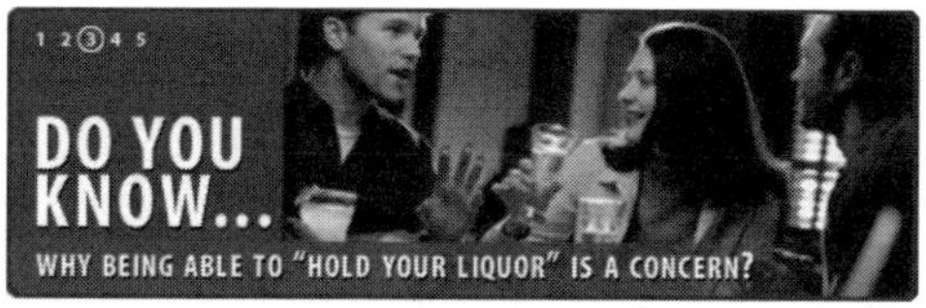
1 2 3 4 5
DO YOU KNOW...
WHY BEING ABLE TO "HOLD YOUR LIQUOR" IS A CONCERN?

http://rethinkingdrinking.niaaa.nih.gov/

What Did My Child Inherit? How Can That Knowledge Help Me?

Gene Basics, Epigenetics, Attachment

Sensory Processing Disorder - Sensory Overresponsivity

Acoustic Startle and PTSD

Impulsivity and Early Sexual Debut

Secondary Disabilities and Inherited Mental Health Issues

Alcoholism, Level of Response, Gene- Environment Interactions

Disclosures

Bias of a Dad:
- -what helps me directly to understand
- -to respond more efficiently
- - to avoid problems that are anticipated

Bias of Doctor
- -understanding Birthparents and their children → will lead to clues for prevention and effective interventions

Genes

46 Chromosomes

½ from mum ½ from dad

Arranged in 23 pairs

25 000 genes – where the genes are and how DNA sequence varies

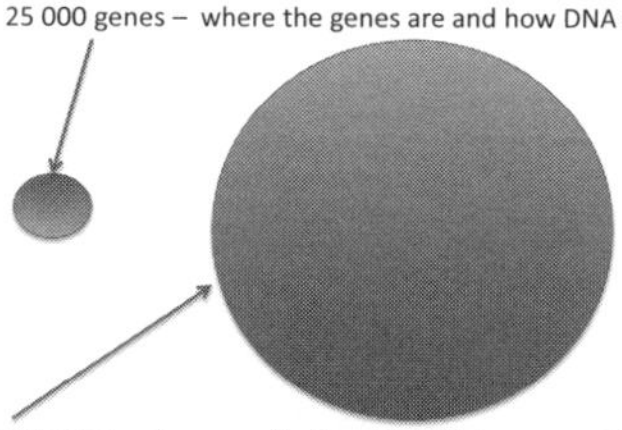

Cloud J. 2010. Why your DNA isn't your destiny. Time. Jan 6, 2010. Available at: http://www.time.com/time/health/article/0,8599,1951968,00.html

EPIGENETICS: turning genes "on" and "off" is key   e.g. Women: "the extra X" is "dormant"

Canadian Licking and Grooming Rats (Michael Meaney et al. @ McGill)...or... We Do Stink Don't We?

Pups handled- have improved resilience to stress when adults!

Q: handling = great for stress?

A: Nope!

Licking and grooming (to get the stink off) is great for stress

Epigenetics, Altered Methylation *and Sperm*

Alcohol's effect on male gametes before conception are consistent with epigenetic effect

Haycock, 2009

Heavy alcohol consumption results in a decreased methylation of normally hypermethylated regions in *human sperm DNA*

Ouko, et al, 2009

Haycock PC, 2009. Fetal alcohol spectrum disorders: the epigenetic perspective. Biol Reprod. DOI 10.1095/ biorepod.108.074682

Ouko LA, Shantikumer K, Knezovide J, et al. 2009. Effects of alcohol consumption on CpG methylation in the differentially methylated regions of H19 and IG-DMR in males gametes-implications for fetal alcohol spectrum disorders. Alcoholism: Clinical and Experimental Research,DOI 10.111/j. 153020277.2009.00993.x

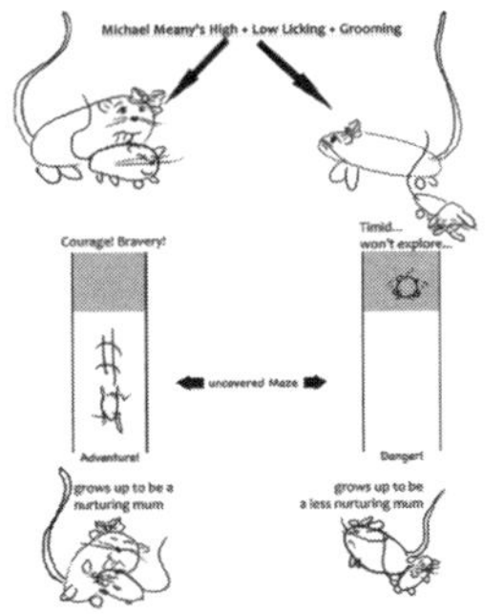

Higgins ES, Gorge MS. The Neuroscience of Clinical Psychiatry: The Pathophysiology of Behavior and Mental Illness. Philadelphia (USA): Lippincott, Williams and Wilkins; 2007, pg. 109

The Pups of High Licking/Grooming Mums

-less (pup) glucocorticoid release after stressed (restraint)

-less CRH messenger RNA in hippocampus (less stress reactivity in hippocampus)

-more glucocorticoid receptors in hypothalamus .. can turn stress down better

-increased resilience, less fear SHOW GREATER WILLINGNESS TO EXPLORE NEW PLACES CURIOSITY (vs. guardedness)

Be vulnerable! explore + learn!

(CRF=CRH=Corticotropin Releasing Factor)

Hormonal Stress System: "<u>HPA</u>" <u>Activation</u>
Stress ⇒ <u>H</u>ypothalamus ⇒⇒ <u>P</u>ituitary ⇒⇒<u>A</u>drenal (Cortex) ⇒⇒
CRF or CRH ACTH Cortisol

Sense of Self – Peter Fonagy

Sense of Self (as a person distinct from your mum)
Sense of Agency (you can "do things all by yourself")

Recognizing / dealing with emotions

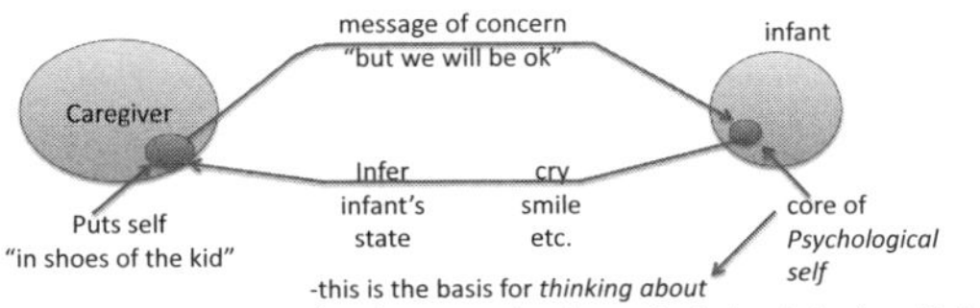

-this is the basis for *thinking about* thoughts or emotions (mentalization) vs. being "engulfed" by thoughts and emotions
-allows you to feel you are distinct from mom/dad/peers

Allen JG, Fonagy P, Bateman AW. 2009. Mentalizing in Clinical Practice. Washington,DC. American Psychiatric Publishing Inc.

Attachment = ⑦ gene systems
Early = Reward Later =Obsession

VTA (ventral tegmental areas is a dopamine – rich area ① which projects to Nucleus Accumbens)

caudate ②

Other Players

-Oxytocin + OTR ③ -in Nucleus Accumbens in an Estrogen ④, Progesterone ⑤ and Prolactin ⑥ Primed brain (in females)

-Vasopressin ⑦ and receptors in ventral pallidum (males)

Attachment can change epigenetic damage!

Higgins ES, George MS. The Neuroscience of Clinical Psychiatry: The Pathophysiology of Behavior and Mental Illness. Philadelphia (USA): Lippincott, Williams and Wilkins; 2007: pg.186

Sensory Processing Disorder (SPD)

- Sensory Modulation Disorder
  - SOR SUR SS/C
- Sensory Discrimination Disorder
- Sensory – based Motor Disorder
  - Postural Disorder
  - Dyspraxia

SOR- Sensory Over-Responsive
SUR- Sensory Under-Responsive
SS/C- Sensory Seeker/Craver

Miller LJ. 2006. Sensational Kids. New York. Perigee Books. http://www.thespiralfoundation.org/

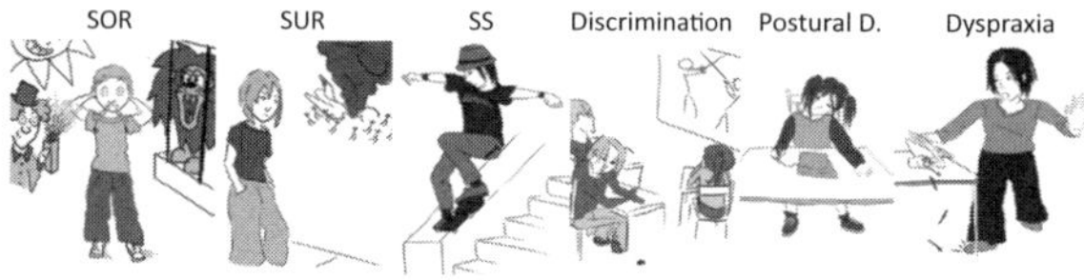

Dr. Joel Paris' ideas re: really volatile people

-see suicidal ideas, self-harm and other crises as "a cry for help" and offer that help; be sure that attention to (albeit necessary) details at a time of crisis, for instance documenting the degree of suicidal intent, planning, access to means, etc., does not distract you from the critical work: which is attending to the "cry for help"

-the *foundation* of any work with volatile or distressed folks is the security of your *relationship with them*...maintaining that respectful relationship is a *primary goal* for without it "helpers" can do *nothing*

-(as a doctor) *NEVER "fire" a* patient (even if provoked by the patient not showing up to appointments, not taking meds as prescribed, or other "no-nos") because often the precipitant for another crisis (of self-harm or similar) is the patient's *perception of being abandoned by a social attachment.* Reasonable boundaries are great but the threat if they are broken must not be severing the relationship for the doctor-patient relationship *is the basis* on which any intervention is built

.....it is all about Attachment

Paris J Personalities Over Time: Precursors, Course, and Outcome. Washington (USA) American Psychiatric Publishing Inc. 2003

Senses

1- Somatosensory (tactile) - deep + light touch, pain, vibration sense, hot/cold
2- Visual - vision and circadian clock
3- Auditory - hearing
4- Interoception - sense of internal body organs
5- Proprioception - where joints + muscles are w.r.t. body
6- Vestibular - where body is w.r.t. gravity
7- Gustatory - taste
8- Olfactory- smell
9- "others"- chemoceptors / eye contact / facial recognition

(4–6: "Internal" senses)

In FASD if there is an "incident" question: overarousal??? Flooded???

Relevant to FASD?

23 year old single mum, 6 year old in care. 2 years ago cocaine, now Esthetics student

-*distressed* by others touching her	SOR (S)
-*has* to have, fidget, wiggle	SS (P)
-tips chair back	SS (V)
-rollercoaster BUT car sick	SS + SOR (V)
-*loves* heavy blankets	deep pressure calms
-*hates* "messy, gooey"	SOR (S)
-bites of lip in lecture	"autoarousal"

... her 6 year old = "the same"

ideas: strattera (atomoxetine), "fidgets", heavy back pack on lap

Acoustic Startle + Abstinence in Women

(post inpatient residential treatment for alcoholism)

	abstinent	not abstinent
Acoustic Startle*	↓	↑
BDNF**	↑	↓

*a marker for SOR also seen in PTSD

**brain derived neurotropic factor – a potent nerve growth factor. (may relate to ↑ neurogenesis activity in hippocampus + prefrontal cortex)

Is SOR (SENSORY OVERRESPONSIVITY) Inherited?

Study: 394 toddler-aged twins

Findings:- ↑ girls with ↑↑↑ tactile defensiveness

Auditory and tactile defensiveness — associated with — anxiety fearful temperament

- "moderate genetic influences"
  tactile > auditory

Goldsmith HH, Van Hulle CH, Arnesa CL, Schreiber JE, Germsbacher MA. A population-based twin study of parentally reported tactile and auditory defensiveness in young children. Journal of Abnormal Child Psychology.2006;34(3): pg.378-392

SOR (esp. Tactile) Has Significant Genetic Component WHAT GENES?

-↑ D2 Receptor binding in the striatum (caudate, putamen and globus palladus) relates to SOR

-ratio of $\frac{\text{D2R binding}}{\text{Dopamine Synthesis}}$ ↑ relates to SOR

... genes: -D2 Receptor (striatum)
-D2R + D1R binding in other areas?
-Dopamine Transporter?

Schneider ML, Moore CF, Gajewski LL, Larson JA, Roberts AD, Converse AK, DeJesus OT. Sensory Processing Disorder in a Primate Model: evidence from a longitudinal study of prenatal alcohol and prenatal stress effects. Child Development.2008;79(1):100-113

Mary Schneider's Alcohol-fed Monkeys, Their Offspring and Short Alleles of the Serotonin transporter

(an allele is a variation in DNA Sequence that occurs at a particular polymorphic site of one chromosome)

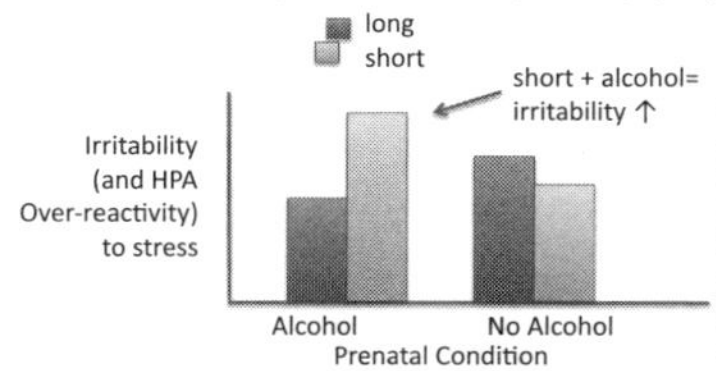

" if individuals carrying the S allele are excluded then the effects of prenatal alcohol exposure on irritability and HPA dysfunction are not statistically significant"

Kramer GW, Moore CF, Newman TK, Barr CS, Schneider ML. Moderate level of fetal alcohol exposure and serotonin transporter gene promoter polymorphism affect neonatal temperament and limbic-hypothalamic-pituitary-adrenal axis regulation in monkeys. Biological Psychiatry.2008;63:317-324

ADHD Heritability (up to 76%)

D4D5 Receptors

Dopamine
Serotonin
Noradrenalin } Transporters

Plus...

Orbital Frontal Cortex
Hippocampus
Amygdala } all project to Nucleus Accumbens

nucleus accumbens focuses attention on more favorable reward

Higgins ES, George MS. The Neuroscience of Clinical Psychiatry:The Pathophysiology of Behavior and Mental Illness. Philadelphia (USA):Lippincott, Williams and Wilkins; 2007

Gene- By – Environment Interaction of the Serotonin Transporter (5-HTT)

("s" allele 25% African → 80% Asian)

1 or 2 copies of the short allele of the 5-HTT (Serotonin Transporter) gene:

- ↑ symptoms of depression with exposure to stress (stress sensitivity)
- ↑ drinking + drug use in college students exposed to negative life events (pacing, diagnose and treat L.D., SPD, ADHD)
- ↑ amount and earlier start of alcohol use in maltreated children (earlier intervention)
- ↑ neonatal irritability in offspring of monkeys who prenatally consumed moderate amounts of alcohol prevent (intense support)

Gelernter J, Kanzler HR. Genetics of Addiction, Chapter 2. In: Textbook of Substance Abuse Treatment 4th Edition. Editors: Galanter M, Kleber HD. Washington (USA). American Psychiatric Publishing Inc., 2008:pg. 17-27

Impulsivity May Relate To FASD

Sexual debut 16 or younger

- -correlates to unintended pregnancy due to ↓ use of contraception
- -immature cervix → ↑ STD, ↑ PID, ↑ HPV
- -20-25% had been drinking
- -if ↑ CD or SUD there is ↑ unprotected sex and ↑ sex in exchange for money or drugs

genetics influence disinhibitory traits: sensation seeking, impulsivity, non-conformity

Cavazos- Rehg PA, Spitznagl EL, Bucholz KK et al. Predictors of Sexual Debut at age 16 or younger [online]. Archives of Sexual Behavior ISSN. Oct 10, 2008: 1573-2800 10p

Dopamine Pathways make sense but ~~proven~~ to play a role in Addiction (yet)

Alcohol → ↑ Dopamine in Nucleus Accumbens=its rewarding effect

↓ Dopamine 2 receptor activity in striatum in withdrawal

-a specific variant of Dopamine 2 receptor gene (DRD2) might be a risk factor for alcoholism...

-if carry A1 allele of DRD2 gene → learning to avoid negative consequences from alcoholism is ↓

-the active genes for this might be DRD2 A1 allele's close neighbor genes:
ANKK1, TTC12, NCAM1

-DAT 1 gene encodes the dopamine transporter (DAT)
DAT1 (A9) variation is associated with more severe withdrawal including seizures!

LeStrat Y, Ramoz N, Schuman G, Gorwoud P. Molecular Genetics of Alcohol Dependence and Related Endotypes. Current Genomics.2008;(9)444-457

ADH (Alcohol Dehydrogenase)

-this enzyme breaks Alcohol down to acetaldehyde

-2 genetic alleles which encode this enzyme:
ADH1B*2
ADH1C*2
are associated with a **faster** alcohol degradation rate are some **protection** re developing A.D.

ADH4 contributes 30% to alcohol oxidizing capacity in liver
ADH7 also affects metabolism, risk of A.D. and personality traits

(AD= Alcohol Dependence)
(AUD= Alcohol Use Disorder)
(SUD= Substance Use Disorder)
(ND= Nicotine Dependence)

LeStrat Y, Ramoz N, Schuman G, Gorwoud P. Molecular Genetics of Alcohol Dependence and Related Endotypes. Current Genomics.2008;(9):444-457

Genes of Alcohol Dependence

Alcohol → Alcohol Dehydrogenase (**ADH**) → Acetaldehyde

Acetaldehyde → Aldehyde Dehydrogenase (**ALDH**) → CO2 + H2O

Alcohol metabolizing genes
enzymes — ADH
ADH1B
ADH1B = ADH2
ADH1C = ADH3
ADH4 – liver metabolism

ALDH
ALDH2 does most of metabolism ↓ = disulfiram
genetic variant in Asian populates

(GABA)A receptor – GABRA2 (chromosome 4)
"within the 3' portion of GABRA2 there is a functional area that changes risk for alcoholism via modulation of the risk factor of anxiety"
(GABRA1 + GABRAG3) GABRA6

Gelernter J, Kanzler HR. Genetics of Addiction, Chapter 2. In: Textbook of Substance Abuse Treatment 4th Edition. Editors: Galanter M, Kleber HD. Washington (USA). American Psychiatric Publishing Inc.;2008:pg. 17-27

ALDH (Aldehyde Dehydrogenase)

-oxidizes acetaldehyde to CO2 and H2O

-blocked by disulfiram (Antabuse)

the syndrome (of acetaldehyde build up, flushing, nausea, palpitations) is also seen in carriers of ALDH2 *2 variant (and ALDH2*1)

note: dopamine→→→→→→→→→→ noradrenilin →→→→→ adrenilin
↑
dopamine beta-hydroxylase (also is blocked by antabuse!)

LeStrat Y, Ramoz N, Schuman G, Gorwoud P. Molecular Genetics of Alcohol Dependence and Related Endotypes. Current Genomics.2008;(9):444-457

Genes of Alcohol Dependence

CHRM2 is the genetic locus for the muscarinic acetylcholine Receptor "M2"

-several SNPs (single nucleotide polymorphisms--"bite sized" pieces of the gene are associated with Alcohol Dependence others – Depression

-several variations predispose to agreeableness and conscientiousness

Gelernter J, Kanzler HR. Genetics of Addiction, Chapter 2. In: Textbook of Substance Abuse Treatment 4th Edition. Editors: Galanter M, Kleber HD. Washington (USA). American Psychiatric Publishing Inc;2008:pg. 17-27

MRS = Magnetic Resonance Spectroscopy: lower Choline Concentration in the Frontal and Parietal White Matter and Corpus Callosum, L. Hippocampus (may relate to lower activity of acetylcholine also).

Astley SJ, et al. 2009. Magnetic resonance spectroscopy outcomes from a comprehensive magnetic resonance study of children with fetal alcohol spectrum disorders. Mag Reson Imaging 27: 760-778

OPIOID Receptors

-OPRM1 is the genetic locus for the mu opioid receptor
-mu and gamma opioid receptor stimulation by alcohol adds to positive reinforcement in the nucleus accumbens

-several SNPs of OPRM1 are associated with A.D. if drinkers have *Asp*40 allele (vs *Asn* 40 allele) Naltrexone treatment helps avoid relapse into heavy drinking (small study)

-opioid kappa receptor stimulation is aversive (not rewarding)
-OPRK1 is the gene encoding the kappa receptor
-some single nucleotide polymorphisms (SNP's) are associated with A.D.
-PDYN encodes the kappa receptors' ligand "prodynorphan"
- a number of PDYN SNPs are associated with A.D.

Gelernter J, Kranzler HR. Genetics and alcohol dependence. Human Genetics 2009;126:91-99

hTAS2R16 Gene On Chromosome 7

-encodes the *"bitter" taste* receptor

-if this gene is expressed ↓ sensitivity to bitter taste stimuli and ↑ maximum number of drinks per 24 hours + ↑ dependence

(avoid "sweet" drinks!)

-HANGOVER / 2NF699 gene polymorphisms are associated with A.D. in Irish patients

-if this gene is expressed tolerance develops

LeStrat Y, Ramoz N, Schuman G, Gorwoud P. Molecular Genetics of Alcohol Dependence and Related Endotypes. Current Genomics.2008;(9):444-457

OPRM1 and Adolescent **A**lcohol **U**se **D**isorder (**A.U.D.**)

SNP: A118G (rs1799971) of OPRM1

AUD	no AUD
52% carry at least 1 G allele	16%

thus a polymorphism of OPRM1 is associated with **early onset** alcohol use problems
- In part by ↑ sensitivity to reinforcing effects of alcohol (naltrexone) (52%)

Miranda R, Ray L et al. Initial evidence of association between OPRM1 and adolescent alcohol misusage [internet]. Alcoholism: Clinical and Experimental Research.Oct.23,2009

Glutamate

-major excitatory neurotransmitter

-GRIK1 is the gene that encodes the GluR5 subunit of the kainic acid glutamate receptor

-variations of this subunit affect Alcohol Dependence

-topiramate (Topamax), anticonvulsant, acts on this area + acamprosate (Campral), GABA agonist and Glutamate antagonist

Kranzler HR, Gelernter J et al. Association of Markers in the 3' region of the GluR5 Kainate receptor gene to alcohol dependence. Alcoholism: Clinical and Experimental Research.2009;33(5):925-930

GABRA2: Odds Ratio of Alcoholism: 1.2, O.R. ~~Married:~~ 2.2!!

(Do you have one or two copies of the High Risk) GABRA2 Allele?

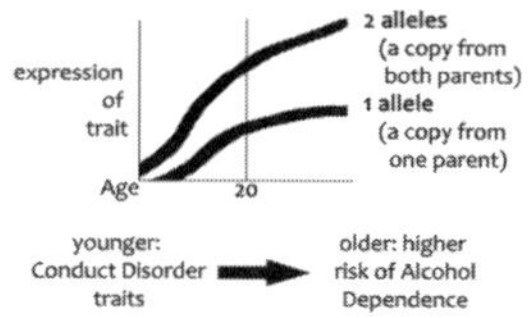

Edenberg H (2009)Symposium 70: Genetic Vulnerabilities for Drug Use and Co-morbid Mental Health Disorders: Genetics of Alcoholism and Related Endotypes (confrence presentation) Americain Psychiatric Assosiation Annual Meeting, San Fransisco

Gamma-Amino–Butyric Acid (GABA) Pathway

-GABA receptor has 5 subunits

2 alpha + 2 beta + one gamma <u>or</u> one delta subunit

-if ↓ GABA activity then withdrawal is worse, GABA activity mediates anxiety

a mutant gamma 2 subunit is associated with worse withdrawal

-Variations in GABRA 2 and GABRA 6 are associated with Alcohol Dependence

LeStrat Y, Ramoz N, Schuman G, Gorwoud P. Molecular Genetics of Alcohol Dependence and Related Endotypes. Current Genomics (9)2008:444-457

GABRA2

- ~~Different proteins~~ made by some SNPs
- Changes how promoters and splicing variants work to change gene expression
- "Severe" "phenotype": alcohol *and drug* dependence, early age heavy drinking, larger binges, worse withdrawal, more CD, ASPD, Depression and "novelty seeking"
- Kids from these families are at ↑ risk

A.D. Can Co-occur:

-with other drug dependences and conduct disorder / anti social personality disorder

-some of this comorbidity is due to shared genetic liability – e.g.. "alcohol dependence" shares genetic vulnerability with other "externalizing disorders" (conduct disorder, ASPD and drug dependence) and this common liability showed

heritability of 80%

-A.D. Also shares genetic risk with Nicotine dependence + caffeine use

Gelernter J, Kranzler HR. Genetics of alcohol dependence. Human Genetics.2009;126: 91-99

Stress Axis HPA Axis

an important mediator of the stress response

CRHR1 encodes the corticotropin releasing hormone receptor 1

2 SNPs: rs 242938
rs 1876831

associated with binge drinking in adolescents and adults with alcohol dependence

Gelernter J, Kranzler HR. Genetics of alcohol dependence. Human Genetics.2009;126: 91-99

Variations in Nicotine Receptor Gene Cluster on Chromosome 15

CHRNA5
CHRNA3 } affect risk of
CHRNA4

developing dependence to
-Alcohol and
-Nicotine

Ghrelin and GHS-R1A Gene Polymorphisms

Ghrelin acts on → **G**rowth **H**ormone **S**ecretagogue **R**eceptors

GHS-R1A

these are in the hypothalamus and reward nodes e.g.. Ventral Tegmental Area

ghrelin activates these reward systems

SNP: "rs 2232165" of GHS-R1A associated with heavy alcohol drinking

Landgren S, Jerlhag E, et al. Association of Pro-Ghrelin and GHS-R1A Gene Polymorphisms and Haplotypes with Heavy Alcohol Use and Body Mass [online]. Alcoholism: Clinical and Experimental Research.Sept. 25, 2008

What Nonsense Can Alcohol Cause In Gene Expression?

can change gene expression in genes that control:

- -neurogenesis
- -cell adhesion
- -apoptosis
- -myelination
- -ubiquitination* (a process of protein modification)
- -cell survival
- -energy metabolism*
- -mitochondrial proteins*

*alcohol also directly adversely affects the *proteins that result* from these genes!

LeStrat Y, Ramoz N, Schuman G, Gorwoud P. Molecular Genetics of Alcohol Dependence and Related Endotypes. Current Genomics.2008;(9):444-457

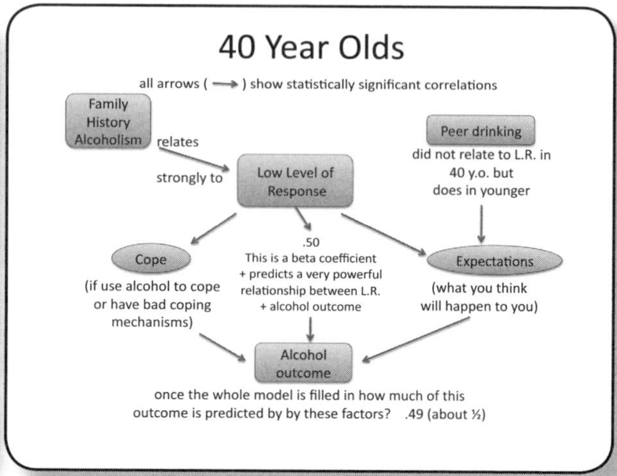

Candidate Genes Associated with ↓Level of Response (LR)

GABRA alpha 6	COMT	5 HTT
GABRG2	DRD2 / ANKK1	ADORA
A5	DRD4	**NPY**
A1		
		ADH1B
KCNMA1	DGK2	ADH1C
CHRNA5	GNAS	CYPZE
	PK	

Schuckit MA. Adolf Meyer Award Lecture. How Alcoholism Develops: Identification of Genetic and Environmental Influences in a 25-year Longitudinal Study. American Psychiatric Association Meeting. 2009.San Francisco

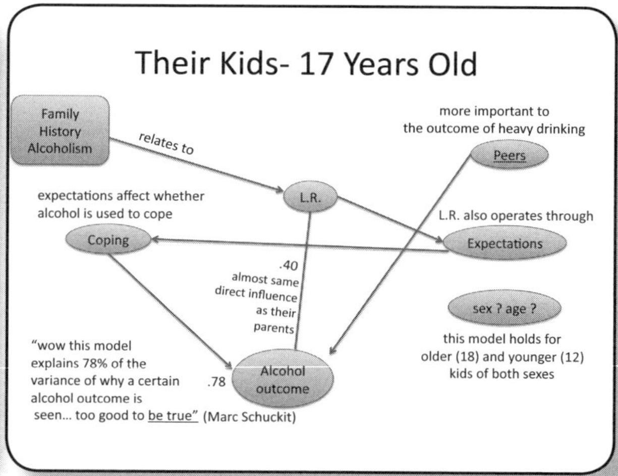

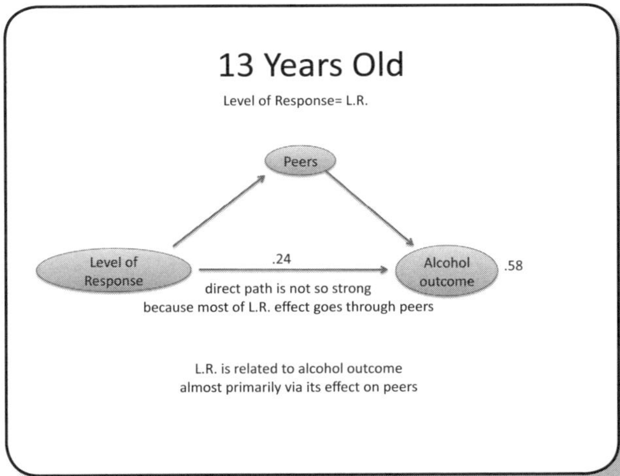
13 Years Old
Level of Response= L.R.
Peers
Level of Response
.24
Alcohol outcome
.58
direct path is not so strong
because most of L.R. effect goes through peers
L.R. is related to alcohol outcome
almost primarily via its effect on peers

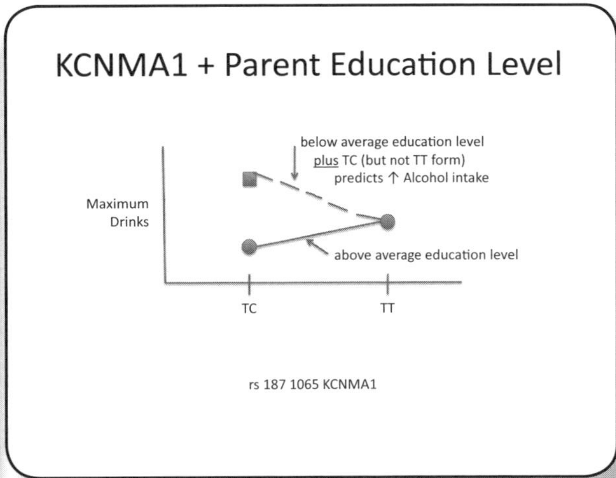
KCNMA1 + Parent Education Level
below average education level
plus TC (but not TT form)
predicts ↑ Alcohol intake
Maximum Drinks
above average education level
TC
TT
rs 187 1065 KCNMA1

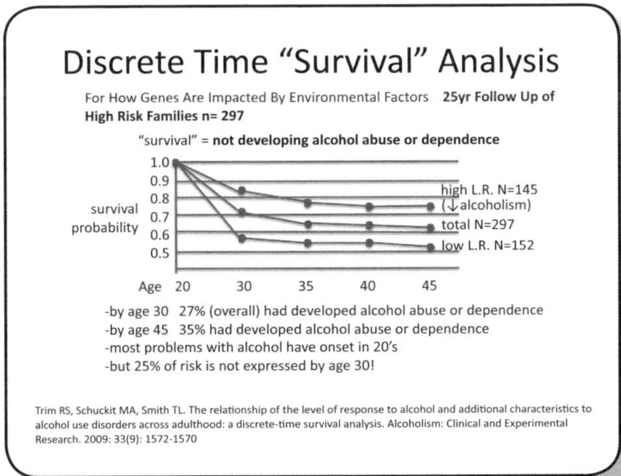
Discrete Time "Survival" Analysis
For How Genes Are Impacted By Environmental Factors 25yr Follow Up of High Risk Families n= 297
"survival" = not developing alcohol abuse or dependence
1.0
0.9
0.8
0.7
0.6
0.5
survival probability
high L.R. N=145 (↓alcoholism)
total N=297
low L.R. N=152
Age 20 30 35 40 45
-by age 30 27% (overall) had developed alcohol abuse or dependence
-by age 45 35% had developed alcohol abuse or dependence
-most problems with alcohol have onset in 20's
-but 25% of risk is not expressed by age 30!
Trim RS, Schuckit MA, Smith TL. The relationship of the level of response to alcohol and additional characteristics to alcohol use disorders across adulthood: a discrete-time survival analysis. Alcoholism: Clinical and Experimental Research. 2009: 33(9): 1572-1570

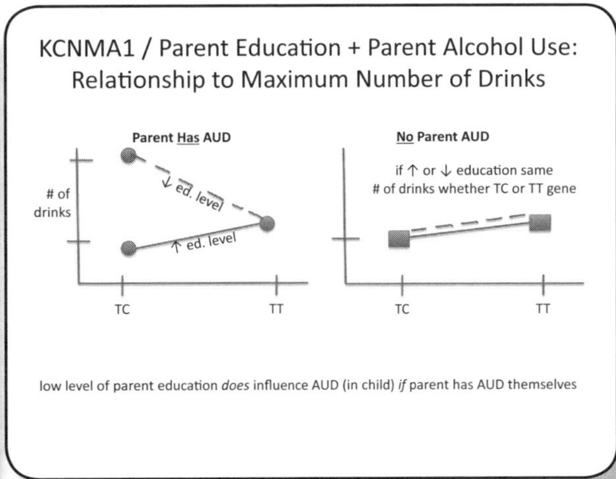
KCNMA1 / Parent Education + Parent Alcohol Use:
Relationship to Maximum Number of Drinks
Parent Has AUD
No Parent AUD
# of drinks
↓ ed. level
↑ ed. level
if ↑ or ↓ education same
# of drinks whether TC or TT gene
TC
TT
TC
TT
low level of parent education does influence AUD (in child) if parent has AUD themselves

Neuropeptide Y Receptor

Variations of Neuropeptide Y and sequence variations in its 3 receptor genes
-NPY1R
-NPY2R
-NPY5R
are associated with alcohol dependence
especially
a severe subtype of alcohol dependence with
-withdrawal symptoms +++ and
-comorbidity with cocaine dependence

Wetherill L, Schuckit MA et al. Neuropeptide Y Receptor Genes are Associated with Alcohol Dependence Alcohol Withdrawal Phenotypes and Cocaine Dependence [online]. Alcoholism: Clinical and Experimental Research.25 Sept 2008

Could *Primary* Inheritance of Mental Health Problems relate to *Secondary* Disabilities

Trait of:	Heritability	Link to?
"Externalizing behaviors"	80%	trouble with law
Impulsivity	50-70%	school drop out
Emotional "dysregulation"	(slightly) less then 50%	anxiety disorder
Bipolar	Up to 70%	mental health, SUD
Alcohol Dependence	50-60%	Substance Use Disorder
Nicotine Dependence	50-60%	Substance Use Disorder

Children with FASD are born with a considerable genetic burden which could emerge as "Secondary Disabilities". As with any inherited traits, our caregivers and professionals must.....BE RADICAL ----EXPLOIT YOUR MEASLEY 20-50% THAT YOU CAN INFLUENCE! "BOTTOM UP REBULILDING JOB" BRUCE PERRY, TRAUMA AND RELATIONSHIPS: DAVE ZIEGLER: RAISING CHILDREN WHO REFUSE TO BE RAISED, EDNA FOA: EFFECTIVE TREATMENT OF PTSD

Environmental Changes Influence *Expression* of a High Risk Gene

"Any <u>one</u> gene only explains **<u>part</u>** of the risk
AND anyhow who wants to change a gene?"*

So *identify* genes that put people at High Risk and then make *robust changes* to environment to help ↓ expression of these High Risk genes

*Schuckit,Marc

Conclusion

"We will never reach a point where we can say we can prevent alcoholism totally but the more we understand about the **risk factors**, the **genes** associated with them and the **mechanisms** through which they work:

for Depression
for Schizophrenia
for Cancer
for MI
<u>AND</u> for Alcoholism –
the better we should be able to provide **early identification** and **prevention** of any disorder"

Marc Schuckit

Understanding Fetal Alcohol Spectrum Disorders (FASD): The Neurobiology for Health Professionals

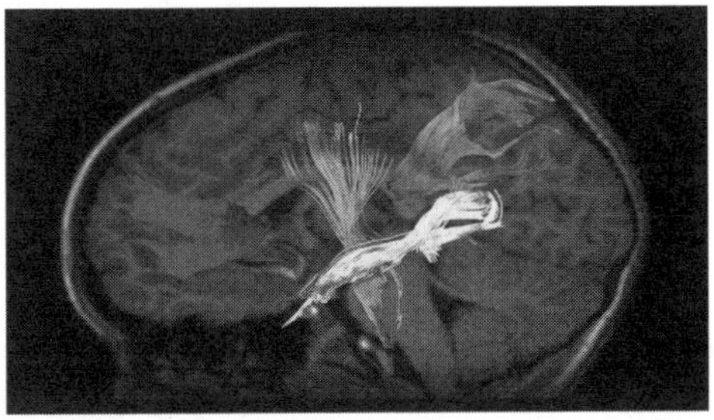

Workshop W16, Canadian Psychiatric Association Annual Conference
Rod Densmore, M.D., Adoptive Father

Psychopathology in Children with FASD

? odds of Axis I and II after controlling for nicotine, THC, gender, placement, low SES, maternal nutrition, FHx psych.alcohol

method: structured interview (C-DISC-IV or K-SADS-PL)

Psychopathology	alcohol exposed n=39	controls n=30
5@ 95%C.I. gp. diff.	age 12.1, IQ 83	age 11.2, IQ 108
ADHD	37 (95%)	9 (30%)
Depressive disorders	7 (18%)	0
ODD	15 (38%)	5 (17%)
Conduct disorder	7 (18%)	1 (3%)
Specific Phobia	9 (23%)	1 (3%)
tic, GAD, soc. phobia	, panic, OCD are all	↑ but not signif.

97% have a psychiatric diagnosis **(Fryer, *Pediatrics*, 2007)**

This Presentation

- Psychopathology in FASD
- Definitions/ Diagnostic Codes
- Brain domains for diagnosis
- Differential Diagnosis
- Prevalence
- Neuroimagining: Cerebellum, Corpus Callosum, Basal Ganglia Thalamus, Frontal Lobes, White Matter Tracts, Hippocampus
- Serotonin- how it relates to Neurogenesis and SIDS
- Sleep
- Shaken Baby Syndrome
- The ADHD of FASD

Also Important

- Attachment
- Social Connection
- Mirror Neurons
- Following Rules
- Alexithymia
- Gifts/ Strengths: Art, Physical Exuberance, Music, Drama, Story-telling, working with animals or the elderly
- Epigenetics: Stress Sensitivity/ Resilience
- Language and Math
- Sensory Processing

Fetal Alcohol Spectrum Disorders include:

- FAS: Fetal Alcohol Syndrome
- pFAS: Partial Fetal Alcohol Syndrome
- ARND: Alcohol Related Neurodevelopmental Disorder
- ARBD: Alcohol Related Birth Defects

4 Digit Code (Astley, 2008)

Severity	1	2	3	4
CNS domains	normal	1< -2SD	2<-2SD	3<-2SD
Craniofacial	normal	in	between	lip 4-5 philtrum 4-5 eye <-2SD
Growth Deficiency	Ht >10% Wt >10%	in	between	Ht <3% Wt <3%
Prenatal Alcohol Exposure	confirmed nil	unknown or not conf.	conf. but ? amount	conf. in high amount

Craniofacial Abnormalities

Lip/Philtrum guides →

Palpebral fissure length

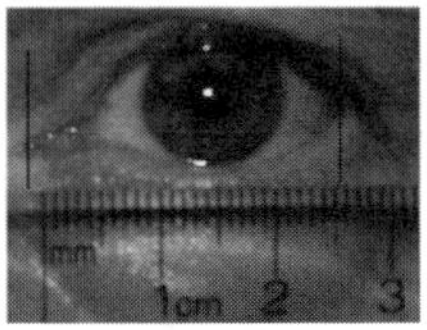

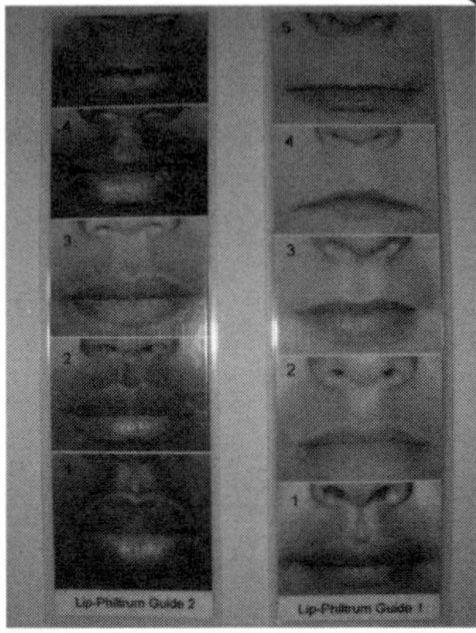

FASD Canadian Codes (Chudley, 2005)

	CNS	Craniofacial	Growth	Prenatal Alcohol
FAS + conf. exposure	3 or 4	4	2,3 or 4	3 or 4
FAS without conf. exp. exposure	3 or 4	4	2,3 or 4	2
pFAS + conf. exp.	3 or 4	2,3 or 4	1,2,3 or 4	3 or 4
ARND + conf. exp.	3 or 4 2 if <6 yrs.	1 or 2	1,2,3 or 4	3 or 4

Alcohol Related Birth Defects

- think neural crest:

craniofacial
- cleft palate/lip
- teeth (orthodontist + weak enamel)
- eustachian tube ...otitis/hearing loss
- sleep disordered breathing

heart septae - VSD, ASD, tetralogy
(do EKG- ?long QT + echo)

eye - next slide

-horseshoe (+ other) kidney problems

-hypoplastic 5th nail/ distal phalanx

Eye - "fuzzy" central processing
(Medina, Krahe 2006)

activity dependent plasticity → establishes cortical functional "Maps"

prenatal alcohol via xs phosphodiesterase type 1 activity:

→ impairs development of maps
→ result = ↓ perception of corners and borders

Vinpocetine - ↓ problems in pups

85% of FASD has **NO DYSMORPHOLOGY**

BRAIN DAMAGE IS **THE most important functional** ISSUE

PROBLEM: If it is a **brain** concern...less research, less focus on the work of Geneticists/ Dymorphologists......
This group has had great difficulty in Clarification of diagnostic criteria

1) We NEED their input for differential diagnosis: Noonan, DiGeorge, DiLange, Dubowitz, Velocardiofacial, Fragile X, Williams, Phenytoin, Lead, Mercury, Accutane

2) Delays in refining DSM or ICD diagnoses **must** end
FAS (not FASD)is being considered by DSM "Condition proposed by outside sources"

Ophthalmology (Stromland, Hellstrom 1996)

n=25 children with FAS (+10 yr. follow up)
all but one had opthal. abnormalities!

-½ visual impairment (<20/100 in 10 eyes!)
-½ hypoplasia optic nerve
-½ ↑tortuosity of retinal arteries
-½ strabismus ?conjugate gaze?

Darren Sass, O.D., Developmental Optometrist (www.insightlearning.ca) College of Optometrists in Vision Development (covd.org) Neuro-Optometric Rehabilitation Association (nora.cc)

birth mum: dead from alcoholism or disappeared 40%!

children with:	
birth mum	16%
dad	24%
foster	52%
institution	8%

If you'd like to provide input to DSM:

http://www.dsm5.org/ProposedRevisions/Pages/ConditionsProposedbyOutsideSources.aspx

BRAIN DOMAINS Canada (Chudley,2005)

1) Hard and Soft Neurological signs

Obvious: CT, MRI, seizure   sensory processing, **fine or gross motor**

2 Cognition (I.Q.)   -FAS= low 70's,   pFAS=high 70's to low 80's

3 Communication   -speech/ writing/ listening/ reading
-auditory processing
Coggins, 1998 < -coherence (infer?, overall plan of a story)
-cohesiveness (get the "gist" of episodes)

4) Academic achievement -math ("primary number sense")
("cognitive estimation")
math < language < hands-on < art/music/drama

Prevalence Large population studies are rare

- Seattle: FAS and ARND 9.1/1000 (Sampson, 1997)
- S. Africa: **FAS** > 4/100 (May, 2000), **+PFAS** 6.8-8.9% (May, 2007)
- N. Canada (isolated): FAS/FAE 190/1000 (Robinson,1987)
- N. Italy: n=543 first grade FAS 3.7-7.4/1000 (May, 2006)

FASD 2.3-4.5/100 overall= 3.5/100

- Western City, USA. (Pilot) n=128 FASD 1.65% (May, 2009)
- Prison: n=106 pFAS/ARND= 10% + "possible"=18% (MacPherson + Chudley, 2007)
- "Juvie" (youth jail): n=287 FASD=23/100 (Fast, 1999)
- "Next" after child with FAS: 771/1000 (Huebert, 1996)
- Homeless (E.Van.): FASD: (est.) 2/3 (Antrobus, 2004)

Likely: FASD: 3/100 (ASD: 1/166)   **>5X ASD**

Brain Domains Canada cont'd

5 Memory -encoding! - for object location (where) is worse than identification (what)

6 Executive Function/ Abstract Reasoning
-working memory/ sequencing/ "cognitive estimation"

7 Attention Deficit/ Hyperactivity
- "is the most frequent presentation of FASD.... FASD's are true clinical masqueraders and ADHD is their most likely disguise!" (O'Malley, 2007)

8 Adaptive Behaviour, Social Skills, **Social Communication**
(Minnesota FASD diagnostic team adds 2 domains)
Maybe in the future:
??processing speed, mirror neurons, alexithymia, ↓"mentalization"

Neuroimaging (Spadoni, 2007)

MRI
- ↓ overall brain volume - parietal (caudate, frontal, temporal)
- regional white matter hypoplasia - posterior parietal
  - posterior temporal
- white/grey matter ratio ↓ esp. inferior parietal

correlations
- ↓ white matter = ↓processing speed
- frontal ⇔ parietal damage = ↓ executive function and ↓ spatial memory

-parietal areas esp. affected = BA 21, 22 language processing
BA 37 object and face recognition

Cerebellum (Spadoni, 2007)

MRI

- ↓ volume, ↓ surface area esp. Ant. Vermis (lobules I-V)

correlates:

- posture, balance, (muscle) coordination

but also.......

- coordination of attention systems (see next slide)

and......

- *"always on-line partial sensory filter which reduces sensory input from self-initiated movement"* (Linden, 2006) (can you tickle yourself?)

- vermis = verbal learning and memory ?DTI is difficult

Corpus Callosum

MRI

- agenesis (2% of FASD) = low rate but 20X normal
- Hypoplasia is common esp.
  - genu (front)
  - splenium (back)

- anterior and inferior displacement of splenium

- "splenium angle" > 90° (Bookstien, 2007)
  n=23 heavily exposed infants and 21 controls
  transfontanelle ultrasound
  12/23 > 90° 1 false positive (Spadoni, 2007)

ATTENDING (overview) (Castellanos, 2002)

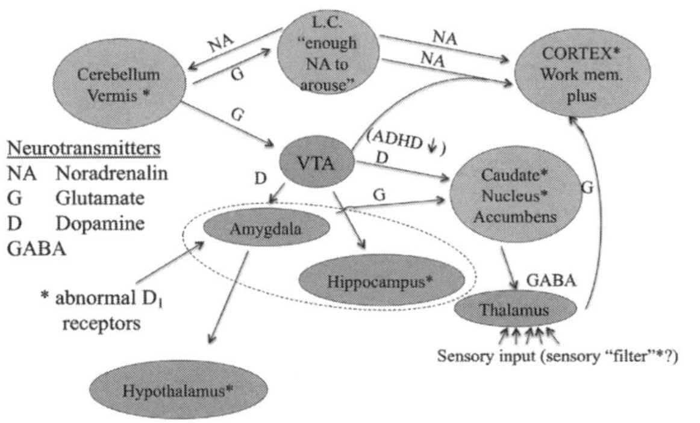

Corpus Callosum

DTI - can see white matter tracts clearly (Lebel, 2008)
- deep grey matter structures Δ diffusion as they develop
- the more developed the cell's microstructure:
  the slower water can diffuse into a compartment

Mean **D**iffusivity (M.D.)
- how easily can water diffuse into a compartment
High = ☹

Fractional **A**nisotropy (F.A.)
- a measure of white matter integrity
High = ☺

↑ M.D. and ↓ F.A. in genu and splenium = white matter microstructure incoherency

Lebel, 2008 Diffusion Tensor Imaging for FASD

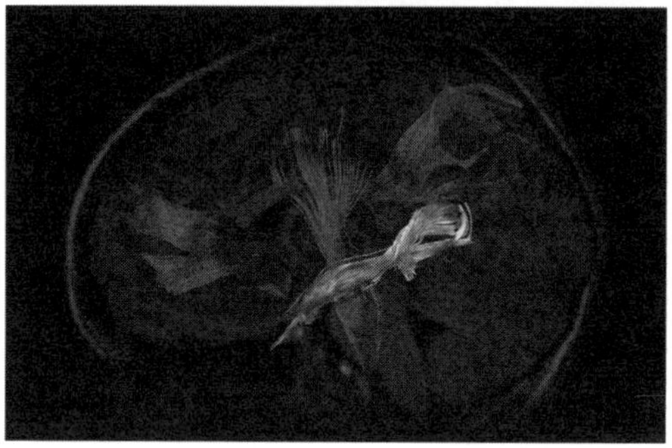

Corpus Callosum (Sowell, 2001)

Correlates

- splenium - displaced (forward and down) and microstructure abnormalities =
  ↓ verbal learning ability
- anterior CC - ↓ projections into frontal regions =
  ↓ executive function
- "thinner CC" - ↓ efficient delivery of information to motor areas = motor deficits
- "split brain" - could this be the basis for "lying"
  - *? "spotty memory" and "filling in the blanks"*
  (Linden, 2007)

Connections ⇒ DTI (Lebel, 2008)

n = 23 children with ARND: differences vs controls ($p < .05$)
"want" ↑ barriers (low M.D.) and ↑ organization (high F.A.)

F.A. changes	Both	M.D. changes
- Splenium (CC)		- Genu (CC)
- R Cingulum*		
- R+L Inf.Long.Fasc.*	- L Inf.Long.Fasc.*	
- R+L Sup.Long.Fasc*		
- R+L Globus Pallidus	- R+L Globus Pallidus	- R Putamen
- L Thalamus		

correlations:

- Splenium = visuomotor integration (Sowell, 2008)
- Inferior Longitudinal Fasciculus (L+R) = visual processing
- Superior Longitudinal Fasciculus (L+R) = language processing
- * = communicates with temporal lobes

Basal Ganglia (Spadoni, 2007 Lebel, 2008)

MRI

- ↓ volume caudate
  but DTI data shows intact microstructure
- putamen, globus pallidus "relatively spared" (volume data)
  DTI data: ↓ integrity (development) of microstructure =
  "↑ dendritic pruning and ↓myelination" (Cortese, 2006)

Correlates

- because of ↓ frontostriatal connectivity:
  - ↓ executive function
  - ↓ "concept formation (caudate ⇔ PFC interplay) (20 Q.)
  - ↓ spatial memory (morris water task)
  - ↓ "set shifting", perseveration

Thalamus

DTI

- L Thalamus ↓ F.A. = ↓ intact or ↓ developed microstructure (Lebel, 2008)

- influenced by stage I I sleep spindles to ↑ sensory "filter" during sleep....result = more easily awoken (stage I I spindles are ↓ in FASD) (Bonthius, 2006)

Hippocampus (Sutherland 2003)

- "**Low dose**" rat study: Morris water task for spatial memory, dams given "nightly drink" @ 2%, 3% or 5% alcohol

BAL undetectable 0.03% 0.08%

trial #2

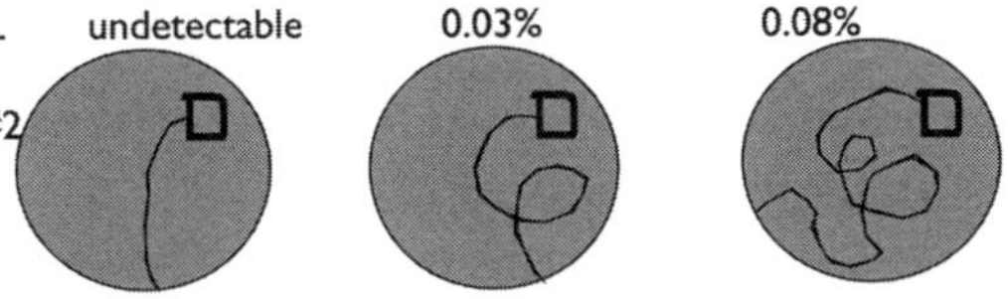

threshold for alcohol-induced spatial memory damage = < 0.03%
= R hippocampus synaptic plasticity ↓, LTP ↓ by prenatal alcohol

approx. ↓ 50% new hippocampal neurons in adults who had prenatal alcohol exposure (encoding)

Frontal Lobes (Malisza, 2004)

fMRI - 10 adults, 15 children plus controls
- push button that lights up (n=0) simple
- push button that lit up *last* time (n-1) = quite hard (50%!)
- push button that lit up *2 times ago* (n-2) = impossible

results

n=0 - ↑ activation and ↑ latency

n-1 - only half could do it
++ activation DLPFC, inferior frontal, anterior cingulate (corresponds to W.M., attention, response selection areas)

vs controls to do basic task of w.m., attention:
- ↑ "work" *so they are tired!! then have to do homework!!*
- ↓ insula (integration) activity (↓ response inhibition/selection) *so they need an "external brain" (Mum!) to assist with choices*
- ↑ errors and esp. ↑ latency *so give them time*

Hippocampus Virtual Morris water task

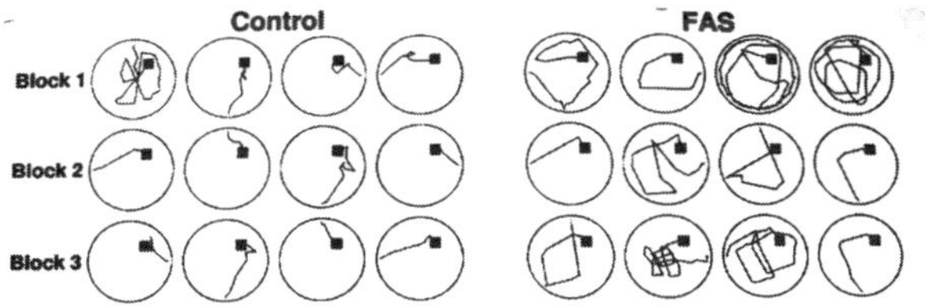

MEG - (dynamic imaging during the task)...only 2/7 showed any R Hippocampus activity during the task (vs 6/7).... this activity correlates with ↓ "initial heading errors"

Frontal lobes (and serotonin)

Serotonin - *fast neurotransmitter*
- *signaling agent for differentiation and maturation*

- 5-HT neurons are esp. vulnerable to prenatal alcohol

- Rat model, exposed 1st and 2nd "trimesters"
    - delayed closure ventral canal (fusion defects)
    - ↓neurogenesis and ↓ differentiation

- most 5-HT neurons are situated in midline raphe' nuclei in the brainstem and from there send projections out to (almost) the entire brain!" (Goodlett, 2005)

5-HT 1A Stimulation

serotonin
5-HT neuron ⇒⇒⇒⇒⇒ **5-HT 1A Rec.** Astrocyte

⇙ S100 Beta ⇙

↑ growth
↑ survival of neurons

Serotonin and Frontal Lobes

5-HT rostral nuclei ⇒ Forebrain (Zhou, 2005)
5-HT caudal nuclei ⇒ (medulla) homeostasis centers

↓ serotonin in development
⇓
"**cascading of deficiencies in forebrain development**"

- there is a **critical window** for 5-HT projections to arrive
- this is seen as a **peak of 5-HT 1A** receptor expression

days 16-20 (Rat) — maturation, differentiation, migration of neurons (with intimate coop. of glia)

Mary Druse - 5-HT 1A ligands *buspirone/isapirone* to ↑ signaling of damaged serotonin system in forebrain

Somatosensory Cortex stained for 5-HT-immunoreactivity (adapted from Powrozek, 2005)

This is a visual image of the impaired touch discrimination subtype of SPD (Sensory Processing Disorder)

SPD is a neurobehavioral disorder that interferes with a person's ability to regulate their behavioural responses to sensory input in a graded manner

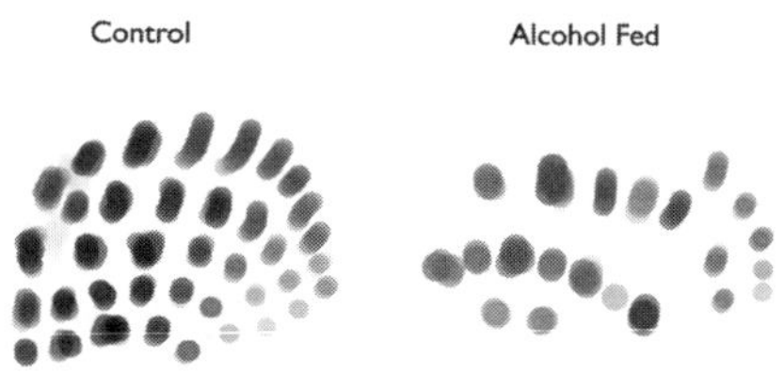

SIDS, FASD and ↓ 5-HT-1A Expression

Hypotonia is common + craniofacial anomalies ⇒ Sleep disordered breathing ⇒ Inadequate rescue response to ↓ O2 or ↑ CO2 ⇒ SIDS death

"ADHD" Spatial Memory L.D.

Hannah Kinney (Harvard): "babies that die from SIDS had deficient neurons in one form or another - at least the 5-HT-1A receptor on those neurons was hypo-expressed

SIDS and Drug Abuse

n = 2143 infants L.A.
mums had substance abuse

19 SIDS 8.9/1000
vs
1.2/1000 in controls

(Ward, 1990)

SIDS + 5-HT-1A (Patterson, 2006)

5-HT neurons in medulla oblongata project to autonomic and respiratory nuclei in the brainstem and spinal cord ⇒⇒ help regulate homeostasis

If ⇓O2 ⇑CO2 ⇓HR ⇨ **prompt response**

"significantly lower density of 5-HT-1A binding sites in all 9 nuclei of medulla involved in homeostasis"
almost **3x lower!**

$\frac{\text{BOY}}{\text{GIRL}} = \frac{1}{2}$ 5-HT-1A binding in raphe' obscurs

explains why SIDS is more common in boys

SIDS Risks and Ideas

Risks
- preterm
- low birthweight
- mother < 20
- less or late prenatal care
- overheating
- soft bedding
- bed-share

(Corwin, 2007)

Ideas

France: attachment videos for higher risk....the new mums sought advice

avoid
- swaddling
- blanket over head
- sheepskin
- polystyrene beads
- bed-share

do
- room-share (5-6 months)
- 18 celsius
- pacifier (> 1 month)
- rule out filicide

SLEEP ARCHITECTURE

Stages: I II III IV

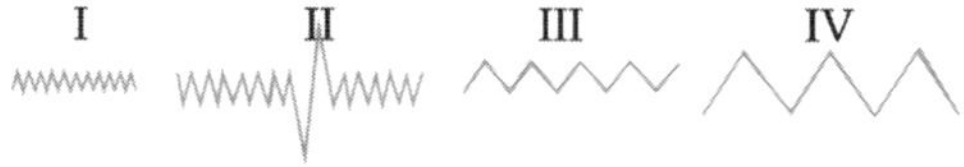

-non-rem "is idling brain in moving body"(Wm. Dement)
-dreams here = like thoughts, as through solving problems

Rapid eye movement (REM): ↑ as night progresses

"active hallucinatory brain in paralyzed body" (Dement)
-dreams more bizarre

I II III IV | R E M | I II III IV | REM | I II III IV | REM | I II III
|←"cycle"→| (5-6 cycles / night)

BAD COMBINATION FOR ATTACHMENT

Baby with FASD
- inconsolable crying, restlessness
- ⇓priming of melatonin receptors
- ⇓able to recognize *cues* for sleep e.g.) it's 9p.m., teeth /story / ⇓ sleep, etc.

Birth/ Adoptive/ Foster Parents
- acoustic startle -infertility
- not like other kids
- "advice" does not work
- ⇓sleep leads to ⇓coping

CIRCADIAN RHYTHM SLEEP DISORDERS

=misalignment of internal clock (SCN) with the social norm
-most common type is: "delayed sleep phase syndrome"
=wake up too early + irregular sleep/wake pattern

Low melatonin < head injuries / alcohol induced brain damage
(if birth mum has Alcohol Dependence)

Fetus -receives melatonin from mum - it primes her MT1 MT2 MT3 receptors

Baby- melatonin is not produced till 2-3 months

Shaken Baby Syndrome (Barr,2006)

Criteria
- subdural hemorrhages
- diffuse, multilayered retinal hemorrhages
- diffuse brain injury

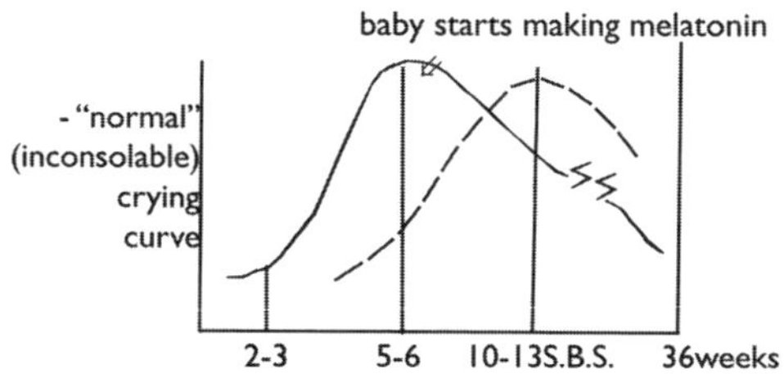

Lag = subclinical shakings?⇒ |← 6-8 →|

Shaken Baby Syndrome

hard to diagnose

- 1/3 missed: "viral gastroenteritis, flu, rule out sepsis"

risks (these are very similar to risk factors of having an alcohol-affected child)

- young parent
- single
- unstable
- interpersonal violence
- ↓ nutrition, housing, $
- ↑ stress
- parental depression
- drug and alcohol abuse
- no job or low hours
- judge baby's crying to be "excessive"

(Christian, 2006)

The ADHD of FASD (continued)

- Earlier onset – often, as infant meet criteria for "Regulatory Disorder" esp. "hard to warm up or difficult to settle" leads to decrease in getting "in synch" with parents (attunement)
- More side effects esp. to Methylphenidate esp. generic
- Methylphenidate should not be used in Native American Children with FASD because of lack of effectiveness and above side effects i.e. growth suppression
- More Psychiatric diagnoses: Depression, Anxiety, and explosiveness
- More common: Complex learning disorders especially math and higher order language

Management: sensory integration, language therapy, special schooling, non-verbal play therapy, medications, parent education, and supportive Family Therapy.

"ADHD IS THE MOST LIKELY DISGUISE FOR FASD…"-(O'Malley, K.)

"Standard" ADHD

- Focus and Sustain worse
- Imbalance of Fronto-Nigro-Striatal Dopamine Pathway (where methylphenidate works)

ADHD with FASD

- Encode and shift worse
- More of a problem of abnormal D_1 Receptors in mesolimbic area

References

Anterobus T (2004) *FASDConnections Meeting*, Surrey, B.C.

Astley S (2004) *Diagnostic Guide for Fetal Alcohol Spectrum Disorders: The 4-Digit Code (3rd edition)*. FAS Diagnostic and Prevention Network, U. of Washington, Seattle.

Barr RG , et al. (2006) Age-related incidence curve of hospitalized Shaken Baby Syndrome cases: convergent evidence for crying as a trigger to shaking. *Child Abuse and Neglect 30(1): 7-16*

Bonthius DJ, et al. (2006) Proceedings of the 2006 annual meeting of the Fetal Alcohol Spectrum Disorders study group. *Alcohol 40(1): 61-65*

Bookstien FL, et al. (2007) Many infants prenatally exposed to high levels of alcohol prenatally show one particular abnormality of the corpus callosum. *Alcoholism: Clinical and Experimental Research 31(5)*: 868-879

Castellanos FX, et al. (2002) "Biological underpinnings of ADHD" in *Hyperactivity and Attention Disorders of Childhood 2nd edition.* (Ed.) Sandberg S. Cambridge University Press, Cambridge, U.K. p 349

Christian C, et al. (2006) Epidemiology, mechanisms, and types of inflicted head injuries in infants and children. *UpToDate 15.3 (medical reference CD-ROM)*

Chudley AE, et al. (2005) Fetal alcohol spectrum disorder: Canadian Guidelines for diagnosis. *CMAJ 172 (Supplement 5)*: S1-S21

Clarren S (2008) Plenary session Canada NW FASD Partnership Intl. Conference on FASD, Banff. (May 22, 2008)

Coggins T, et al. (1998) Analysing Narrative Production. *Linguistics and Phonetics 12(3)*: 221-236

Cortese BM, et al. (2006) Magnetic resonance and spectroscopic imaging in prenatal alcohol exposed children: preliminary findings in the caudate nucleus. *Neurotoxicology and Teratology 28(5)*: 597-606

Corwin MJ (2007) Sudden Infant Death Syndrome. *UpToDate 15.3 (medical reference CD-ROM)*

References slide 2

Fast DK, et al. (1999) Identifying fetal alcohol syndrome among youth in the Criminal Justice System. *Journal of Developmental and Behavioral Pediatrics 20(5):* 370-372

Fryer SL,et al. (2007) Evaluation of psychopathological conditions in children with heavy prenatal alcohol exposure. *Pediatrics 119(3):* e733-e741

Goodlett CR, et al. (2005) Alcohol teratogenesis: mechanisms of damage and strategies for intervention. *Experimental Biology and Medicine 230:* 394-406

Huebert K, Raftis C (1996) *Fetal Alcohol Syndrome and other Alcohol-related Birth Defects (2nd. edition)* Alberta: Alcohol and Drug Commission

Jan JE. (2008) Personal Communication

Lebel C, et al. (2008) Brain diffusion abnormalities in children with Fetal Alcohol Spectrum Disorder. *Alcoholism: Clinical and Experimental Research 32(10):* 1-9

Linden DJ (2007) *The Accidental Mind: How Brain Evolution has given us Love, Memory, Dreams and God.* Belknap Press, Harvard U. Press, Cambridge, Mass.

MacPherson P, Chudley AE. (2007) FASD in a correctional population: preliminary results from an incidence study. Presented at Fetal Alcohol Canadian Expertise 2007 Meeting. downloaded from http://www.knowledgenetwork.ca/fasvi/webcast/index.html

Malisza K. (2004) Evaluation of executive function of FASD. Presented at Fetal Alcohol Canadian Expertise 2004 Meeting. downloaded from http://www.knowledgenetwork.ca/fasiii/index.html

May PA, et al. (2000) Epidemiology of fetal alcohol syndrome in a South African community in the Western Cape Province. *American Journal of Public Health 90:* 1905-1912

May PA, et al. (2006) Epidemiology of FASD in a province in Italy: prevalence and characteristics of children in a random sample of schools. *Alcoholism: Clinical and Experimental Research 30(9):* 1562-1575

May PA, et al. (2007) The epidemiology of fetal alcohol syndrome and partial fetal alcohol syndrome in a South African community. Drug Alcohol Depend 88: 259-271

May PA, et al. (2009) Prevalence and epidemiologic characteristics of FASD from various research methods with an emphasis on recent in-school studies. Developmental Disabilities Research Reviews15: 176-192

Medina AE, et al. (2006) Restoration of neuronal plasticity by a phosphodiesterase type 1 inhibitor in a model of fetal alcohol exposure. *Journal of Neuroscience 26(3):* 1057-1060

References slide 3

O'Malley KD. (editor) (2007) *ADHD and Fetal Alcohol Spectrum Disorders.* Nova Science Publishers, Inc., New York

Patterson DS, et al. (2006) Multiple serotonergic brainstem abnormalities in Sudden Infant Death Syndrome. *JAMA 296(17):* 2124-2132

Powrozek TA, Zhou FC. 2005. Effects of parental alcohol exposure on the development of the vibrissal somatosensory cortical barrel network. Brain research. Developmental brain research 155(2): 135-146

Robinson GC, et al. (1987) Clinical profile and prevalence of Fetal Alcohol Syndrome in an isolated community in B.C. *Canadian Medical Association Journal 137:* 203-207

Sampson PD,et al. (1997) Incidence of fetal alcohol syndrome and prevalence of alcohol-related neurodevelopmental disorder. *Teratology 56(5):* 317-326

Sowell ER, et al. (2001) Mapping callosal morphology and cognitive correlates: effects of heavy prenatal exposure. *Neurology 57(2):* 235-244

Sowell ER, et al. (2008) Abnormal cortical thickness and brain behavior correlation patterns in individuals with heavy prenatal alcohol exposure. *Cerebral Cortex 18:* 635-639

Spadoni, AD, et al. (2007) Neuroimaging and Fetal Alcohol Spectrum Disorders. *Neuroscience and Neurobehavioral Review 31:* 239-245

Stromland K, Hellstrom A. (1996) Fetal Alcohol Syndrome- and opthalmological and socioeducational prospective study. *Pediatrics 97(6):* 845-849

Sutherland, RJ. (2003) Prenatal alcohol exposure neuropathology and cognition: integrating behavioral and neural approaches in rats and humans. Presented at Fetal Alcohol Canadian Expertise 2003 Meeting. downloaded from http://www.knowledgenetwork.ca/fasii/index.html

Ward SL, et al. (1990) SIDS in infants of substance abusing mothers. *Journal of Pediatrics 117(6):* 876-881

Zhou FC, et al. (2005)General discussion at the Fetal Alcohol syndrome Symposium. *Experimental Biology and Medicine 230:* 407-412

Chapter Four

Relevant FASD brain biology differences to consider when viewing Dr. Gordon Neufeld's "Vital connection" attachment-parenting DVD series

I sought further training from Dr. Gordon Neufeld because I think his attachment-parenting videos are among of the most constructive, practical, empowering resources available for parents of any children. Several years ago, Dr. Neufeld and his faculty trained me as a facilitator of this video course and since then I have presented it to numerous parent and professional groups. To use Dr. Neufeld's concepts with children who have FASD, I find it helpful to keep in mind the relevant FASD-specific brain differences presented in this chapter.

The chapter is based on an 8-session DVD set called: "Power to Parent- Part 1 of a 3 part Series: *The Vital Connection*" which can be obtained from: http://www.gordonneufeld.com/products Readers may want to check their local public library because many hold Dr. Neufeld's books and DVDs; additionally, many parent support organizations use his materials. In preparing this chapter, I used the most recent version of *The Vital Connection* (released in 2010 - yellow cover). If readers locate the older version of the DVD series, this chapter will still serve as a useful study guide. Although the times will differ slightly in the older DVD, Dr. Neufeld discusses the same concepts in each session.

I am grateful to Dr. Neufeld for his permission to use his materials in this way. He just said, "Be sure to make it clear what's mine and what's yours!" Thus, I have separated his comments from mine. It will take readers 55 minutes each to look at each of Dr. Neufeld's sessions - and, additionally, about 30 minutes to review my comments on each session.

This is a significant study time commitment, but feedback has been very positive from parents who have taken the course. If you are a bewildered, depleted parent caring for a child with FASD and it's not going well - this chapter is for you. If you are a professional struggling to help families that are stuck in conflict and estrangement, this chapter is also for you. Despite the rants in Chapter One, I am not really a strident pushy fellow - on purpose - because I want you, the reader, to take notice when I do stand on a soapbox. I'm doing that now. I've been both a depleted parent and a struggling professional; Dr. Neufeld's ideas - integrated into our family's situation - have given hope. It does take a while to get your head around this material but I know you'll find the effort more than pays off.

I encourage readers to peruse the poster about this facilitated DVD course that I presented to the Fetal Alcohol Canadian Expertise (FACE) Meeting, September 14th, 2010 in Vancouver.

This is the content of the poster:

(Poster title) Restoring Hope: An Adapted Attachment-Parenting DVD Series Empowers Caregivers of Children who have FASD

Introduction: Why "The Vital Connection" is a suitable psychoeducational support/tool for caregivers of children who have FASD

Dr. Gordon Neufeld is a Developmental Psychologist who taught parenting and child development courses at UBC for many years. His concepts aim to keep the attachment connections between children and their parents *thriving and vital* despite many stressors (exhausted parents, post-partum depression, strange or even threatening child behaviour, or brain injury [including FASD] in kids or parents). I have found all eight of Dr. Neufeld's concepts to be of great help as I struggle to be the most effective Dad I can be for my own family. My wife and I have 4 children: 3 have ADHD, one has a Traumatic Brain Injury and one has FAS. I have not seen most of these concepts outside of Dr. Neufeld's work.

I have undertaken "Facilitator Training" so I am authorized to present his material. "The Vital Connection" is part one of Dr.

Neufeld's DVD series. I find that discussion of FASD-related brain biology differences helps parents apply Dr. Neufeld's concepts to their family situation if their kids have had prenatal alcohol exposure.

Key concepts in The Vital Connection (part one of Dr. Gordon Neufeld's Power to Parent attachment-parenting DVD)

1. Handling ***Aggression*** - "The Traffic Circle"
2. "***Counterwill***" - "talking back," refusing to listen to parents, etc.
3. Understanding "when you are with Dad you resist Mum," "when you are with peers you resist parents," and other competing or ***polarized attachments***
4. Guidelines for handling a ***crisis*** or "***incident***"
5. Six ways of becoming attached/ stages of attachment
6. "***Collect***" the child ***before*** you "***direct***" or "***correct***"
7. Helping an ***Alpha child to quit trying to control you - and depend on you instead***
8. Being "***Spoilt***" often means the child cannot accept failures and then re-direct his/her energy into problem solving

Participant feedback: spring 2010/fall 2009 Vital Connection courses: Usefulness of specific concepts for your family:

1.	Aggression/ "Traffic Circle"	n=10	3.8
2.	Counterwill ("Talking back", etc.)	n=10	3.8
3.	Polarized attachment	n=11	4.0
4.	Crisis Management	n=11	4.0
5.	Stages of attachment: senses, loyalty, significance, etc	n=11	3.7
6.	Collect before direct	n=7	3.7
7.	Alpha kids (that want to be "in control")	n=7	3.7
8.	Spoilt kids	n=7	3.7

Scale: 1=not helpful 2=helps a bit 3=helpful 4=very helpful

This feedback confirms that course content of "*The Vital Connection*" is perceived by caregivers to be practical and relevant.

Methods

Dr. Densmore provided facilitation of the 8-session Power to Parent - The Vital Connection DVD course to two different parent groups in the fall of 2009 and spring of 2010. Each session lasted 2.5 hours. The DVD took 55 minutes; the balance of course time was devoted to explaining Dr. Neufeld's concepts so they "fit" the specifics of each family's situation. Some parts of Dr. Neufeld's ideas need to be adapted to work well with the brain biology of children who have FASD - Dr. Densmore took about 20 minutes of each session to explain how the concepts could be applied for children affected by FASD. Sessions are designed to teach skills *not just present information*.

Courses were held at the Shuswap Children's Association in Salmon Arm, B.C. (population 17,000) and the Urban Native Health Center in Kamloops, B.C. (population 86,000). A total of 12 parents/ grandparents/caregivers (including 2 social workers) completed the course. 8 parents/ grandparents cared for a total of 11 children who were diagnosed with or suspected of having FASD. The remaining 4 parents/grandparents cared for 7 children who had various physical and mental health issues: 2 were diagnosed with ADHD, 2 had Traumatic Brain Injury (TBI), 2 were recently adopted from out of the country and 3 of the kids resided part-time with each of their parents who were in the midst of acrimonious marital breakdown.

Caregivers were surveyed to see what course content items were most helpful and to learn what changes in attitude, skills and confidence course attendance had achieved.

Results: Survey of caregiver responses before and after the 8-session facilitated DVD

PARENTING GOALS	# Responding	Before course	After course
Feeling empowered as a parent/ grandparent	11	2.2	3.4
Sense of confidence as a parent/grandparent	11	2.4	3.4
Sense of being able to cope with behaviours*	7	1.9	3.4
Being able to share feelings about parenting with someone who has gone through similar experiences*	7	2.9	3.7
Sense of effectiveness as a parent	9	2.5	3.6
Ability to understand your child's thoughts and behaviours*	11	2.2	3.7
Ideas that help if your child is upset or acting strange*	7	2.6	3.4
Ability to have realistic expectations re: behaviour and thinking of your child*	5	2.5	4.0
Ability to modify your response to the child's behaviour	4	2.0	2.9
Peace of mind	4	1.25	2.5

Scale: 1=very low 2=low 3= OK 4=optimal

* Denotes criteria from the list of "The Top Unmet Important Needs from Caregivers Raising Children with FASD and Behavior Problems" [3]

Limitations

It is appreciated that these caregiver groups were *not* homogeneous; not all were looking after children affected by FASD - nevertheless, in *real life* "Small Town" or "Medium-sized-city" Canada most support/psychoeducation initiatives are taught to caregivers who look after a heterogeneous group of children. Furthermore, Heather Carmichael Olson's recent review suggests that caregivers' most vexing child issues are not unique to FASD. [2] Parental stress was highest in families caring for children who more extreme levels of: 1) "externalizing" behaviour, 2) "internalizing" behaviour, 3) adaptive function problems and [especially] 4) more executive function problems. These four traits are not "FASD-specific" but are often seen in kids affected by ADHD, TBI, and attachment issues or living in a chaotic environment ("diagnoses" present in the 7 of my course participants' children *who did not* have FASD).

This small, unfunded study would also be improved by assessment of a control group - I cannot see how this could be done in a rural setting where overwhelmed parents are often desperate to try to get some answers and access any resources - but perhaps in a larger center control groups would be feasible. Also, a larger sample size would allow more confidence in results.

Not all who started the course could complete it - life was too chaotic for one divorcing couple to continue to attend. Dr. Neufeld's material is not "prescriptive" - parents first learn the concepts and then develop their own ways to apply the ideas to their family's specific situation. Overwhelmed, depleted parents sometimes just want to "be told what to do" and sometimes are too exhausted to "figure out what *that* behaviour means." This course is "too contemplative and analytical" to be immediately helpful for parents "in crisis." Two Mums who were just "swamped" by ongoing crises left the course after 2 or 3 sessions. If caregivers possess written/spoken language comprehension skills below grade 9-10 they struggle understanding parts of Dr. Neufeld's content. One Dad quit the course after three sessions because the language content was pretty challenging for him but found the aggression and polarized attachment concepts very helpful when I taught them to him "1 on 1." *Getting to* such a course could be problematic - lack of *transportation* or *childcare* were insurmountable barriers for several parents who wanted to attend. *Timing* was another limiting issue - the Kamloops course, taught at night, allowed more Dads to attend; the Salmon Arm course, taught Friday mornings, allowed easier attendance for caregivers of school-aged children.

Discussion

This small, unfunded study suggests that isolated, inadequately supported rural or smaller-city caregivers can significantly benefit from this facilitated 8-session attachment-parenting programme.

Olson and her group at the University of Washington, Seattle have recently underscored the central importance of good family function and a high-quality caregiving environment in achieving favorable long-term outcomes for individuals with FASD. [1] Caregiver resilience relates to a sense of satisfaction and efficacy in parenting. [2] Caregivers must be provided with adequate tools and resources to be able to effectively problem solve. No one expects a plumber to fix a sink without his wrench - or a surgeon to operate without her nurses or anaesthetist! Yet every day parents are expected to nurture, support, understand and advocate for their children who have special needs - this is an infinite job - no less demanding than the surgeon's or plumber's! And, having been an Adoptive Dad for 15 years to a child with FAS, I know caregivers are under-resourced - my hope is that educational initiatives such as this DVD course can be part of a solution.

Success is *undermined* if solutions are not found to the **"Top Unmet Important Family Needs from Caregivers Raising Children with FASD and Behavior Problems"[3]:**

1. Discuss feelings about my child with someone who has gone through the same experience*
2. Have help in preparing for the worst
3. Have enough resources for myself or the family
4. Have help in remaining hopeful about my child's future*
5. Get a break from my problems or responsibilities
6. Have complete information on my child's thinking problems*
7. Be reassured that it is usual to have negative feelings about changes in my child's behavior
8. Be shown what to do when my child is upset or acting strange*
9. Be told why my child acts in ways that are different, difficult or strange*

10. Have different professionals agree on the best way to help my child
11. Pay attention to my own needs

Does this facilitated DVD course address: "Top Unmet Important Family Needs from Caregivers Raising Children with FASD and Behavior Problems"?

As a clinician (and father of a child who has FASD) I'd love to be able to offer support for *all* these unmet needs with this modest intervention (the Neufeld DVD series). The five needs marked above with * (needs **#1, 4, 6, 8, and 9**) appear to be helped by the intervention. (See: RESULTS) I believe parental indications of increased confidence suggest that they have acquired some additional "tools" or "knowledge resources" so need **#3** may have been partially addressed by the course. Anecdotally, I can say that need **#7** (validating parent's negative feelings about their child's [mis]behaviour) was addressed. Both Dr. Neufeld and I gave numerous examples of when we personally "blew it" and reacted harshly when provoked by our kids. Malcolm Forbes' maxim, "Failure is success - if you learn from it," comes to mind!

I honestly did not fully consider "Preparing for the worst" (need **#2**) when I surveyed course participants - perhaps I am overly optimistic but I'd prefer to be that way - besides, believing (sometimes against considerable odds) in a positive outcome is good for your health. [4] Not disregarding the challenges of caring for children with cognitive and behavioural problems, Dr. George Singer *de-emphasizes* direct expression of emotion and the sharing of emotional support. Yet his psychoeducational groups parents (of children with Traumatic Brain Injury) "do talk openly about their feelings, and are often highly expressive, *but the (educational) context places emphasis on effective ways to cope with adversity and take care of oneself in the middle of extremely challenging circumstances."* [5] I support Dr. Singer's model for parent education groups.

Effective respite is needed to address need **#5** (getting a break). Need **#10** (professional agreement) requires a cohesive interprofessional "team" and need **#11** (caregiver self- care) requires parents to step back and partially "separate" or disengage themselves from the "crisis of the day" for long enough to actually lower their stress level - I often recommend psychologist, Dr. Alice Domar's book: *Self Nurture: Learning to Care for Yourself as*

Effectively as You Care for Everyone Else (Penguin Books, New York, 2001) - this fine read offers a wealth of self-care ideas in a practical format.

Conclusions

A commercially available DVD series (designed to equip caregivers with some skills to enrich or even reclaim vital attachments with their kids) appears to be a successful intervention for parents and grandparents of a mixed group of children. More than 65% of course participants were caring for a child with FASD. More than 60% of the children cared for were suspected to have or were diagnosed with FASD. I "added" enough information about the brain biology of FASD to facilitate adaption of course content for children affected by prenatal alcohol exposure.

Parents liked this course - some participant feedback:

- "This course has given me the ability to be more proactive than reactive."

- "I also like Nathan Ory's book, *Working with People with Challenging Behaviours*; Nathan's book and Gordon's course really help me when dealing with my son [who has FASD]."

- "I am really impressed with how helpful the ideas of polarized attachment are; they have helped me gain a constant closeness with all of my children - these ideas have helped me tremendously, and I see results in my children every day - especially through the difficult times. This class should be offered on reserve because it made so much sense and it was not confrontational at all. Thank you very much."

- "I appreciated the extra info directed at FASD; the 'Aggression' unit was useful and so was info on attachment."

- "A spoilt child is one protected from his own failures - now I know what to do for my daughter!"

- "This is such an excellent course, we wish it could be available and taught to all teachers, social workers and as many parents as possible."

- "Now I understand how to deal with toddler's tantrums - now I have ideas to test out"

- "This course improved relationship with my child and resulted in more harmony in the home; I can see a reduction in the incidents of friction or conflict."

- "I wanted more understanding of complex behavioural issues - this has happened and can be measured by seeing our way of parenting change when we have a deeper understanding of where the behaviour originates."

- "I hoped to become more proactive and less reactive - it has happened."

- "I hoped to better plan crisis management in advance [so as not to be "thrown off" by the next crisis] - this has happened."

- "This was a great course - good set up and discussions; I'd recommend it for all parents."

- "I don't always remember in the heat of the moment what I SHOULD do or say but now I have a reference to look at; I've used it."

The future

Dr. Neufeld's DVD Series is titled: *The Vital Connection* (part 1 of the 3 part *Power to Parent* Series) It is available for purchase from his website: http://www.gordonneufeld.com/products

Interested readers can obtain any of Dr. Neufeld's DVD's from his website but about 50 facilitators of these DVD courses have been trained. There may be a facilitator in your area - if so - attending a facilitated DVD course will likely be more helpful than just perusing the DVDs on your own. Facilitators have several hundred hours exposure to Dr. Neufeld's concepts and additional training in helping participants apply course content to their family's particular situation. A list of Facilitators can be found at: http://www.gordonneufeld.com/people/facilitator

I would like to design an FASD-specific caregiver education module to include:

1. Dr. Neufeld's ideas on restoration and preservation of robust relationships between caregivers and children (as taught in this parenting DVD)
2. Dr. Bruce Perry's model of how to optimally influence brain development for at-risk children (his "Neurosequential" model) [6]
3. Dr. Lucy Miller's understanding of sensory processing differences and therapies [7]
4. Concepts of recovery from trauma presented in the recent book edited by Dr. Edna Foa [8]
5. Dr. Gilles Julien's concepts of proactive "Social Pediatrics" [9]
6. Recent understandings of how brain biology is changed by prenatal alcohol exposure [10]

These six models for making sense of some of the issues encountered by kids affected by FASD and their families are simply the most helpful I have seen. I use these concepts every day in my primary care physician work with patients who have FASD.

I hope this modest presentation on *The Vital Connection*, (part 1 of Dr. Neufeld's parenting DVDs), can be of some assistance to those researching effective caregiver support strategies - and especially for the families they seek to support.

References for poster:

[1] Olson HC, Oti R, Gelo J, Beck S. 2009. "Family Matters:" Fetal Alcohol Spectrum Disorder and the Family. Developmental Disabilities Research Reviews15 (3): 235-249

[2] Olsen HC, et al. 2009. page 238

[3] Olsen HC, et al. 2009. page 242

[4] Waytz A. You have superpowers: How to tap the strange power of being wrong. ScientificAmerican.com. downloaded (August 15, 2010) from: http://www.scientificamerican.com/article.cfm?id=you-have-superpowers

[5] Singer GHS, Glang A, Williams JM. 1996. Children with Acquired Brain Injury: Educating and Supporting Families. Baltimore: Paul H. Brookes Publishing. page 239

[6] Perry BD. 2006. The Neurosequential Model of Therapeutics: Applying principles of neuroscience to clinical work with traumatized and maltreated children. In: Webb NB editor. Working with Traumatized Youth in Child Welfare. New York: The Guilford Press. pp 27-52

[7] Miller LJ, Fuller, DA. 2006. Sensational Kids: Hope and Help for Children with Sensory Processing Disorder (SPD) New York: Penguin Books

[8] Foa EB, Keane TM, Friedman MJ, Cohen JA, editors. 2008. Effective Treatments for PTSD, Second Edition: Practice Guidelines from the International Society for Traumatic Stress Studies. New York: The Guilford Press

[9] Julien G. 2004. A Different Kind of Care: The Social Pediatric Approach. Montreal: McGill-Queen's University Press.

[10] Norman AL, Crocker N, Mattson SN, Riley EP. Neuroimaging and Fetal Alcohol Spectrum Disorders. Developmental Disabilities Research Reviews15 (3): 209-217

Thanks for having a look at the poster, above. If you'd like to now start on the DVD series, a table with running times of each DVD session is presented next. The table includes a brief summary of Dr. Neufeld's concepts at each specific time along with my suggestions of relevant brain biology to consider when applying the concept to a child who has FASD.

Session One: Our Hidden Source of Power

Time 7:25

Dr. Neufeld's Statement: Attachment power gives us influence and authority to allow us to do the job of parenting

FASD-specific Comments: The strength of attachment depends, in part, on the child's *perception* of attachment signals of others (esp. parents). In FASD many of the parts of the brain's attachment and sensory perception "hardware" can be altered. An example is the mirror neuron system, which allows us to know quickly, accurately and automatically what other people *do* and what they *feel*. In FASD, one can imitate others' movements easily ("motor" mirror neurons usually work well) but often there is great difficulty in understanding others' emotions (problems with "emotional" mirror neurons).

FASD has two truths:

1) It really *is* permanent and serious brain damage but also (according to educator, Brian Redman)

2) Caregivers will *never cease to be amazed* at what their kids can accomplish!

There is, however, a severe dilemma: since kids with FASD take longer to mature, they need assistance and guidance from parents and other caring adults longer - maybe forever - but forming and maintaining these attachments is harder because of damage to their perceptual and attachment systems.

Dr. Neufeld says to the extent we are not mature we depend even more on attachments to caring adults to shoehorn ourselves into adulthood. Parents of older kids with FASD are painfully aware of this: the kids need attachments to caring, mature adults to negotiate life;

yet, at the same, time they resist parental involvement, "because I'm *19 - I'm an adult* now, Dad!" The *only* way parents and caregivers can influence outcomes for their kids is to have good communication - this requires an open channel, a conduit of connection between children and parents. This vital conduit is the result of deep, secure attachment.

TIme 15:00

Dr. Neufeld's Statement: These qualities in a child make that child easy to parent.

FASD-specific Comments: I think this is a great list to strive for in FASD but some items will be harder to attain. For instance: "Seeks our help" - implies that the child *knows* they need help with a given task. The self-awareness needed to know you are getting off-track is a prefrontal cortex/ sequencing/ executive function issue and this area is especially impaired in FASD. "Listens and attends to us" depends on accurate perceptions (of seeing and hearing your parents); this might be difficult if you had *visual or hearing oversensitivity*. Some kids with FASD have marked *touch oversensitivity*; hugs may be over the top; others cannot tolerate *direct eye contact* - especially if mum is mad at them! Such sensory differences can make deep attachments harder to achieve.

Time 21:46

Dr. Neufeld's Statement: Must have the heart of the child...

FASD-specific Comments: The unfortunate reality is that often kids with FASD experience multiple placements - they are often in and out of foster care as their birth parents attain abstinence and then relapse. Kids often come to expect impermanence - this can affect their ability to trust deeply and make it harder for them to attach - especially at the "give your heart away to" or "deep emotional connection to" levels.

I have also seen superficial "bond to anyone" behaviour in kids with FASD. The most profound example of this strong but indiscriminate and superficial attachment pattern is found in Williams Syndrome

- this disorder affects facial recognition - and in FASD some of the same areas are affected (Fusiform Gyrus and Superior Temporal lobe) but, I believe, to a lesser degree.

Time 29:45

Dr. Neufeld's Statement: To walk on your own two feet, to think for oneself, to have good boundaries

FASD-specific Comments: Really, *none* of us are truly *independent* - we are all interdependent. In FASD adaptive function and independence skills are often *profoundly* affected despite minimal (or even no) impairment in I.Q. - thus a core problem: kids can pass a test but flunk at life (skills). They look better than they can act or understand.

As Dr. Neufeld says, if children are not independent we need to facilitate their dependence on caring adults or they will fill an "attachment void" with peers. We have found that all aspects of our child's life have been enriched by support and tutoring from Deedee the landlady, and time spent with Uncle Garth, Auntie Anne, Gramma, Big Sisters, and Church youth group leaders. Sometimes when our child is in no mood to accept ideas from Mum or Dad, Deedee or Anne might be able to get through. Supervision and guidance is needed - the bigger the group doing it, the less onerous a task it is.

Time 40:00

Dr. Neufeld's Statement: Get on with the job of being "the answer" for your kids

FASD-specific Comments: I think this idea is even more important for kids who have FASD and/or posttraumatic stress disorder (PTSD) and/or Traumatic Brain Injury (TBI) and/or chaotic early social lives - any of these conditions dramatically increases a child's level of stress and stress reactivity. Psychiatrist Dr. Bruce Perry notes that FASD, neglect, abuse and chaos all overstimulate the body's stress system (Hypothalamic-Pituitary-Adrenal [HPA] Stress Axis). Kids so affected need to learn to tone down their level of stress even more than typical children or they will literally be going through the day in a state of "fight or flight or freeze!"

Young or immature kids don't calm down by themselves; they 1) first, link emotionally with mum or dad in an "attachment dance," and then 2) let the parents calm them down. This beginning stage of self-regulation of emotions depends on attachment. The firm base is even more important for kids with FASD - they have so much more stress and less self-regulatory brain hardware.

Session Two: Becoming Attached

Time 5:00

Dr. Neufeld's Statement: Children initially "keep parents close" by keeping them in sight, by smelling them, by touching them - through senses...

FASD-specific Comments: Susan Fleisher's NOFAS-UK caregiver's group and I spent several hours thinking about how bonding via senses would be affected by sensory oversensitivities/ sensory processing problems. Examples from this groups' kids: a 23 year-old who could not tolerate direct eye contact, an 8 year-old who would arch and pull away from a hug (touch oversensitive), many kids with poor coordination of eye muscles and slow reading/poor reading comprehension (visual discrimination problem) - all these sensory issues interfered with "getting in synch" with caregivers. Prenatal alcohol exposure can contribute to the cause of these sensory conditions that impair attachment. Additionally, exposure to trauma and resultant posttraumatic stress disorder (PTSD) is associated with startle reactions (oversensitivity) to, especially unexpected, touch, noise and smells.

Time 10:00

Dr. Neufeld's Statement: Electronic devices that facilitate attachment such as cell phones, text messaging and Skype ...

FASD-specific Comments: These can be very addicting. However, because they largely facilitate attachment at the most superficial levels, they usually cannot satiate or "fill up" attachment needs. Kids with FASD, yearning to fit in and connect, can spend literally all day using these devices. It is wisest to try to set up rules, habits, structures that everyone in the household can live with re: these devices: e.g. no cell phones/texts during meals, ½ hour of screen time *after* 1-2 hours of homework or reading.

Time 11:00

Dr. Neufeld's Statement:...By age 2, if all goes well, kids can attach by "sameness"

FASD-specific Comments: If vision is distorted, for example by double vision or other eye tracking problems, and hearing discrimination is poor, then *being able to imitate your parents* - essential for learning language - will be slower and more difficult.

Time 15:00

Dr. Neufeld's Statement: "Belonging" ... this is *my* Mum!...

FASD-specific Comments: If it is harder to *form a representation of another person (or object)* it would harder to "hold on to mum" when she's not there. Being connected to you mum when not right next to her depends on you forming a picture of mum in your mind and holding on to that picture while you are physically separated from her. Knowing "that iPod is mine" requires you to form a picture of the iPod in your mind (a representation) and then hold on to that picture when you are in a different room. Being connected to another or having ownership of an object *when you are not right next to or with the person/ object* requires you to form and hold on to a representation of the person/object. I have not seen studies on causes and underlying brain biology of representation formation in FASD, but many of the kids I see have great difficulty in this area.

Time 18:00

Dr. Neufeld's Statement: Be significant to... "You matter so much to me"

FASD-specific Comments: In FASD *concepts of quantity or amount* can be difficult. Unlike their unexposed peers, toddlers prenatally exposed to alcohol did not fix their gaze on a puppet show when the number of puppets changed - thus, researchers believe that prenatal alcohol exposure impairs primary number sense. To make "how much I love you" easier to understand it is wiser *not to talk about it*! It is better to give some concrete visual cue (e.g. hold your arms wide) - then "I love you this much" is easier to understand for someone who has difficulty forming concepts of quantities in their mind.

Time 24:00

Dr. Neufeld's Statement: When kids give you their hearts...

FASD-specific Comments: This zeros in on one of the most difficult parts of parenting children who have special needs. One mum, describing her son (who has FASD) said, "We adopted him when he was 5 years old - the first time he snuggled in close and tucked his head under my chin was when he was 12!" Especially if children have been exposed to multiple placements, chaos, or trauma, developing the deepest levels of attachment (psychological intimacy--that is, sharing secrets/ being known--and "giving your heart away") can be delayed. David Ziegler's 2000 book, *Raising Children who Refuse to be Raised: Parenting Skills and Therapy Interventions for the Most Difficult Children*, (Phoenix: Acacia Press) has been a helpful resource for many families in their quest to connect with previously traumatized kids.

Time 30:40

Dr. Neufeld's Statement: Deeper levels of attachment expose vulnerabilities

FASD-specific Comments: Sometimes, *especially if you have been exposed to neglect and abuse*, letting down your guard is so stressful (causes such a flooding of stress hormones such as adrenaline and cortisol) that you move to protect yourself by *refusing* to let yourself be in a vulnerable position.

Time 33:00

Dr. Neufeld's Statement: If the vulnerability is too much to bear, we move to defend ourselves.

FASD-specific Comments: In FASD the influence of the brain's main self-regulation centers (the prefrontal cortex and the hippocampus) are diminished because of direct brain damage to these structures and their communicating pathways. This means that there is less power to rein in impulses and less ability to talk down to strong emotions and calm oneself. If we genuinely want to help kids affected by FASD *everyone involved with them* (parents, teachers, child welfare workers, etc.) must strive to reduce stress whenever possible - otherwise the kids will send much of their lives emotionally overwhelmed (living in perpetual "fight/flight/and freeze" states).

Time 36:15

Dr. Neufeld's Statement: Some kids are born so sensitive...

FASD-specific Comments: Dr. Kieran O'Malley, in his 2007 book *ADHD and Fetal Alcohol Spectrum Disorders (FASD)*, (New York: Nova Science Publishers) says many babies with FASD have a high degree of oversensitivity to touch, noise, and smells. They startle excessively and have such great difficulties with feeding that they meet diagnostic criteria:

- *sensory* problems such as needing music or white noise to settle

- *motor* issues such as requiring rocking or jiggling to settle and

- *behavioural* issues such as extreme fussiness or irritability

for *regulatory disorder of infancy.* Regulatory disorder of infancy is a diagnostic category in the DC:0-3R, a diagnostic manual used by infant mental health clinicians. Kids affected by FASD are often born overly sensitive - caregivers need to decrease over-stimulation. Dr. Lucy Miller's 2006 book, *Sensational Kids: Hope and Help for Children with Sensory Processing Disorder (SPD),* offers some wise guidance for parents with overly sensitive children. (New York: A Perigee Book). I have included a narrated power point about understanding and developing strategies for sensory problems in this book.

Time 38:00

Dr. Neufeld's Statement: Peer interaction is a major source of wounding

FASD-specific Comments: Peers matter too much for many kids affected by FASD. They ache for acceptance; they are *devastated* by ostracism. The stigma of being different and not fitting in is crushing. (Stigma is such a crippling, injurious *problem for anyone with mental health issues* that the Canadian Psychiatric Association devoted the entire 2008 year to addressing this issue.) As Dr. Neufeld says, for anyone, peers can be a major source of wounding - and being well attached to caring adults can help buffer the damage. In FASD, it is *even more* important to link our kids to caring adults because *they will* suffer a lot more than average kids from peer rejection.

Time 44:30

Dr. Neufeld's Statement: What my dad (and other adults) think of me and how they interact with me protects me from bullies

FASD-specific Comments: Knowing you are loved and valued by parents - at exactly the same time as you are being ostracized by peers - depends to a degree on your working memory holding strong messages of adult acceptance and support "online" whilst you are dealing with peer rejection. Working memory functions are amongst the most damaged by prenatal exposure to alcohol. To help our kids remember adult support it may be wise to give them a concrete reminder, such as a locket that says "I love you" or lots of pictures to keep in familiar places that show hugs from grandma, trips with grandpa, etc. These reminders will help compensate for smaller capacity working memory.

Being deeply accepted ("really rating with") a caring adult is a potent protective effect for mental health. Its opposite, invalidation and social rejection, is toxic. Diane Malbin, a social worker and mum in Portland, Oregon, presents FASD: *Into Action* training courses. At one such course I attended, a lady from the back of the class started crying. "I get it," she said: "I am the very first adult that ever really cares, that ever really gives a s__ about this 25 year old guy in my care!" She was his parole officer. The whole class cried. Isn't it beyond sad to think of growing up without adult acceptance? No wonder this fellow was in jail. What is gratifying, though, is that even at the advanced age of 25, when the parole officer made efforts to concern herself with and give a damn about this young man in her custody he was able to make great progress towards accountability and self-care.

Time 47:00

Dr. Neufeld's Statement: If I get close I expect to get hurt

FASD-specific Comments: Handling emotional intimacy can be bewildering for many of us - but kids with FASD, because they have difficulty understanding non-verbal information (body language), can suffer extremes of social awkwardness. Alternatively they can try to over-control the situation by being the class clown, the cool risk-taker, the generous guy that buys pot or drinks for his "friends," etc.

Dr. Neufeld suggests that adults can help impart social skills to less mature folks by 1) getting in a caring "right" relationship and then 2) once the young people are receptive and listening, by *scripting how to relate to others*. E.g. "I like boys too - to talk with them stand about an arm's length away. Ask them a question and if they turn away or ignore you don't worry - just go ask someone else."

Session Three: Harnessing the Power of Attachment

Time 9:30

Dr. Neufeld's Statement: Many people don't have a sense of whether they are "invited to exist in another's presence" or not - they don't "do this dance" very well

FASD-specific Comments: Two comments re: FASD:

1) Often reading body language, gestures, and non-verbal communication are areas of great difficulty - problems here lead to difficulties keeping friends and social ostracism.

2) Eye contact, though not often as threatening as it might be for a child who has autism, can still be uncomfortable. Forcing kids to look at you, esp. when you are angry with them, can put the kids into a "fight, flight or freeze" mindset. In this case they have virtually no language processing - talking to them will not calm the situation, resolve anything, or teach anything. One mum who forced her son to look at her when disciplining him changed this practice - and estrangement that had lasted for years ended when she made this change. Direct eye contact, in Dr. Neufeld's words, was a "vulnerability too much to bear" for this lady's son. He moved back home after his mum no longer insisted he look at her when she was angry with him.

Time 22:00

Dr. Neufeld's Statement: "Hurry up - you've got to do this..."

FASD-specific Comments: It's variable, but often, in part because of sensory processing issues, kids with FASD can take a long time to get revved up enough to start their day. *Alerting activities* like taking a shower, brushing their hair, or a pillow fight with Dad, *heavy work activities* such as wheelbarrow walking, and *deep pressure activities* like a big bear hug or maybe a story while you are wrapped up in Dad's arms with a heavy quilt wrapped around you can be ideal ways to get the "arousal level" set to a high enough energy point to function.

People unfamiliar with sensory processing and muscle coordination difficulties may mistake slowness in the morning as an attitude problem. Personally, I struggle to get going (and even to have proper muscle coordination) first thing in the morning and, believe me, these issues have *nothing* to do with lack of willpower or desire to improve!

Time 24:50

Dr. Neufeld's Statement: The ratio of 2 positive interactions to each "directive"...

FASD-specific Comments: FASD makes life really difficult. Kids make *many* mistakes; they experience many failures and need many corrections. They become defensive and fed up with failure.

In FASD, corrections are needed even more frequently. It becomes even more vital to maintain a viable communication channel so such information can be listened to and acted on rather than defended against and ignored. I think that for kids affected by FASD, the ratio needs to be a bit higher - 3 or 4 positives for each negative or directive comment.

Time 31:30

Dr. Neufeld's Statement: Warmth, delight, enjoyment

FASD-specific Comments: Depletion in caregivers is the rule rather than the exception. Depletion is a barrier - it requires energy (that you might not have) to look at kids and maintain a feeling of warmth, delight and enjoyment when you are worn out. Parental weariness may result in harshness. This makes it more difficult to prime receptiveness in the kids.

Much of the time, interaction with our kids proceeds *without* a sense of connection; our interactions are *not* characterized by warmth, delight and enjoyment. Is it any wonder that the outcome of many such interactions can be described as "unproductive head-butting?"

Time 40:00

Dr. Neufeld's Statement: The issue is: does the child *want* to do it herself?

FASD-specific Comments: In FASD, I think very often children *do* want to do a task *but have struggles figuring out how to get started*. It is helpful to think of "bookends" - how to get started and how to know you have completed a task. If we coach our kids on these bookends, more often than not we will see that they just need a bit of help figuring out how to get started, and then they can do the task. Later, a bit of coaching re: whether the child is "done" (or what is needed to complete the task) can be very helpful. Assume the child *does* want to do a task and try these coaching ideas and you will meet with more success.

Time 41:30

Dr. Neufeld's Statement: To resist dependence is to encourage the transference of dependence to others

FASD-specific Comments: Unfortunately, kids with FASD don't often succeed on their own - if they are not linked to caring adults they will flee to others (such as not-always-wonderful "boyfriends" on the internet, peers or gangs) to be taken care of. It is hard work, but maintaining connection with a team of supportive adults can be a key for successful transition to adulthood.

Additionally, Dr. Neufeld points out that if young people can connect with an established *role* such as being a mother, being an employee at A. &W., being a singer, etc., such a role can help "shoehorn them into adulthood." (Source: Dr. Neufeld's DVD Series: Making Sense Out of Adolescence)

Time 44:00

Dr. Neufeld's Statement: You are her compass point...

FASD-specific Comments: In FASD, linking with trusted people to help you make sense of your world is needed for a longer time - often forever. Frequently, non-FASD-aware programmes provide wonderful support for a year or two, and then end for arbitrary reasons. Programme directors are mystified when progress is not sustained after support has ended - they don't understand that the success was *due to the support.*

I would love to know of some way of growing better adaptive function. Avoidance of trauma, extreme stress, and substance abuse helps adaptive problem solving become as good as it can be - but often folks with FASD need an external trusted person to bounce ideas off in order to avoid blunders. Authoritarian or judgmental attitudes kill the trust required for such a relationship.

In British Columbia, the Representation Agreement programme aims to honor folks with FASD and other disabilities by having them appoint trusted friends or family as spokespeople that have authority to interact on their behalf with virtually anyone - lawyers, bank officials, Government officials, etc. This programme extends the concepts of "a trusted adult to act as a disabled person's compass point and help him or her make sense of life events" in a more formal way. Otherwise, as my family has found, officials have no problems with matters of confidentiality *when they want you to pay for something* that your (over 18) child has signed up for (like a loan or a course at college or some credit card or cell phone matter), but they have *endless* problems "because he is an independent adult and I can't tell you that and violate confidentiality" answering any of your questions! (Yes, I *am* just a bit bitter!)

45:00

Dr. Neufeld's Statement: Provide more than is pursued

FASD-specific Comments: Kids (especially if they had to contend with early abuse, chaos or neglect as well as FASD) may wear dark colored "glasses" that won't let them see good things that are done for them and good will that is extended to them. Kids can perseverate on how hard done by they are and what monsters their parents are for not letting them communicate with that friendly guy from Utah on Facebook, etc. In FASD, outward signs that kids perceive how much caregiver love is poured in can be frustratingly minimal - at times parents doubt that their efforts sink in.

If I had not been a parent for nearly 18 years I might not really know that long-term optimism *is more realistic* than being discouraged - kindness and support really do register eventually. One idea that helps is to be sure, especially in volatile teen years, that kids have connections to other adults that are connected with you - coaches, youth group leaders, aunts and uncles, etc. Go out of your way to facilitate these connections - the effort will pay off.

Time 48:40

Dr. Neufeld's Statement: Be "alpha", be the answer to their attachment needs

FASD-specific Comments: In FASD often parents are depleted and cannot find the energy to act like they are "alpha" and in charge. I understand this; I've been there. Nevertheless, as Dr. Neufeld says, if you cannot present yourself as "the child's best bet," your kids will have less ability to depend on you and you will have less control of them. The quest is sometimes to find your alpha, "I can take care of you", protective instincts *in spite* of being depleted simply because, to be blunt, you, as a caregiver of someone who has FASD, don't have time to fiddle around being ineffective!

Dr. Dave Ziegler describes this dynamic as "fake it 'till you make it!" Dr. Sterling Clarren adds: "Raising a child who has FASD (profoundly) grows *us* up also!"

Especially when overwhelmed I find Dr. Neufeld's concept, that *parents should be "a place of rest,"* to be a good "pole star" to aim for. At times, parents need to be actors (of confident characters) in order to be effective. It'd be nice if this was not so, but to be effective, often in daily life, we need to rise above our feelings - especially our hurts.

54:00

Dr. Neufeld's Statement: Steer into the skid

FASD-specific Comments: Dr. Dave Zeigler expands on the above concept with these comments: "If mum and dad 'win' - everyone wins; if the kids 'win' everyone loses." One of Dr. Zeigler's methods of steering into the skid sounds like this: "It usually takes William 2.2 minutes after we get home 'til he starts to hit Suzie - lets' see how long it takes him today!" (Concept: Mum is in charge, not William's impulses)

Session Four: Competing Attachments

There are several features of this course I find helpful for families raising kids who are affected by FASD - but these concepts of divided attachment energy and how to redirect it towards more constructive patterns are particularly valuable.

Time 14:10

Dr. Neufeld's Statement:...Gaze aversion in delinquents...

FASD-specific Comments: In the few studies done on the topic, about 25% of the youth held at juvenile detention centers were found to have FASD. Few youth detention centers or adult jails recognize or diagnose FASD in their inmates. Often incarcerated youth have chosen affiliation with peers - sometimes in a gang - over attachment to parents. Not infrequently, attachment with parents is strained because parents were not always supportive or even safe to be with.

Williams Syndrome is a rare (1 in 10,000) neurodevelopmental disorder caused by gene deletions on chromosome 7. It is characterized by *indiscriminate friendliness* towards strangers. At the level of forming distinct representations of the faces of familiar people (versus strangers) - the brain hardware of individuals with Williams Syndrome is flawed. Many kids with FASD I have worked with are unable to draw differences between their mum and sister (or - of more concern - which boys in their class they could trust they'd be safe with and which ones might take advantage of them) in art therapy. Whether this is due to flaws in facial recognition systems in FASD-affected individuals is not known as far as I know. However, I believe, at least for some, very serious "brain hardware" issues exist in areas devoted to facial recognition and areas that decide that "this is a friendly face so I ought to approach" versus "this is a threatening face so I ought to get away from him/her." My point: for biological reasons, I think kids affected by FASD often have reduced abilities to visually perceive potential ill will in others. This problem would increase the likelihood of potentially dangerous choices of friends.

Time 21:30

Dr. Neufeld's Statement: Can't be close with both at the same time.

FASD-specific Comments: This might be even more of a factor in FASD because of reduced working memory capacity. Thus, your ability to hold "online" your affection for your mum when you are with your dad (and vice-versa) would be diminished.

Time 28:00

Dr. Neufeld's Statement: (Immature) individuals have difficulty thinking about more than one person or one thing at a time

FASD-specific Comments: In FASD, diminished abilities to consider more than one point of view, or to be able to feel close to more than one person at a time, *may persist into adulthood*. These abilities require:

1) Flexibility - of being able to switch from one thought to another and

2) A good working memory

Both these functions are problematic in FASD.

Time 29:40

Dr. Neufeld's Statement: Deeper attachments are more resilient

FASD-specific Comments: But deeper ways to attach - being *significant* to the other, *giving your heart* to the other, and sharing secrets/being fully known to the other - are all more abstract, less concrete concepts. Those with FASD struggle more with understanding abstractions, so likely they will have more problems trying to forge deeper levels of connection. Even attachment at the level of the senses might be problematic because of sensory hypersensitivities or sensory discrimination problems.

So, what are caregivers to do? Brian Redman, who taught a work placement programme for youth affected by FASD at Franklin Pierce High School in Seattle, has helpful pointers: "Never hold a kid back because they don't have formal pre-requisites - with support, they'll often be successful. Two things are true: FASD causes real brain damage - but also, *I never fail to be amazed at the great things the kids can accomplish.*"

Time 38:00

Dr. Neufeld's Statement: It is good to keep all you care about on one side of the "attachment magnet"

FASD-specific Comments: Many families with kids who have FASD suffer social dysfunction and marital breakdown. Dr. Neufeld suggests "when the kid looks to you, if he can also see in you the conduit - the way he can connect to your ex-spouse - then he will not be pulled apart by competing attachment energy." In my observation, this dynamic is very powerful and - when utilized - has led to much healing in families who participated in this course.

Time 39:40

Dr. Neufeld's Statement:...Mistaken assumption that kids need their peers...

FASD-specific Comments: Because kids with FASD face ostracism parental support is even more important. Caregivers are wise to connect their kids to a network of caring adults - and to keep the lines of communication open with these supporters so they'll know what is actually going on when your kid claims how mean you are because you keep him 'caged up' and won't let him have any freedom like all the other kids have (translation: go to parties with underage drinking). Correct response from Uncle Joe: "Bummer! My mum wouldn't let me drink when I was 15 either!" Dumb response from Uncle Joe if he doesn't have any communication with you: "Gee whiz - your parents are over-controlling!" Point: communicate with your support network.

Time 43:00

Dr. Neufeld's Statement: To become one's own person, i.e. to develop an identity of your own

FASD-specific Comments: It may be achingly difficult for kids affected by FASD to emerge into adult personhood and then be able to engage with peers without a loss of identity.

Kids with FASD yearn for peer acceptance but are often taken advantage of, for example by being used as the "fall guy" by a gang. As mentioned, they'll be more resilient if they have good attachments to mature adults and a defined role such as being a singer, a painter, a musician, a mother, an employee at the Dairy Queen, or having a role at church. But often, kids bend over backwards to be with a boyfriend or girlfriend who parents think is bad news.

Question: What do you do when your daughter is smitten with a nasty guy that you know is up to no good? Answer from a very astute mum (oh, how I wish I was this smart): "Invite him to dinner, give him 2 hamburgers off the barbeque, always answer the phone before your daughter does and be interested in him - how is the brake job coming on your Cobalt? Etc. etc. - it'll drive a nasty guy NUTS and he'll move on - YAY! And if the guy turns out alright, he'll wonder what she's talking about when your daughter 'disses' you."

Time 49:00

Dr. Neufeld's Statement: Surrogate aunts and uncles

FASD-specific Comments: At the peak of teen angst, peer rejection, and teen rejection of parents - for our child age 15 - Lillis Bremnes, a youth group leader, was able to keep a close connection, listen to hours of whining and complaints, and steer our child back on track lovingly but firmly. Lillis was killed in a car accident, but not before she may well have saved a life - our child's. We are forever in her debt. We can never pay her back for these deeds of selflessness - but we will strive to pass on her kindness. Anyone who thinks this is overstated or melodramatic doesn't know what our child experienced at that age.

Time 51:00

Dr. Neufeld's Statement: Adoption

FASD-specific Comments: You can defuse competing attachments if you can be seen as the *conduit for communication to the other*. That might look like, "Well, it's your birthday so I bet your birth mum will be wanting to know you are okay. Even though we know she died a couple of years ago maybe we can write her a letter and put it in the fire and send it up to her in heaven so she can know you are safe..."

53:20

Dr. Neufeld's Statement: When the child looks to you he sees both (you and the competing attachment)

FASD-specific Comments: Kids with FASD, by definition, have *birth mothers* - and those individuals have a staggering burden of social and mental health issues:

-1/3 are dead or missing within three years of their children being diagnosed with an FASD

-They have an average of 4 DSM-4 Psychiatric Diagnoses - few, though, are actually diagnosed and fewer yet are appropriately treated

-The burden these mums face is beyond comprehension for the average person

-I have never met anyone who intentionally set out to harm their child by drinking while pregnant

-I believe caregivers should help their kids develop respect for their birth mums - if more saw the dignity of birth parents' struggles and supported funding for real solutions to the actual causes of their plight - such as inadequate housing and inadequate resources to help stop domestic violence - there'd be less FASD and the world would be a more civilized place. Point: don't diss birth mums - it is ignorant and, if you are a foster parent or adoptive parent, it is the opposite of Dr. Neufeld's concept of connecting to potentially competing attachments.

Time 56:00

Dr. Neufeld's Statement: Cultivate a deeper attachment

FASD-specific Comments: Tragically, some kids grow in utter social deprivation. Even in some unbelievably extreme situations of deprivation - such as an 11 year-old who was so neglected he could speak only unintelligible sounds - there were ways to attach through noticing preferences and helping the child learn about things he enjoyed. This would communicate significance - he *mattered* to you. Point: even in extremes, there are some ways of connecting and attaching that can be workable - and there is great benefit in finding them.

Session Five: Preserving and Restoring the Ties that Empower

Good for you! - You are half way through!

Time 6:20

Dr. Neufeld's Statement: The child should not be responsible for *my* feelings

FASD-specific Comments: Recognition of, naming, and dealing with feelings are areas of particular challenge for kids who have FASD. *Alexithymia* means "no words for emotions" - there is a chapter reviewing this issue in FASD in Kieran O'Malley's 2007 book, *ADHD and FASD*. A difficulty in identifying and processing emotions harms one's abilities to deal effectively with frustrations. Resilience and ability to adapt are reduced. Yes, impaired language ability can certainly make it difficult to accurately name and process emotions, but we need to assume that kids *deeply feel* all kinds of events - they just have trouble sorting out their feelings. Again, I would like to emphasize the importance of good attachments. A well-attached child will look to you to help them sort out their feelings and emotions - to act as their compass point. At school, programmes such as social circles can help.

Time 16:50

Dr. Neufeld's Statement: Relationship is more important than conduct

FASD-specific Comments: Foster or adoptive placements are common for kids with FASD. Unfortunately, the multiple placements that these kids often experience can profound harm a child's ability to develop a sense of permanency. An attitude of "if this dad doesn't work out, no worries, I'll just get another in a week or two," is a tragedy and a child protection system failure. Such a shallow sense of belonging handicaps development. Nevertheless, I've seen Dr. Neufeld's concept of bridging problem behaviour - "No worries, we'll figure out what to do, that was not a good morning but we'll be okay" - to have a huge impact even for kids with FASD who have been subjected to multiple placements. This message of unconditional support seems to cut through the façade of kids not caring.

If you are a frayed parent, separating the behaviour from the child will be something you know you *should* do but it will be difficult to not lose your temper when provoked. Many families live - at times - in a state of crisis and can't keep a neutral, positive tone. Respite, until parents can adopt a non-blaming tone with an emphasis on relationship, is sometimes necessary.

Time 25:30

Dr. Neufeld's Statement: Attraction to peers

FASD-specific Comments: As mentioned in Session Four, people with FASD have difficulty discriminating between who is a safe person to be with and who might be dangerous. Protecting kids from harm requires a level of supervision that might look invasive to people who do not understand FASD. Such supervision *allows* our kids to be as successful as they can be - and as safe from harm as they can be.

Time 27:20

Dr. Neufeld's Statement: Give them something of yours to hold on to during an absence

FASD-specific Comments: "Bridging" when you are physically separated from your child is a concept Dr. Neufeld believes to be very powerful - parents in courses I have taught have tried it to good effect. E.g. From a birth mum whose child went into foster care for several weeks whist she recovered from surgery: "I used my old T shirt as a pillow cover - it helped my daughter to stay connected even though I did not see her for 2 weeks."

Time 30:00

Dr. Neufeld's Statement: Be the answer for attachment hunger

FASD-specific Comments: A 25-year-old patient of mine truly has heart-wrenching struggles with knowing how to be a caring parent. He has FASD, and a terribly abusive mum who repeatedly abandoned him as a small child. She is addicted to cocaine, incessantly bugs her son for money and constantly voices disapproval: "You *still* don't have (full time) custody of your son?" His estranged partner, his child's mum, is in jail. He is striving to be a good father to his 4 year-old son; he has weekend custody. Problem: he has no useful model for how to parent or how to make good decisions re: rearing the child. Here's what we have tried to set up as best we can with no money!

1. Weekly meetings with trusted mental health counselors or me - mostly simple trouble shooting and topics such as easy food preparation ideas that kids like, fun kid activities, what to do if some nice man or lady says she'll watch your kid for an hour (how to decide if the offer of help is well-intentioned or potentially dangerous), how to cheer up your kid when he's dejected, etc.
2. Emergency on-call "external brain" numbers to call to talk with one of four trusted friends for advice if parenting problem-solving is needed and there is not time to wait to discuss it at the next meeting. Foster Mum is part of the on-call group. Model: Grandma's emergency phone

numbers that her medic alert gadget calls if she falls while she is alone.

3. Encourage this dad to do activities *that he is good at* with his son - such as music (to try to help bolster Dad's confidence in himself and his parenting)

Point: even this dad, with his unfortunate lack of positive parenting models, can be the answer to his child's attachment hunger. (Result: it is working!)

Time 31:45

Dr. Neufeld's Statement:...Give and give yet somehow it does not sink in...the child needs a softer heart

FASD-specific Comments: This can be a core issue in caring for kids with FASD - and can lead to parental burnout. We, and other parents, have learned that sometimes we need to "adaptively detach" (just a bit) so we don't burn out and so we can objectively make decisions - but not from a place of utter depletion and stress overload. Don't wait until all is well before doing restorative, creative activities such as taking flute lessons, joining a choir, taking painting courses, getting together with friends or spending a weekend just with the two of you. These activities help caregivers avoid burnout.

A problem is that sometimes in FASD, as psychologist Nathan Ory puts it, parents can try too hard - and even if they strive to assist or guide or correct their child still harder (leading to even quicker burnout), their kid often resists changes that would actually be helpful for him or her. Paradoxically, backing off can help break the impasse sometimes. Maybe, with backing off comes a new energy that Dr. Neufeld would see as newfound confidence to "be the child's best bet" - and this energy helps kids "let down their guard and follow the lead."

Time 33:30

Dr. Neufeld's Statement: Structure and ritual are important

FASD-specific Comments: If kids struggle to develop concepts then there are additional challenges adapting to new demands throughout the day. Rituals and traditions can reduce the number of choices that must be made and decrease the number of uncertainties that must be figured out.

Time 35:50

Dr. Neufeld's Statement: Don't let technology rule your family

FASD-specific Comments: As mentioned previously, kids with FASD find text messaging and other social networking technologies *irresistible*. Rules and rituals like these might help: nobody answers a phone or text during meals; violent video games or porn serve no useful purpose and are not viewed by anyone in the household; if budget allows: interesting biofeedback video games that promote self-regulation such as "The Wild Devine" are practiced; screen time is limited to ½ an hour - after chores and homework.

Time 38:30

Dr. Neufeld's Statement: The softer the heart, the deeper the attachment will become

FASD-specific Comments: Prenatal exposure to alcohol causes overactivation and oversensitivity of the body's stress system. A smaller degree of stress will cause a larger release of stress hormones for longer. This overreactivity is life-long, but recent work by Canadian Michael Meaney at McGill University has given us hope - nurturing interactions with caregivers can literally grow "off" switches for children's hyper-excitable stress systems. Point: I think kids with FASD have stress system overexcitability, which makes it even harder than for typical kids to let down their guard and become vulnerable enough to have a "soft heart" - yet I have seen, with gentle caregiver persistence and always in the context of safety, many examples of "kids" in their late teens and 20s become very open to direction from trusted adults.

Improvements in rigidity and refusal to become vulnerable have a biological basis in nurturing caregiving - this is Michael Meaney's message - so the faith of a dad that said, "we live by hope" at one of my courses has been borne out by recent scientific developments.

Time 39:10

Dr. Neufeld's Statement: Shield the child with a deep emotional attachment that is free from wounding

FASD-specific Comments: They will be taunted and teased...this is even a harder thing to deal with for kids with FASD - in part because they have fewer cognitive tools to defend themselves with, but also because they experience more disappointments and failures that could lead to ridicule. Calgary-based clinical social worker Liz Lawryk says that prenatal exposure to alcohol can damage so many different body and brain areas at so many different stages of gestation that generalizations about specific patterns of impaired function are impossible, but 100% of the people with FASD she works with have one crippling problem: low self-esteem. Resilience against further wounding experiences is very limited.

In his 2006 book, *Social Intelligence* (New York: Bantam Dell), Daniel Goleman points out that social ostracism is the *most* wounding (and stress provoking) of all experiences (page 231). Let's not gloss over this finding: shunning, rejection, snubbing, and ostracism of our kids by peers or adults causes massive release of stress hormones such as cortisol; flooded with stress, our kids cannot think properly and may fall prey to a gang or someone that would exploit them, or may self-harm. Playground bullies that abuse developmentally disabled classmates, or those that bully caregivers by intentional stonewalling or minimizing caregivers' concerns - or, even worse *blaming* us for our children's problems - ought to be dealt with harshly, for we all pay too high a price for the social ostracism they mete out.

Time 52:00

Dr. Neufeld's Statement: Flight from vulnerability/ emotional desensitization

FASD-specific Comments: In FASD you already have difficulties recognizing, naming and regulating emotions. Dealing with feelings is difficult to start with, which makes it even more important not to add on the additional problem of separation-induced emotional desensitization.

Time 57:30

Dr. Neufeld's Statement: Create an attachment void you are the one answer to

FASD-specific Comments: Creative ideas that parents of kids who have FASD have tried: "forgetting" the cell phone charger while on vacation, camping where there is no internet or cell phone coverage, canoeing, etc. As Dr. Neufeld suggests: arrange a situation where the kids *must* depend on you; for example, take a one-on-one trip - but make it several days not just a weekend. Try to get some habits started such as a movie night on Tuesdays, support the child's interests - if your child loves cars, try going to the next town just to kick tires.

Time 59:40

Dr. Neufeld's Statement: Hold on to your kids until they can hold on to themselves

FASD-specific Comments: I wish it was different, but no matter how optimal their family, many people with FASD need ongoing supervision and support as adults. Lucky ones may find a supportive, loving spouse. Most can benefit from a controlled environment where there are not too many choices, group social activities such as youth groups, regular get-togethers with supportive adults and basic jobs if the boss is supportive. Habits, routines, and reminders (such as putting appointments in your cell phone) can help.

Example: A pleasant 30 yr-old mother of two kids who had FASD herself. This lady lived on a US Army base with her family. This housing was ideal because she used the base store, did not have to drive, and could easily attend two women's/young mums' groups per week. This situation was excellent but her husband's job transfer forced the family to moved to a new town where housing was off the military base. In the new town, she had to drive everywhere. Planning, making meals and social life - in her words - "went to hell." She became very unhappy, quite irritated and grouchy with her kids. Moving a third time - back to living on base (more structure/ less choices) - resolved her problems with meal preparation, planning, social life and caring for her kids.

Session Six: Handling Aggression

Time 1:20

Dr. Neufeld's Statement: Imposition of "consequences" exacerbates aggression

FASD-specific Comments: We know a minimum of 1 in 4 - likely 1 in 3 - young offenders has FASD. Unrestrained aggression may be part of the reason they are in custody. Applying this session's methods for de-escalating aggression can be regarded as some of the most indispensible work caregivers can do.

Time 6:00

Dr. Neufeld's Statement: It might be your back that does not work

FASD-specific Comments: Consider sensory changes in FASD, specifically *poorly perceived messages from the body* (medical term: impaired interoceptive discrimination) A typical child, noticing a tummy ache, would see his mum and get soothed (or taken to emergency if it was severe.) A child with impaired body perceptions caused by FASD is not as able to grade the extent of the tummy ache and not as able to be soothed by his mum's reassurances. He is more distressed because the upset from the tummy ache causes a bigger release of stress chemicals like cortisol and adrenaline - this can lead to even higher levels of frustration. Though he may not be as fully aware of the exact causes of bodily distress because of impaired sensory discrimination, FASD causes overreactivity of the stress system so he will be more upset for longer by any given stressful issue - such as a tummy ache.

Point: Kids with FASD have many sensory perception and sensory processing reasons to have increased stress and frustration compared to their typically developing peers.

Time 7:50

Dr. Neufeld's Statement: We are looking for some story...

FASD-specific Comments: Kids with FASD are often unclear what the root cause of their frustration is. Often, they can recall just parts of an event ("spotty memory") and fill in the blanks by weaving a "creative" narrative (confabulation) between the small episodes they recall.

The uninitiated (to FASD) accuse our kids of lying - reality is more complex, though. Creative narrative *should* undergo an editing and correcting process *if the left brain narrative center can ship its "draft story" to the right brain's "editing areas."* Problem: in FASD impairment in corpus callosum function reduces the ability of the two sides of the brain to "cross-talk". The result: "unedited confabulation" - but it is *not* lying because the individual is genuinely trying her best to weave the items she remembers into a coherent story.

Ok, what might we do?

1. *Don't* ask, "What is your story, Billy?" when you see him fighting on the playground. You'll get a great story and your head will hurt trying to sort out what actually happened.
2. *Do* get "outside" corroboration, decide on a fair way to resolve the matter, and try to change the environment so a similar sequence of events is less likely.

Time 28:50

Dr. Neufeld's Statement: This is the path of tears...

FASD-specific Comments: To let themselves shed tears (either "for real" or symbolic tears) can be too threatening for some kids, especially if they have been abused. Rather than let themselves be vulnerable by admitting mistakes, sometimes kids will stick to their plan whether it is patently silly or not - they can become almost glued to an unworkable idea, a wrong-headed point of view or an unworkable plan. It is almost like an obsession with the absurd! Confronting doesn't work.

Example: an 8 yr-old boy who continued to insist he had not (repeatedly) taken his sister's iPod even though it was in his pocket. Plan: He was given a small amount of paroxetine, an SSRI antidepressant (the target was to reduce obsessive thought patterns), and his parents applied Dr. Bruce Perry's concepts of regular, rhythmic, repeated, age-appropriate fun activities (30-40 minutes a day trampoline, skipping rope, drumming). After a few months, self-regulation improved and paroxetine could be stopped with no return to previous obsessive-like behavior.

32:40

Dr. Neufeld's Statement: If there is any numbing out or tuning out of feelings it is harder to have tears of futility

FASD-specific Comments: I think alexithymia (reduced capacity for emotional processing) in FASD impairs recognition of and ability to cope with strong feelings. Touch oversensitivity might impair "attachment via the senses" and make it harder to relax into Mum and Dad's arms and be soothed. Parental burnout might further impair attachment.

Point: In FASD, brain biology predisposes to numbing out/ tuning out and impaired ability to attach - both these factors make it harder to have tears of futility. I wonder if lack of tears explains a portion of the *profoundly impaired adaptive function* that is almost universally found in FASD.

Time 34:29

Dr. Neufeld's Statement: When we have an impulse to attack we are supposed to have mixed feelings - these let us call forth reasons why acting on an impulse is not a good idea

FASD-specific Comments: In FASD the working memory area (where you hold an impulse on line while you consider the implications of acting on that impulse) is impaired. Even compared to other executive or prefrontal cortex functions, working memory is more profoundly impaired.

If the problem is reduced working memory capacity, one solution is to provide external structure. I find that when patients have a chance to actually see the implications of an action, most of the time they make good choices - impaired working memory just means they can't consider all relevant parts of a situation in their head.

Example: "Jason bugs me - I want to hit him."

	"Hit"	"Don't hit"
Advantage	It would feel good	I'd stay out of trouble
Disadvantage	I will end up in the principal's office and not have recess outside**	I'd bottle up all my feelings and explode and make a big mess all over the classroom! *

* I have found saying something silly and a bit off the wall gives everyone a giggle and brings out better problem-solving energy.

** Psychologist Nathan Ory suggests that for individuals with FASD the disadvantage (*what they will lose* if they do a certain thing) is a more potent motivator than the more abstract *advantage* they will gain by staying out of trouble."

Most often, when I show folks with FASD this little advantage/ disadvantage chart they make good decisions. Please try this with your kids. Marsha Linehan's Dialectical Behavioural Therapy uses similar tools.

Time 44:30

Dr. Neufeld's Statement: That's not how to share your frustration...

FASD-specific Comments: In FASD, meltdowns or incidents often follow:

1. An unanticipated transition
2. Sensory overload
3. Being cornered or coerced
4. A perception of being abandoned or separated from a social attachment
5. Out of the blue aggression might be due to a previous traumatic brain injury

As Dr. Neufeld suggests, kids in the middle of an incident are not processing subtle language. If they also have FASD then language comprehension will be *profoundly* impaired mid-crisis. *Try to use as few words as possible*, use gestures.

Useful ideas *to reduce incidents* follow 1) through 5) above. If you think the child reacted because of:

1. A transition - give her more warning, maybe a "visual time line" on her desk, etc.
2. Sensory overload - figure out her sensory profile and make changes based on this - talk to her Special Education teacher re: sensory tools. Look up: http://www.thespiralfoundation.org/
3. Being cornered - don't corner or coerce, review Dr. Neufeld's information on counterwill (Session Seven)
4. Abandonment - try to avoid separations and prepare for transitions, for instance when there is a new counselor, by ensuring there is an adequate introduction. From the 2008 UBC Developmental Disabilities Conference: The most common cause of an incident in group homes that house developmentally disabled mentally impaired adults? Perceived social abandonment.
5. Unrecognized traumatic brain injury - in my clinical work I see many patients with these issues. A useful approach is to look at Dr. Daniel Amen's assessment tools and advice: http://www.amenclinics.com/clinics/information/ways-we-can-help/agression

If you are worried your child might have a brain injury discuss this with your doctor; maybe take along a completed questionnaire (especially the temporal lobe section) from Dr. Amen's website to the appointment.

Time 45:58

Dr. Neufeld's Statement: That is when we are the least creative...

FASD-specific Comments: *Our kids* will find it difficult to creatively problem solve (or learn) mid-crisis also. It is silly to try to settle a dispute or teach a lesson in moments of upset. This is even more important in FASD. Think of the overactive stress response system and the excessive stress hormones - they sabotage memory, learning and language processing so that learning your lesson in the middle of a catastrophe is unlikely!

Time 50:40

Dr. Neufeld's Statement: Reduce separation-based frustration

FASD-specific Comments: Problem is, caregivers are overwhelmed - that's what this course aims to try to alleviate. Parents complain, "Dr. Neufeld says to not send my child to her room but I get so wound up that I might yell or worse." Dr. Neufeld suggests that *you*, the caregiver, might need some time out to cool down - you can almost always go to the bathroom, etc. - but if you send your kid to his room as a penalty you will further increase his frustration by imposing a separation.

Time 53:30

Dr. Neufeld's Statement: Facilitate safe eruptions of foul frustration

FASD-specific Comments: In our household often our child would come home utterly spent, steaming mad, ready to attack. *Words* did not calm but playing foosball worked! You could almost see the distress flowing out. Before long there was some laughter - and then you *could* talk about the frustrations. I *used* to let my kid beat me - but now I usually get trounced!

Time 55:10

Dr. Neufeld's Statement: You can't manage an emotion you don't have a relationship with

FASD-specific Comments: Several times, I've commented on impairments of emotional recognition and processing in FASD. Caregivers will find more success if they just "think younger and more concrete." Parents might approach a 9-year-old *as if* he was a 6-year-old; "You have lots of hits in you, eh William?"

"How does your engine run?" is a helpful programme for young kids. "If your engine is too hot you gotta let it cool down or it'll burn out." More info:

http://www.alertprogram.com

Time 59:00

Dr. Neufeld's Statement: Soften the heart

FASD-specific Comments: A lot of the time this can be accomplished in FASD by *validation*. In my clinical work sometimes I don't agree with what a patient has done, but saying, "I can see why you'd be so upset - anyone would be really angry in that situation," is very powerful. Validation melts hardness.

Session Seven: Handling Counterwill

Time 7:20

Dr. Neufeld's Statement: None of us likes to be pushed around...

FASD-specific Comments: Being pushed around is *pervasive* for kids who have FASD. They are often taken advantage of by "friends" and can't seem to live up to peer expectations. Caregivers, weary of behavioural challenges, can become rigid and controlling, sometimes micromanaging the kids in a bid to keep them out of trouble.

Time 23:30

Dr. Neufeld's Statement: Attachment is meant to preempt counterwill

FASD-specific Comments: In FASD, attachment, especially at deeper levels, is difficult. There are often more superficial levels of attachment. Result: It can be difficult to achieve powerful enough degrees of attachment energy to counteract the counterwill instinct.

Example: Special Education Teacher taking about a grade 9 boy (who has FASD): "Getting along with him has been a constant struggle *for years*." Her plan: "If it takes from now 'til Christmas - even if some curriculum must be set side - my goal is going to be to get a really solid connection and attachment with him *whatever it takes to achieve that!*" Result: the best year of school ever, *much* better cooperation and learning.

33:40

Dr. Neufeld's Statement: We need words to become conscious

FASD-specific Comments: But in FASD poor language ability and comprehension impairs ability to make meaning from words. Difficulty understanding the gist of a situation makes life much harder to negotiate.

Ideas to increase comprehension:

1) Keep words simpler, i.e. not too abstract
2) Don't talk and talk - avoid too many words
3) Never "teach" if you are upset (the message *will not be learned*)
4) Use repetition; use hands-on teaching methods

Time 39:40

Dr. Neufeld's Statement: Child has an alpha complex

FASD-specific Comments: In FASD, what looks like alpha behaviour (taking charge of a social situation) might be an attempt to not embarrass yourself. Slow language processing speed means you might be trying to figure out a sentence your classmate said while he is already 3 sentences ahead in the conversation. Asking him to slow down and clarify exposes you to ridicule for looking slow.

Poor understanding of non-verbal body language and gestures makes it hard to follow the gist of a conversation - why not take charge of the scene by being the class clown or talking constantly? Controlling a conversation means you don't have to respond; you can avoid misreading situations and looking clueless to your peers.

Time 43:00

Dr. Neufeld's Statement: A child is released from attachment hunger - he is filled up, satiated

FASD-specific Comments: Parents report their kids can be likened to "spaghetti colanders with holes that are too big." You can pour in support and hugs and other positive energy, but "it's hard to fill them up." Kids can have a "Cinderella complex:" "I have to work *all the time* but my sisters *get everything* and I *get nothing*!"

If you can't seem to fill up your kid Dr. Neufeld's ideas about "softening their hearts" might help. In FASD, parents have had some success writing positives down (make it concrete) - "Oh, it looks like you actually received *more* than your sister last week!" and enlisting help from uncles or aunts - "Oh, your dad makes you rake the leaves - bummer! But if you lived with me you'd need to cut the grass and do the edges also!"

Time 44:30

Dr. Neufeld's Statement: Taking charge of my own environment

FASD-specific Comments: Dr. Neufeld calls this taking charge energy "emergent play:" "let me do it my way, let me 'take the steering wheel', it's okay Mum - I can do it myself."

Emergent play depends on confidence in oneself. Emergence is not common in FASD. Creating nurturing relationships and building self-esteem will develop emergence as far as possible.

Time 46:00

Dr. Neufeld's Statement: If we see counterwill as "being on purpose"...

FASD-specific Comments: "FASD 101" (Chapter One of this book) starts with Dan Dubovsky's silly little acronym, **NURMU**. *If caregivers view* kids as Noncompliant, Uncooperative, Resistant, Manipulative or Unmotivated - especially if we are a bit exasperated or tired - our buttons get pushed and we get ticked off" with them.

Even if (parts of) NURMU are true, if we see our kids this way *the ensuing interchange will seldom progress beyond a head-butting session!* Even Mother Theresa would struggle to "collect before direct" if she was convinced the child was NURMU! To make progress, banish NURMU from your vocabulary! This is hard...but if you want to improve your happiness and your child's success do it.

Time 47:50

Dr. Neufeld's Statement: It provokes our alpha instincts and as a result we attack

FASD-specific Comments: If we can see preservation of relationship as a main priority and if we can allow ourselves to get curious about why our child has misbehaved in a certain way (see the neurobiology section of "FASD 101"), we can rise above the urge to attack or push back. Parents struggle with, "but I cannot let him *get away with that!*" I agree. You can't. But you have finite energy and time. Don't waste it on a strategy doomed to fail. Without the conduit, the channel for communication that comes from a viable relationship, *you cannot have any influence over your child*. If you want to be able to influence, you cannot characterize your kid as NURMU because you will sabotage your relationship and torpedo communication channels.

Time 50:00

Dr. Neufeld's Statement: Repair - when you blow it

FASD-specific Comments: Parents, including me, report great results from honest apologies when they are needed. Dr. Neufeld's example, "That did not go very well; sometimes I lose my temper too, but don't worry, we are okay and I'll figure it out" is a great model because:

1. It is honest
2. It conveys your regret
3. It leaves your dignity intact
4. It shows you care about your child's hurt feelings
5. In Dr. Neufeld's terms - it conveys that the relationship can take upsets and still survive

Time 52:35

Dr. Neufeld's Statement: GO FLUSH THAT TOILET RIGHT NOW!

FASD-specific Comments: Most of us, hearing this would have a surge of "counterwill energy." An additional factor in FASD is the easy startle with unexpected loud sounds (including yelling). Result: Kids are automatically flooded by excessive stress and enter a state of "Flight, Fight or Freeze." Children in these states can't think or process language (for instance, your command!) They take off (flight), yell back (fight) or curl up in a little ball (freeze).

Time 53:30

Dr. Neufeld's Statement: Refrain from SHOULDs

FASD-specific Comments: Humourist and stress expert (who consults on anxiety and depression issues for Massachusetts General Hospital) Loretta LaRoche says, "Don't Should on yourself or anyone else!"

Time 57:00

Dr. Neufeld's Statement: Pink pajamas or blue pajamas?

FASD-specific Comments: Giving kids choices - either of which we could live with - is a potent tool for our families. Kids with FASD have difficulty coming up with new ideas; that is, they have impaired concept formation. But they usually know which of two choices they'd prefer.

Making choices helps to build a sense of effective control over your life - self-efficacy. If we as caregivers generate possible options and then ask our children to select their choice, we can work around our kids' concept formation problems and empower them with a sense of some self-control. Being in charge of your own destiny - insofar as that is possible - builds *identity* and self-esteem.

Example: Mum's directions to her 11 year-old in Wendy's: "I am going to the bathroom so get whatever you'd like for yourself and a Taco salad for me." On her return, her child had purchased the Taco salad but nothing for himself. (He could easily order what she had requested but to formulate his own choice [i.e. develop the concept of what he wanted and then order it] was much more difficult) When his mum asked, "Would you like the hamburger or chicken burger, he immediately said, "The chicken burger."

This strategy of empowerment by giving choices - but keeping folks out of trouble by ensuring the choices offered to them are viable and safe - is a powerful way caregivers can help FASD-affected people *of any age*.

Session Eight: Guidelines for Discipline

Time 4:00

Dr. Neufeld's Statement: You may feel guilty about the times you've been trying to find consequences that you now know could increase separation between you and your kids

FASD-specific Comments: I have followed Gordon Neufeld's and Barabara Coloroso's teachings for over twenty years. Barbara is the author of *Kids are Worth It.* For as long as I can remember, she, and many other parenting experts, have advocated for appropriate, natural and swiftly imposed consequences for misbehavior.

But two years ago I attended a daylong workshop with Barbara Coloroso. "Don't praise, don't invent and impose consequences - these ideas won't pay off," she said.

We don't need to invent more consequences. Gordon Neufeld often says that life is a series of consequences. We'd assist our children's development better if we came alongside and coached them on how to deal with life's consequences.

Time 8:20

Dr. Neufeld's Statement: A primary challenge is our self discipline

FASD-specific Comments: Parents must release their urges to micromanage; yet keep their "natural and healthy arrogance" ("I am your best bet - you can depend on me") that Gordon Neufeld talks about. It's quite a dance to achieve this balance! Personally, I have probably made most every mistake that is possible in parenting - but once in a while I get a glimpse of this wonderful sweet spot - *the right amount of concern but not so much as to make kids feel over controlled.* Kids respond. Good things happen in the family.

For *parents* to grow into the resilient, non-reactive, validating, constructive people that their children need them to be is one of the biggest challenges in FASD according to Stirling Clarren, developmental pediatrician and CEO of the Canada Northwest FASD Research Network.

Time 14:00

Dr. Neufeld's Statement: Deeper layers of attachment are the roots of the child's desire "to be good for you"

FASD-specific Comments: Many of my "FASD-specific" comments address the difficulty that kids with FASD have in attaching (especially at deeper levels) - but pessimism is not my goal. It's just that building strong attachment *takes longer* and *requires more persistence*. Though I know it'll break your heart, try not to be frustrated if your child cannot seem to attain one of the deepest layers of attachment (such as sharing secrets). Choose the goal of helping your child attach as securely and deeply *as is possible*. By doing so you will help them develop *as far as possible*.

Time 16:50

Dr. Neufeld's Statement: Kids try as much as they can to measure up to expectations.

FASD-specific Comments: With language processing difficulties, *accurate understanding* of expectations becomes more difficult. Reduced working memory capacity makes it *tough to hold expectations on line* while being bombarded by impulses.

Kids with FASD don't willfully decide not to fulfill expectations. They *can't* fulfill expectations as easily as some of their peers - but if caregivers can appreciate the dignity of their struggles, our validation will help them achieve all they can.

Time 18:00

Dr. Neufeld's Statement: Collect before direct

FASD-specific Comments: If the situation you are in are in with your FASD-affected child isn't working ask yourself, "Is she collected?" My hunch is, more often than not, you'll pinpoint the problem. You are not reading this to review my failures in parenting, but when I find that my kids are being ridiculous, more often than not, they are not collected.

Time 19:30

Dr. Neufeld's Statement: Cannot control a child who cannot control himself

FASD-specific Comments: Self-regulation skills develop and grow in those affected by FASD, but not as easily and quickly as everyone would like. Dr. Bruce Perry's notions help guide caregivers:

1) The brain develops in a predictable sequence from lower (urge) areas to higher (able to suppress an urge) areas
2) Regular "doses" of rhythmic, repetitive, age-appropriate, fun exercises helps to calm stress and prime brain development
3) These exercises and supportive social attachments help grow brain circuits of self-regulation

More info re Dr. Perry's approaches is available at: http://www.childtrauma.org/

Time 22:55

Dr. Neufeld's Statement: Work with the child's memory of the incident

FASD-specific Comments: I don't want to disagree with trying to work with your child's recollection of an incident, but just need to point out that kids with FASD have spotty memory and creatively try to weave the parts of an incident they recall into a coherent story.

Sometimes making an educated guess what caused the incident (Probably Bill hit Sally because she teased him) and trying to develop habits or structures to prevent recurrences ("If others tease you, come talk to me") is the best way to go.

I've seen programmes such as "Circle of Friends" - info: social/circle/lecture01.html

And "Social Stories" - info: http://www.autismnetwork.org/modules/social/sstory/index.html

help build social problem solving skills in children affected by FASD.

Time 23:30

Dr. Neufeld's Statement: Delinquents with FASD

FASD-specific Comments: It might be best to wait a while to debrief - there are several FASD-related factors to consider:

1) Less effective self-regulation of the stress caused by upsets
2) Slower wind-down of the stress system
3) Impaired language processing
4) Ability to understand words and problem solve using words *is even more impaired if still upset*

Don't ask, "Do you understand?" or "Do you have any questions?" To oblige and to try to avoid embarrassment most kids with FASD will say, "Yes" (I understand) and "No" (I don't have questions).

If you want to know whether you've been understood, ask kids to explain the concept in their own words and coach them until they can apply the concept to some topic in their life. Three things will happen: you'll see how hard it is for the kids to make sense of what is going on; though it is a tedious process, the kids will have much better understanding; and - if you can be patient - the coaching role will deepen the relationship between you.

Time 25:20

Dr. Neufeld's Statement: Don't let anything sever the relationship

FASD-specific Comments: Malcolm Forbes says that *failure is success if you learn from it.* Solid relationships are the keys to letting ourselves become vulnerable enough, to let down our guard enough to be able to learn from failures. Without viable relationships, our ability to learn from mistakes and failures is diminished.

Time 26:30

Dr. Neufeld's Statement: Once we see the child as immature we are moved to assume responsibility

FASD-specific Comments: In FASD this concept may still apply even if the "child" is 20, or 25. By this time, many parents are burned out and passively capitulate to demands such as supplying money for an apartment (so their son can move in with a bad-news girlfriend), cosigning a credit card application, and so on. Parents think, "Well, he *has* to learn." The danger is that even if he gets a sexually transmitted disease from the bad-news girlfriend and gets his (or your) car repossessed to pay off credit card debt, *learning* from these blunders is not a given. What if he gets HIV?

I think parents should actively try to protect their FASD-affected kids from anticipatable harm as long as they possibly can. People who don't understand FASD may think you are over controlling, but in fact you are trying to help your kids be as successful as they can be.

Let's call this honestly - allowing FASD-affected adults to blunder into harm's way when others can anticipate the harm is *abusive*. Some would state, "you cannot infringe on his rights - he's an adult." I suggest he has the right to dignity as a person, to be as fully developed in his personhood as is possible - if he has HIV or must pay 55% of his meager monthly income to the Royal Bank to just meet the interest charges (at 18% per year) on his VISA card debt his quality of life will be drastically affected. (Both these issues - HIV and [Royal Bank Visa] credit card debt that can never be paid off and impoverishes families - have affected patients I see.) Forcing non-swimmers into the deep end of the pool is unthinkable - so why do we tolerate abuse of people with adaptive function impairments. Society needs to look out for them - we'd all benefit.

Useful ideas to support your adult-aged kids:

- Representation Agreements - info: http://www.rarc.ca/PDFs/RA_now_Dec_04.pdf

- Adult college programmes which offer support for kids affected by FASD such as those at the College of New Caledonia - info: http://www.cnc.bc.ca/Campuses/Lakes_District_Campus/Children__Family_and_Community_Programs/Supported_Work_Placement.htm

- A supportive boss, landlady, youth group leader or coach can help older kids stay on track. Try to facilitate your child's connections to these people.

Time 35:50

Dr. Neufeld's Statement: Use structure and ritual

FASD-specific Comments: Establish household rules and traditions about screen time, "safe sites" and devices at meals. Start early, before your kids are using many devices regularly.

Homework is just part of life for any kid but sometimes an unfortunate pattern happens in FASD. Trying to complete *all* the work that is not completed at school can turn home into a battleground *not* the attachment oasis and place of restoration it is supposed to be. Kids' MRI scans have shown that almost the whole brain lights up for even basic tasks in FASD. Our kids work harder to do a given task than their neurotypical peers. At the end of six hours of this they are pooped! They need rest and restoration. Eventually, my wife and I and our kid's teachers saw that more was learned overall with *no* regular homework but scheduled after school activities such as dance, youth group, bowling and music.

38:20

Dr. Neufeld's Statement: Scripting is the primary intervention for the immature

FASD-specific Comments: Effective self-directedness is really a struggle for many with FASD (even in their 20s). To help:

1) Collect first - then, once you've got a receptive audience, you can:

2) Provide a basic script that will help them function e.g. "This is how to talk to a policeman" or "This is what to say if a stranger asks if you want a ride."

Time 43:40

Dr. Neufeld's Statement: Help the child find his sadness when encountering futility

FASD-specific Comments: When our kids are upset their already imperfect ability to understand (especially abstract) language is further compromised. Try to give reasons using simple unambiguous words. Don't get into long explanations.

Time 50:00

Dr. Neufeld's Statement: When we become the parents our children need, it grows us up!

FASD-specific Comments: True for all parents, I think this statement is even more applicable if kids have FASD because they are less mature for a longer period, have less insight, are more reactive, and have more difficulties attaching on sensory, sameness, loyalty, being significant to, and sharing secrets levels. Parents need to be more involved for a longer time than they anticipated.

One of the most difficult issues is that at times it seems there is less reciprocity - less return of the love you pour in. At the end of the day, if you have done all you can to connect and encourage, you've done a lot. Having been an adoptive dad now for 15 years I can say I am more optimistic now than at any time about my relationship with my child.

Time 50:20

Dr. Neufeld's Statement: Find tempering elements

FASD-specific Comments: Use this concrete little line diagram as an external working memory aide (see also: Session Six - Aggression (time: 34:29)

	"Hit"	"Don't hit"
Advantage	It would feel good	I'd stay out of trouble
Disadvantage	I will end up in the principal's office and not have recess outside	I'd bottle up all my feelings and explode and make a big mess all over the classroom!

Time 56:10

Dr. Neufeld's Statement: Solicit a good intention

FASD-specific Comments: "I'd really like to quit snitching iPods," he said. "Great," said his mum. Now she can change from the role of policewoman, judge and jury to coach - and she can coach him on how to overcome barriers that get in the way of his intension.

One of my favourite researchers in this dynamic is Dr. Mark Ylvasaker. Sadly, Mark died of cancer May of 2009. He spent his career refining best practices for optimal rehabilitation of children with brain injuries. A good intention suggests a "buy-in," a choice to pursue a certain activity. Mark takes this idea further: "There is something that I say a lot in rehabilitation - **In the absence of meaningful engagement in chosen life activities, all interventions will ultimately fail."** (Message: work within the intentions, dreams, goals and actions your child chooses, and your interventions are more likely to succeed.)

I will finish these comments also with a quote from a letter Mark wrote me in response to my questions re which of his ideas might be most helpful to address self-regulation issues kids who had FASD:

"I am sure there is lots of overlap between FASD and TBI [traumatic brain injury]. My experience is that, in many cases, the most valuable contribution we might make is to present ourselves as roll-up-your-sleeves collaborators with parents in figuring out how best to help the kids. In particular when kids have executive function/self regulatory problems (common as you know in FASD and TBI) then the trick is to design everyday routines of interaction and support at home (and at school) consistent with the child's difficulties but also with a view to long term maturation in these areas."

To summarize, Mark suggests that kids set goals consistent with their dreams and caregivers (and their supporters) act as "roll-up-your-sleeves" coaches to help them accomplish what they can. The context of this work is everyday routine things we all have to do: get to school or work on time, remember to take our books, get to appointments on time, eat properly, figure out what the teacher or boss wants and try to do it, try to figure out why the dog is sick - the everyday stuff of life. So our job is to help our kids negotiate and make sense of life. As we plug away at this job some magic is happening - new brain circuits for self-regulation, self-esteem and identity are growing (even for kids with brain changes caused by trauma or prenatal exposure to alcohol and even in their mums and dads!)

Chapter Five

Music and FASD

For heights and depths no words can reach
Music is the soul's own speech

--Author unknown

Grief

A beloved cousin of mine died tragically last summer. He was only thirty-five. He and his wife had a baby on the way.

The words: shock, desolation, overwhelm, and devastation *do not begin* to describe our family's anguish and emptiness. Yet somehow music allowed us all - bumbling in our grief, not knowing what to say because words were so inadequate - to touch feelings that we really wanted to express. Of course, the melody is important also, but the lyrics to *Lay Your Hands* from the Canadian Catholic Hymnal were both poignant and healing:

Lay your hands gently upon us,
Let their touch render your peace,
Let them bring your forgiveness and healing
Lay your hands, gently lay your hands.

Lord we come to you through one another.
Lord we come to you in our need.
Lord we come to you seeking wholeness,
Lay your hands, gently lay your hands.

---Lyrics: Carey Landy

After 9/11, society, collectively, was at a loss. I don't remember a lot of the details from CNN reports of those times but, like many others, recall the moving rendition of *Amazing Grace* that Renee Fleming sang on Oct 28, 2001 from Ground Zero:

Amazing Grace, how sweet the sound,
That saved a wretch like me...
I once was lost but now am found,
Was blind, but now I see.

Through many dangers, toils and snares...
We have already come.
T'was Grace that brought us safe thus far...
And Grace shall lead us home.

A renowned opera singer, Renee Fleming explained her personal thoughts as she sang for the World Trade Center Memorial Service:

" ...and then I turned around and saw the faces of these nine thousand people who had crowded into this extremely narrow space.

...in their grief, trying to connect to the spot, to what we were doing...

It was definitely the most difficult thing I've ever had to do in terms of singing. Normally it's my job and joy to connect with the audience. I had to look above the audience because I just knew I would not be able to go on. It was the children..." [1]

Renee Fleming - at this time just barely able to hold on to her composure - was able to touch *core feelings* of longing and grief and *core needs* for connection, transcendence of suffering and hope with her singing. Somehow she channeled her inner struggles into emotional expression that helped her music access her listeners' deepest anguish. Her audience *was* not passive. Rather, they were swept along with the profound emotions found in Renee's singing as she struggled to reach beyond 9/11's tragedy for meaning and reassurance. Through active engagement with the music, her audience was transformed.

Lyrics are important but there are, arguably, even more vital forces at work within music. Also to assist people after 9/11, Leonard Slatkin conducted the BBC Orchestra on September 15, 2001 in honor of those who lost their lives a few days prior. They selected Samuel Barber's very evocative Adagio for Strings, op. 11. The performance can be watched at: http://www.youtube.com/watch?v=RRMz8fKkG2g

The combination of tight harmonies and simple, slow melody that gradually increases in pitch and strength takes listeners on a sad, intense journey, "full of pathos and cathartic passion, rarely leaving a dry eye," as Alexander Morin comments. [2] Adagio creates "an uneasy, shifting suspension as the melody begins a stepwise motion, like the hesitant climbing of stairs," adds Johanna Keller from The New York Times. [3]

After 9/11 people did not need an erudite treatise on some academic aspect of grief - they needed action - to be tangibly touched right down where it hurts, and then transformed. Music had and has the power to engage us - and then reshape us.

Music gives another avenue for expression

For everyone, grief is very real but it's difficult to process by talking about it - grief is just too big. In FASD, a lot of things happen to you that you cannot easily express. Arthur Sullivan introduces the concept of alexithymia (difficulties naming and processing emotions) in FASD. He explains that emotions need to be dealt with in some way or mental health issues are more common. [4]

I think music opens up potent pathways for processing and making sense out of strong emotions. Music's alternative pathways for emotional recognition and processing can "work around" some of the limitations of alexithymia.

"Music can name the unnamable and communicate the unknowable." ***---Leonard Bernstein***

Beauty - The piano in the lobby

Last December my wife and I heard a piano in a hotel lobby. After listening to some wonderfully played versions of familiar (and some new) Christmas songs for half an hour, I felt differently:

I was calmer, more focused, more grounded, able to think more clearly, at peace.

How could music do that?

From where does music derive its power?

More learned music lovers than I debate about the sacrilege of breaking music down into its elements. We will look at some of music's components but only with an understanding that, when combined, the sum of music's elements create something much bigger.

Overtones are important components of the over-arching feel of music. *Live acoustic* music can create even richer layers of overtones than amplified music. In the last few years our little church has organized a series of Christmas concerts. The place is small so no amplification is needed. We've been blessed by the participation of local musicians playing a variety of acoustic instruments including guitar, cello, Celtic harp and *4*-stop button accordion. When considering overtones, that accordion is interesting because with four stops each melody key actually plays four different sets of reeds. The top set is pitched two octaves above the bottom set. In addition, there are two sets of reeds pitched at the middle octave but tuned ever so slightly apart - so played together they "ring" with a beautiful series of overtones. Beyond the beautiful Christmas tunes, audiences comment on how uniquely rich and lush the sound is in that small space. I think overtones from the combination of acoustic instruments playing together are what make the sound so full. This year I played a hammer dulcimer with the other instruments. I'm not very good at playing fast yet, but am captivated by the *resonance* - that rich sound that gives me a tingle down the spine.

Several years ago I attended a Montreal Symphony Orchestra concert. I've always enjoyed symphony orchestras and have heard a number of them. But Montreal's was different - the sound was so full; it was *lush*. I think this difference comes from subtle adjustments in tuning (such as playing a minor third just a little bit sharp and playing a major third just a little bit flat so that chords will ring). Not all orchestras have the experience needed to make each chord ring - but when they do, I think rich layers of overtones create that lush sound.

Overtones arise from interacting sound waves and are defined as any frequency higher than the fundamental frequency of a sound. [5] Overtones create timbre - that discrete quality that makes one guitar "the one that sounds *just right*," and causes a note played on this favourite guitar to be heard differently from the same note played on a trumpet. Overtones can make our bones rattle the right way! Overtones are one reason why music can touch us so compellingly.

Getting back to that piano in the lobby - Shannon and I were impressed that simply listening could energize us and improve our moods for the whole morning. It sounded *so* beautiful. If it could so powerfully affect us, we wondered how much more it could do in a women's shelter or downtown drop-in center. I thought of several patients I see who live lives filled with such misery - violence, deception, poverty, invalidation - that concepts of beauty, of some realm beyond their suffering must seem impossibly distant. There is nothing beautiful in their day. Maybe someone reading this will decide to donate their piano to the local women's shelter and hire music students to play there on Friday mornings. Maybe the music will reduce suffering, and inspire someone to touch the divine/ the transcendent or to step outside his or her little slice of reality:

"Music washes away from the soul the dust of everyday life" ***---Berthold Aurbach***

"We need magic, and bliss, and power, myth and celebration and religion in our lives, and music is a good way to encapsulate a lot of it." ***---Jerry Garcia***

"Music at its essence is what gives us memories." ***---Stevie Wonder***

Phrasing

My trombone teacher at the University of Alberta Music School, John MacPherson, was one of the most musical guys I've known. One day, we looked at phrasing of two lines of music for *two hours*! A phrase must, above all, be natural. For example a slowing (a ritardando) must be like a car coming to a stop sign. At first the slowing is subtle, almost imperceptible, but then gradually the slowing will gather more and more momentum until one arrives at the pause. The slowing is not contrived and linear, it is much more in accord with natural phenomena.

A phrase begins with a breath and that breath is the start of the music - a fast breath suits fast music but a slower breath is required for slower passages.

The more the phrase resembles a natural breath, a smooth curve, and a natural occurrence, the more successful it'll be.

Stand like Pavarotti; *plant* your feet; let your belly go out when you take your breath. The first breath is the first thing you play - do it in time. If you run out of wind and need to sneak a breath, do it naturally, without interrupting the energy or the flow of the phrase.

After a couple of years of John's teaching I could see phrasing and smooth natural curves in painting, sculpture, literature, designs of highways - everywhere! And I could hear his comments (in my mind) when piano players cut chords off too quickly - but I also began to realize why I like Sarah McLachlan's singing so much: elegant phrasing.

My musical journey

I have been passionate about music since I was a young child. I think my major musical setback involved mum. She should have never forced this *non-morning person* to practice piano before school! After completing several years as one of John MacPherson's students I had a pretty good idea of what it would take to be a professional musician - but that involved brutal amounts of night work, and often being away from your family. So I became a physician and faced even more night work and constant uphill battles trying to balance work and family time! Go figure!

Anyways, I enjoy regular gigs with trombone in a jazz band, French horn in a concert band and every second Sunday I do music for a small community church using button accordion, Irish flute and hammer dulcimer. I never cease to be amazed at how worn out I can be, barely able to "drag my butt" into Thursday night practices, blow my heart out for two hours on the trombone and emerge refreshed and energized.

"Music is spiritual. The music business is not!"
---Van Morrison

Goofing around in the back row: an ode to Murray

Murray and I sang baritone in a choir - and we were a bit naughty. We chatted when the conductor was trying to explain something and circulated a teasing "straining/strident/way-too-serious" sketch of the lead tenor. Nevertheless, that choir made wonderful music.

Kids with FASD often have difficulties trying to engage in social situations "one-on-one." They may do better with "parallel play" activities, such as singing in a choir, working alongside others in a friendly way. Helping our kids discover engaging leisure activities - that involve friendly, natural "rubbing of shoulders" with others - is a powerful gift parents can offer. Trying different musical possibilities until one "clicks" is a great idea.

Sensitivity to sound can sometimes be a barrier, but can be overcome. One of my patients liked drumming but the First Nation's drumming circle she was invited to participate in was too loud. We got her some of "those really cool earplugs that rock musicians wear." Now, she is not overwhelmed and has enjoyed drumming with others.

When we make music *with others* - in a choir or a band or a drumming circle - our brain starts to fire in synchrony with our neighbour's brain. This might explain the camaraderie of many musical groups...and why I liked goofing around with Murray so much!

Music causes neuroplastic changes in the brain

Musicians develop enhanced circuitry in the motor cortex and the cerebellum. [6]

Motor planning areas and cerebellar procedural memory circuits are often damaged by prenatal alcohol, so, if people with FASD have any musical interest, I strongly encourage them to learn an instrument or sing, especially in a group. Musical activities can be a fun, engaging "therapy" of sorts for some of the areas that prenatal alcohol affects. If you wanted to design activities that promote new nerve cell growth in parts of the brain most likely to be compromised by prenatal alcohol I'd suggest you place playing an instrument, singing and dancing "at the top of your list."

Kicking butt; talking back to oppressors but not getting into trouble for doing so

Have you ever been unfairly treated, abused, or had your rights trampled? Ever wanted to seek revenge? I wish those events had not happened to you - or me. People with FASD often feel coerced and invalidated. Music is not alone as an artistic retort or "push back" against tyranny and oppression. The northwest corner of Musee' Orsay in Paris contains a collection of perhaps a dozen little busts - elegant little sculptures of the heads of prominent Parisian politicians of about 200 years ago. Each is so intricately and delicately crafted that viewers are at first entranced by the magnificent craftsmanship and beauty of the creations. That was the sculptor's plan! Looking a bit closer, the snub, the mockery, the buffooning of these obnoxious pompous characters becomes obvious. This one's nose is a little too big, that one has an Ebenezer Scrooge sized scowl and that one is just too full of himself...but they are of such quality, that the officious people being teased probably did not even know others were snubbing them.

Protest songs did not force the US government out of Vietnam, but at a certain point it "became politically untenable to fight the war." [7]

Daniel Levitin explains that during the 1960's a build up of public resentment against the war was fuelled and cemented together by a series of unforgettable songs including: *Where Have All the Flowers Gone, Give Peace a Chance, Universal Soldier, Ohio* and others. [7]

Songs can plant ideas in our brains. A "meme" is an idea spread from mind to mind.

Kayne West and John Legend are two popular singers that create a very personal link with their audience and then pour in honest and sustaining ideas with their lyrics. They demonstrate the best in this musical way of spreading messages.

" Music expresses that which cannot be said and on which it is impossible to be silent"
---Victor Hugo, author of Les Miserables

We are rhythmical creatures

Biologic rhythms govern all creatures, including us. People vary, a bit, in resilience to disrupted biological rhythms. Some can fly from North America to Europe and adjust after a day or two. Others - those who have less adaptable circadian rhythm biology - suffer "jet lag" until they return home.

Ellen Frank has linked disrupted biological rhythms to mental illness and also restoration of those rhythms to recovery. Since I heard Dr. Frank speak about the pattern of health disruptions caused by interrupted biological rhythms I've been asking my patients:

When do you go to bed?
When do you get up?
When do you first talk to a human being (not a computer) each morning?
When and what do you eat?

Often, whether my patient has FASD or not, I get answers like:

Bed? - maybe 3 or 4 (A.M.), whenever I get tired
Get up? - maybe 2 (P.M.)
A Person? - well, I text all kinds of people but I don't actually meet them very often
Eat? - well, whatever my brother makes for me, whenever he gives it to me

These social cues - bed, other-contact, eating - help to "set" our biological rhythm "clocks." Disrupted patterns of social cues can induce severe mental illness as Dr. Frank saw when she studied patients with Bipolar Disease several years ago. Since then, she's found success in treating depression (in various groups including young adults) by working alongside patients to develop more stable, predictable sleep/social contact/eating patterns. [8]

Pediatric psychiatrist, Bruce Perry suggests that by participating *in rhythmic, regular, repetitive, age-appropriate, fun, engaging activities* children (even those with FASD, chaotic early home life or abuse histories) can find solace and eventually learn to self-regulate. To effect neuroplastic changes that can lead to increased self control requires practicing these activities 40 plus minutes a day, 3-5 times a week for several months. Especially if rhythmic activities are performed at a 40/60 or 80 beat per minute speed patients will find them comforting and grounding because of associations with fetal or infant rhythms. Mum's heartbeat (usually at a 40/60 or 80 beat per minute cadence) was associated with being warm, fed and snuggled in the fetal and infant environments. Activities done at this same cadence seem like an artificial strategy but Dr. Perry has found very encouraging levels of neurodevelopmental progress have resulted. Activities a school-aged child might try include walking, strumming a guitar, dancing, martial arts, trampoline, horseback riding, or drumming. [9]

Surviving terror

Patients disclose the most difficult stories. How some find the strength to go on is a testimony to human resilience. One young woman's story I heard several years ago in Ontario took my breath away. Let's call her Elly. "Growing up" with an abusive crack-smoking drug dealer for a mum, she was mostly ignored, except for when the mother's "boyfriends" molested her. This young woman, who has cognitive difficulties caused by prenatal alcohol exposure, was forced to live in such hellish circumstances until age sixteen when she conjured up enough resolve and stole enough money to run away. Life on the streets wasn't much of an improvement. Eventually she met a supportive boyfriend but the legacy of her abusive past still intruded daily.

As a child, shutting herself into a closet in a bid to keep out of sight of her mother's boyfriends, Elly would pass hours sitting - rocking back and forth and *singing*. She actually had, and has, a great voice, but she never had enough confidence to sing out at school. Predictably, she quit school in grade 9. Academic work was "boring." (Translation: [Which was proposed after she was evaluated for sensory processing difficulties by an occupational therapist] Elly had such levels of touch and visual sensitivity that she could not comply with her teacher's requests to sit still and concentrate - I wish one of her teachers had noticed her singing.)

Elly sounds like Beyonce or Jem, a famous Welch singer. Last year I heard she won a province-wide singing contest and cut a CD. Elly may have been able to rise above her sexual, physical and emotional abuse by escaping into music, by singing in the closet. The music that started as an escape may continue to help her transcend her disabilities. But more importantly, Elly can define herself as a successful and talented singer, not by her abuse and difficulties. Go Girl!

"Music has healing powers that can bring peace to a stressful mind." **---Daniel Amen**

"Music was my refuge. I could crawl into the space between the notes and curl my back to loneliness." ***---Maya Angelou***

"It's the music that kept us all intact, kept us from going crazy." ***---Lou Reed***

References

[1] Fleming R. 2001. Excerpts from: PBS-Frontline: Faith and Doubt at Ground Zero. Accessed on You Tube Jan 15, 2011 using this link: http://www.youtube.com/watch?v=87BxqK7KKCc

[2] Morin A. 2001. Classical Music: Third Ear: The Essential Listening Companion. San Francisco: Backbeat Books. p. 74

[3] Keller J. March 7, 2010. "An Adagio for Strings, and for the Ages". The New York Times. http://www.nytimes.com/2010/03/07/arts/music/07barber.html?_r=1&ref=arts Retrieved 2011-01-14.

[4] Sullivan AK. 2007. FASD in the Adult: Vulnerability, Disability or Diagnosis - a Psychodynamic Perspective. In: O'Malley KA, editor. ADHD and Fetal Alcohol Spectrum Disorders (FASD). New York: Nova Science.

[5] Wikipedia: http://en.wikipedia.org/wiki/Overtone Retrieved 2011-04-14

[6] Doige N. 2007. The Brain That Changes Itself. New York: Penguin Books p. 287

[7] Levitin D. 2008. The World in Six Songs: How the Musical Brain Created Human Nature. Toronto: Viking Canada. p.72

[8] Frank E. 2005. Treating Bipolar Disorder: a clinician's guide to interpersonal and Social Rhythm Therapy. New York: The Guilford Press.

[9] Perry BD. 2010. Introduction to the Neurosequential Model of Therapeutics: Application in Children Impacted by FASD. 2010 Alberta FASD Conference: Promising Practices, Promising Futures. Feb 8, 2010, Calgary

Chapter Six

Insights from FASD Stakeholders

A variety of people from the wider community have a keen interest in, and work directly with individuals who have FASD. We'll call this group FASD *Stakeholders*. As a father of a young adult who has FAS, I have another name for FASD Stakeholders: my helpers and my heroes! Over a number of years, as I seek answers and resources for my family members and patients, I've come to know a very diverse group of wise and resourceful stakeholders. I asked them each two questions:

1. What do you wish you'd known sooner about FASD?
2. What would you like others in your line of work to know about FASD?

This chapter presents their responses.

Stakeholders:

Family:

1. Leesa and John -Childcare / Preschool Owner, Foster Parent, and Adoptive Parent
2. Kassie –Sibling

Family Supporters:

3. Henry Sundquist –Executive Director of Kindale Developmental Association, Residential Care Administrator, Advocate for Developmentally Disabled Adults
4. Dawn Grunert and Alison Gaul –Coordinators of: Respite services for Families
5. Krystal Oleson – Parent Educator

Direct Supporters of FASD-affected Individuals:

6. Grace Gerry –Social Worker and Coordinator of an FASD Assessment Clinic for adults
7. Ron Jorgenson –Educator, Counselor, Community Developer
8. Larry Keats –Music Therapist
9. Mary Culshaw –Occupational Therapist

Physicians/Medical Office Receptionist:

10. Renata Johnson –Medical Office Receptionist
11. Rod Densmore –Primary Care Physician
12. Jonathan Down –Developmental Paediatrician

Family

1. **Leesa and John** - Childcare / Preschool Owner, Foster Parents and Adoptive Parents

What I Wish I Had known about FASD - Written by Leesa

I *thought* I knew a fair bit about FASD and other special needs. I had taken many courses and attended seminars and read books on the subject. My staff and I developed an integrated centre model to provide childcare for kids with a variety of needs. My husband and I also fostered older children with emotional needs. I was the primary care giver to children with a parent (usually the mother) in a rehab or other mental health program with an average duration between four to six months.

The first thing we learned is that it is possible - for, maybe, four to six months - if one has the patience of Job, to survive. However, as an adoptive parent without respite (never knowing if and when you could get a time out), patience becomes a quantitative dynamic. Over time one becomes socially isolated and with isolation comes a sense of abandonment. The lack of understanding (from peers, professionals and family) of the intense day-to-day pressure has an adverse effect on one's self-esteem and confidence. As a foster-parent respite is part of the package but an adoptive parent is treated as a failure when he/she seeks respite.

We found many adults failed to recognize these are not BAD kids just ones requiring constant supervision. They also failed to accept that many, parents of FASD-affected children are not poor parents by choice but become so as a result of never getting a chance to recharge their personal batteries.

One of the biggest surprises to us was the profoundly unsupportive attitude that we encountered from Social Workers because our children were foreign adoptees. One Social Worker even harshly asked, "Where would we be if every middle class family adopted a FASD child and then asked for supports?" My reply, "We would have a world without starving and dying children trapped in orphanages!" My reply was not appreciated.

When discussing our daughter with FASD at a team conference (IEP) at her new school, a teacher declared that I was ridiculous to suggest that my very blonde blue eyed daughter could have FASD because she was not native! However, my dark haired, dark eyed son - presumed to be native - could have supports! Needless to say, this teacher and the other equally "FASD-aware" school team members did not follow through to provide the class supports or school adaptations that the psychologist had recommended. How do we help society to understand FASD is not isolated to race or socioeconomic conditions, but can affect any and all of society?

We wished we had fully appreciated the FASD brain's difficulty in perceiving and processing concepts of truth. I often joked that "Truth" and what my youngest children said where not even distance cousins… these kids' statements reminded me of the old school game of "a line of whispers." Remember, as a kid, when you started with a whisper of a short statement in the first set of ears and eventually saw what long convoluted sentence would arise at the end of the line of your classmates? With the FASD brain, kids can come out with an entirely different version of what they think you said (compared to what you know you did say) and they will swear they have it correct.

A great deal of time and emotional effort was taken on our part to understand our kids' propensity for manipulation, half-truths and their inability to comprehend abstracts and absolutes. I cannot say that as young adults these problem areas are resolved, but our responses have changed. We seek confirming independent sources. We expect that each time we disagree or correct then retaliation will occur. We do our best to protect ourselves, our marriage and our other birth children from the fall out.

We learned that what we considered to be "stealing," they considered as "taking." My husband wishes when we adopted the children we had begun a "legal fund to save for the day that their actions were no longer accepted or excused by teacher, stores, police officers, etc." Sadly, the time comes when they cannot reap the dividends of being young and cute.

I wanted a hand out or letter from an M.D. or Psychologist that explained my child's diagnosis and the associated behavioural and cognitive problems so that I would not need to explain the situation over and over again to other adults. I formed a relationship with the police. I advised them about our children and our family's situation. I spoke with new officers transferring into our community. This helped in a variety of ways. Firstly, the police knew the situation and did not jump to the conclusion that we were bad, or disinterested, parents. We were simply *very* experienced and burned out.

When one of the children had skipped off, or had gone for a wander (my daughter's term for running away impulsively and without any obvious reason), they had her picture and would advise the bus and train. This helped to contain her to our small geographic area. It also increased our chances of recovering her without undo harm.

Our son loses belongings (including his ID) frequently. He suffers from seizures and is non-communicative. Our *prior* communication to the police ensures that we will be called if they find him wandering somewhere. Unless the police were spoken to ahead of time, they would likely assume he was on drugs. What else could they think when confronted with a spaced out, nonverbal adolescent?

One of the behavioural problems we found the *very* disconcerting was that of self-destruction and self-harming. We have consulted many professionals and have yet to understand this component of FASD. For example, our daughter, with no warning or provocation, grabbed a carving knife from the drawer and cut her face. On other occasions she would stab herself or slit her wrists, choke herself until she passed out. The only explanation we have been given was that it was related to the "impulsivity factor"... the inability to understand action and consequence. *Parents* suffer emotional trauma from these actions of their kids. Additionally, parents sense that they could never turn their back - not even for a moment.

The most devastating example of this type of destructive judgment for me involved a new Social Worker who came to our city. He blamed me for being responsible for the scars on her body. It took years of court battles and a great deal of financial expense to prove that I was innocent. Sadly, in foster care during this time, my daughter attempted suicide by overdosing and cutting her wrists. Why ever did social services not understand her self- harm (when she was with us) was a plea for help and assist us in recognizing that plea and addressing it - for the plea just got louder in foster care. That escalation of self-harm did not have to happen. Our family did not need that trauma of being falsely accused of causing harm. Finally, social services recognized the problem that we had been seeking help for since we adopted her at age two. With help of medication this problem is now under control. I ask myself why as parents we could not get the professional help required even though we *sought* many professional's assistance. Only when social services could no longer blame a parent did they acknowledge a problem and apply a solution.

As a mother, I would say, "You appear to have a big owie on the outside, do you have one on the inside you would like to talk about?" Then I just listened. The hard part is self-loathing after an episode of harming, impulsivity or other destructive behaviours. She wants so much to understand herself and asks why, oh why do I blow up my life when it is going good? We have no answers.

One night in the hospital, at three a.m., after a running away, drinking and drug overdose adventure, I sat alone in the waiting room feeling sorry for myself. I called out to God, "Why me? You promised me the desires of my heart. You lead us to adopt but why must it be this hard?" The reply from the Lord was, "What makes you think it was your hearts' desires I was fulfilling? What about the little lost girl in the orphanage who cried for a mother to love her, care for her, one who would be there through thick and thin?" It was at that moment that I felt humility and gratitude. There was nothing my children could say, do, or be that my love for them could not surpass.

Attachment Disorder

We expected attachment disorder in our adoptive children, as they were two and a half and four years old when they came to live with us. The fact was that the children had been institutionalized for the majority of their lives, and had been exposed to multiple caregivers some of whom had been abusive added an additional challenge.

We accepted that a full bond might never be achieved. We sought to create as successful a bond as possible. We assumed that the adoptive children would have a natural bond from their shared experience of being adopted at the same time. My husband states that our family fell into a parents (us) versus adopted kids (them) scenario.

Our family created successful bonds with foster children (many who are still like family) and daycare children who continue relationships with us even as young adults. We took for granted our ability to create bonds with our adoptive children.

Our naivety at the full extent of the ramifications of FASD on the ability to bond on the children's parts surprised us. For example, our children appear capable of only one attachment at a time... "serial bonding." Our daughter will detach from me and choose another adult female ("mom" figure) to attach to. These attachments are predominantly obsessive; emailing and phoning the person fifty or more times per day, not even choosing what to wear or eat without her impute and approval. Then she will meet another woman, be it a teacher, friend's mother, youth group leader or the like and will behave so outrageously as to drive the previous woman away. This pattern repeats itself for a father figure as well. Our son demonstrates this with male friends, brothers or brother-in-law, but never more than one at a time. He shows no attachment to parents, teachers or other authority figures.

"Natural consequences for their actions" have been a difficult area. For example, a typical kid leaves a new bike in the driveway. You remove the bike and the privileges associated with riding. They learn to care about and for their possessions. A person with attachment issues who forms little or no bond to humans also forms no bond to items, toys etc. Depriving them of time with friends or items does not result in deterring unwanted behaviour.

In an adoptive FASD relationship gratitude, love or acceptance are not expected. One can expect anger and resentment. We recommend doing your best to inform the adults who may be the object of infatuation or (other-than–parent) attachments about this disorder. People see a child who appears unattached and possibly hostile to their parents. They assume the child has a valid cause such as abuse. Do not be the subject of the uninformed public or misinformed professionals' judgment. We have been. It is painful.

Unrequited love is always a pain-filled experience be it a romantic relationship or a parental one. If you are an overly sensitive person who is not capable of true unconditional love then my husband's advice is GET A DOG. They are always happy to see you. They are loyal. They never hate you. They never lie about you - and they live for twelve or so years so long-term burn out is not an issue.

Foster parents and adoptive parents: pray no one judges you by your child's label and assumes you are an alcoholic and spread rumours to this effect. Always give love support and encouragement to FASD birthparents.

What gets me through the tough times of being a parent of children who have FASD is remembering my worst day as a passenger on the roller coaster of their lives will never be as bad as what it feels like for them, never being the owner and operator of their own roller coaster. They will never fully understand why they are the way they are. Living with the judgment and condemnation of others must be so difficult for our kids.

P.S. Give away prepaid phone cards to those young people who are obvious runways. Encourage them to phone home. When your FASD-affected child/adult has gone for a wander and they do phone home - always tell them you love them. They can get back on the wagon at any moment. Unconditional love, acceptance and understanding are the greatest gifts we can give them.

2. **Kassie** - Sibling

How does one go about describing life with a person who has FASD? Where is the dotted line to cut along, the line that would separate my sister, Natasha, from the effects of her birthmother's drinking? How do I discern which characteristics are inherently hers and which were altered while she was still in the womb?

With FASD, unlike a brain injury resulting from an accident, there is no before and after to compare. The effects are pervasive, seeping into every thought, action and decision until it becomes too easy to see the problem, the diagnosis, and miss the person living underneath.

When my baby sister joined our family at three and half years old her luggage included big blue eyes, an impish grin and the ability to charm the socks off anyone who crossed her path. What we didn't know at the time was that along with a taste for borscht and the ability to swear like a sailor in Ukrainian, she also brought the legacy of a culture fraught with alcoholism.

So what did and does it mean for me, having a sister with FASD?

When we were young it meant making her bed because she couldn't remember from day to day that this was the rule. It meant reminding her over and over of the same things and then watching her confusion over the resulting consequences of her inaction. It was peeling her off the walls when she got too wound up and intervening when she missed social boundaries. It meant living with a fun-loving little girl who could switch between activities like a butterfly in fast-forward.

Living with FASD meant watching Natasha, a bright girl, struggle in school. It meant watching her compare herself to her friends and knowing that, in her mind, she was always falling short. It meant seeing her grow to distrust herself after a series of bad decisions, the reasoning behind which she was at a loss to explain. Living with Natasha meant biting my tongue when she got involved with the wrong people or into bad relationships.

Living with FASD meant enjoying the good days of relative peace and tranquility, storing up strength for the bad days, when our family was more like a warzone populated with weary combatants.

It meant and still means loving her so much wihout knowing how to help.

Living with a person with FASD, in a lot of ways, was like living with a chameleon. This person who could show a different face to everyone in their lives, changing their colours to suit the surroundings. Each reincarnation of themselves is wholly believable, intended to make the other love them more, pity them more, admire them more, fill some void in their lives. But, like pouring water into a sieve, no matter how much was given, it was never enough to fill it up.

It also meant living with a person whose skills of manipulation were on par with a political head of state, a person who would tell any lie to serve his or her own short-sighted purposes. It meant watching helplessly as those lies grew and engulfed our family, destroying what wouldn't be bent. It meant driving my baby sister to her foster home when my parents, finally broken, had given up. It meant vomiting into a ditch under the effects of the emotions from having to drive away and leave her there.

It meant and still means loving someone who can hurt you so badly.

Having a loved one with FASD meant lying awake at night, worried that Natasha had exhausted every relationship and burnt every bridge in her life. It was wondering where she could go next? Would she be opening the door to our home?

It meant and still means never giving up hope that this time will be better.

Having a sister with FASD meant finding all the empty bottles after she moved out. Those bottles seemed to mock your optimism. It meant learning to look past failure to marvel at the successes she was and **is** achieving. It meant knowing that for her, success and failure always come together.

It meant watching Natasha blow her life into little bits every time things started to go well, with bad decisions, lies, manipulations and unhealthy relationships as the fuel for the bomb. But, it also meant watching her struggle repeatedly to put it back together again, each rebuild a little stronger, a little better, and a bit more solid.

It meant and still means always wondering if this blow up is the last, if this rebuild is the one that will hold.

Having FASD in our family has meant watching Natasha grow up, slowly and painfully. It has meant watching her learn to embrace herself, FASD and all. It has meant quietly rejoicing when she enters a positive relationship and cheering her on when she achieves new goals.

It meant and still means knowing a beautiful, strong, resilient young woman who I am proud to call my sister.

Family Supporters

3. **Henry Sundquist**, Executive Director of Kindale Developmental Association, Residential Care Administrator, Advocate for Developmentally Disabled Adults

Henry works at building communities of social support around people with FASD and their families.

When one is building support systems, one is always searching for alternatives to create as many options as possible for parents and individuals. Drained people need to know the way out.

Having a group of professionals from various backgrounds facilitates effective ideas to accommodate diverse individual needs. Working together is at times difficult, but this group model generates the best strategies. Like puzzle pieces, one professional's ideas might be bigger than the rest but their *single* approach doesn't make the whole puzzle. Enduring solutions result from diverse, complex thinking.

While working with people who have FASD, one might ask who are the scientists who can help? It's really just been within the last ten years that professionals have turned their focus on FASD. Because of the different symptoms of FASD, there are so many different types of science that can help. Studies on brain, physiology, hearing and visual processing can be applied to FASD.

As for those who have FASD, some IQs are 100+ but social skills are much lower. It's easy to be deceived by the "look." They know how to "talk the talk" and appear as if they are having no problems. Some of them have a hard time living with a "label". The key here is to be sensitive.

No "one size fits all" formula applies to helping people with FASD. The support "recipe" for every person is different.

One must be interested in individual talents. Many times the focus is on negative incidents. *Support systems work best with a positive, "look for the gifts, not the disabilities."* We must use what they are good at to help them succeed. We must create a positive vision for future success knowing that success leads not only to their own favorable outcomes but also empowers individuals who have FASD to become leaders and self-advocators.

People with FASD need to build trust with people-peers, parents and mentors. They need personal relationships with people who understand the difficulties in maintaining relationships that are experienced by those with FASD. Supporters must let FASD-affected people know that they are accepted and help them accept and believe in themselves - especially youth.

Relationships with professionals also work best if built on trust and reliability. Professionals must not make promises they do not intend to keep. Professionals must know their clients by name not by a number. When building familiarity and trust, one cannot be a "paid person" all the time - it is about honest connection.

Support people must be creative in how they work with people who have FASD. They must use theories of gentle teaching - thinking of dream boards, things to work towards and steps to get there. They should ask enough questions to ease people with FASD towards the answer rather than giving the answer to them. They should create comfort. "Natural" consequences are not understood. A reward system is solid gold! For example, rewarding good redirections after mishaps, trying to catch the "downs" and help point folks in the right direction. Consistency is key.

Parents need to know they are not guilty. They are not alone. Support people must be a "buffer" for complicated government "support systems" and other systems that are not user friendly.

When one finds the right system, the perfect puzzle, it is like a breath of fresh air for everyone.

4. **Dawn Grunert and Alison Gaul**, Coordinators of Community Respite, Victoria B.C.

The Community Respite Service for Families has spent 20 years defining and refining our values and mission statement. We expected that our 2 year FASD Respite Demonstration Project would carry on in a manner of "business pretty close to usual". What we discovered when we started supporting families raising children or youth with FASD was that our values were tested…and confirmed. Our bright ideas were adapted…and revised. Our beliefs about respite remained solid.

We believe trust, respect, open communication and confidentiality are essential.

For the first time in the history of our service…we were meeting families that hadn't been connected to our organization. We were meeting families that had never had any kind of respite before. We had to earn trust. We had to earn respect. We had to establish open communication in a way that we had previously taken for granted with families. *We wish we'd recognized that it would take longer to build relationships.* It would take longer than anticipated to assure families that their confidentiality would always be respected.

We believe that individual family strengths and differences are respected.

We learned that some of these families have NOT been respected. They have lived through grief and loss and fear of judgment. These powerful emotions had a very real impact on the families…and their stories had a very real impact on us. We wish we'd been better prepared for our reactions.

We believe that parents are the most important members of the training team.

This has been a core belief for our service since its inception in 1989…but to some families, this statement was totally new. We shared in the experience of helping them make choices around their children's' caregivers for the first time. We also shared in the joy from the sidelines as families allowed respite workers into their lives and shared the experiences and skills they have learned themselves.

We believe that respite needs to be flexible, convenient and affordable for families to access it.

Our flexibility was tested in every way possible. With timelines, with meeting dates, with training…we became known as the "Plan B" girls at work as we struggled to revise and regroup at every level.

We needed to recognize the importance of FASD specific training for the respite workers. We needed to understand the unique challenges for Birth families, Grandparents, Adoptive parents and Foster Families raising children and youth with FASD. We needed to adapt and find ways to continue to support children as their own living situations changed.

We learned that poverty is a barrier to accessing respite even if the respite worker's salary is paid. We also re-confirmed for ourselves that Respite workers couldn't take the place of childcare, intervention or therapy. For respite to truly offer a break, the family's most basic needs have to be met.

We believe that respite facilitates the growth and well being of families and gives every family member the chance to broaden their experiences and develop relationships with other people.

We knew this to be true. We expected this result. I don't think we could have expected so many respite workers and families' to share so much of this with us. We have heard about youth connecting with their home territory for the very first time. We have heard about parents reconnecting with friends and family members. We have heard about swimming, skating and mountain climbing adventures.

We believe that respite workers grow from this work.

We have always loved watching young respite workers learn and grow and go on to careers in similar professions. With this project we also watched them grow into strong, determined advocates alongside the families they work with.

This Two Year Respite Demonstration Project quickly turned into a Three Year Demonstration Project…and business was not so "usual" at all. We were fortunate to have this opportunity to display the positive impact that quality respite can have on families raising children with FASD.

There are things we wish we'd known at the start. There was a good deal of learning and growing along the way. Unquestionably, the journey has been worth it. We would be happy to be contacted as resource people for others who endeavor to develop and/or provide respite support in their own communities.

5. **Krystal Oleson**, Parent Educator

When I became a certified Parent Educator who facilitates video-courses by Dr. Gordon Neufeld, I never dreamed I would find myself working with many adoptive/foster families of children with FASD. Now I wouldn't have it any other way. I have such incredible respect for these parents because I see their commitment to their children despite the frustrations they feel. The focus of these video courses is attachment, relationship, development and maturation, all of which are often a challenge for kids with FASD. We are constantly faced with the fact that even though their bodies tell us they are a certain age, they remain impulsive, poor decision makers and often appear to be resistant to authority. These attributes make parenting/teaching them very frustrating and the parents in my class often express this by asking questions like "Is he ever going to mature?" or "Is she always going to be so impulsive?"

My own son struggles with and is in the midst of being diagnosed with sensory processing sensitivities, ADHD, OCD, anxiety and possible asperger disorder. Many of his symptoms look like FASD, but I know for certain that I never drank during my pregnancy. His behaviours often move me to a place of anger and wanting to give up. My frustrations can be over the top some days especially when I am tired and feeling alone in my struggles. I know if I can switch my focus from trying to change his behaviours to seeing his frustrations that drive his behaviour that I will move back to a place of softness and invitation where he can rest and his behaviours soften.

Such limited understanding of FASD today result in huge judgments from mainstream society about the 'way' someone is parenting. That alone can leave a sense of burden and guilt on the already overwhelmed parent. Parenting is difficult enough, throw in FASD or any other brain sensitivity that causes a child to be over sensitive, vulnerable, impulsive, volatile, mean, etc. and you have a parent that soon becomes tired and grasping for control.

I see parents who are exhausted and at their wits end because there is very little effective support and understanding for families living with FASD. I work with some agencies that do provide support and education on FASD, but that is only a small part of the child's life and sources of interactions. There are many directives that support the 'tough love' and 'let them learn the hard way' methods when dealing with teenagers and young adults. The 'don't let him get away with that behaviour' comment is so often heard. Intuitively, these parents know that methods using bribes and punishment are not going to work. They often backfire causing more problems. They are also at a loss to discover what does work and are often trying to figure it out alone.

Throughout my classes, we talk about the importance of self-care and the possibility that the care provider can lose sight of their relationship with the child, especially when the care provider's own frustrations and exhaustion has taken over the driver's seat. Burnout can render them blinded to the daily frustrations and vulnerabilities that their child with FASD has to live with, and keep them focused on the child's behaviour and how to fix it. When the care provider (parent) can find a place of support and hope, they can let down their own defenses (hardened by sheer exhaustion), can again see how important they are to their child and can find strength to be the person they need to be in order for their child to succeed. This isn't easy and exhaustion is sure to surface again which is why a supportive community of understanding people, professionals and respite is so very much needed.

Direct Supporters of FASD-affected Individuals

6. **Grace Gerry**, Social Worker, and coordinator of the Victoria FASD Adult Assessment Clinic

What I wish I had known sooner as a social worker: My training in FASD started long before I ever became the social work coordinator for a 3 year pilot in Victoria BC for the assessment of adult women with FASD in 2008. It actually started back in 1999 when my husband and I made the life changing decision to foster which led us into the world of FASD.

From this decision, we unknowingly climbed onto a roller coaster of intense experiences that took us up and down as we adapted to living with FASD. Over and over we learnt to adjust our expectations as parents. We did our best to teach other professionals who were sometimes resistant to the lesson; we supported each other nightly with long debriefing sessions after the children were asleep. At the end of each day we would fall into bed exhausted only to get up and start the adventure again the following day.

When I joined our multi disciplinary FASD adult assessment team, it wasn't my 25 years of social work experience in Ireland, England and Canada that I drew on, but the years as a foster parent living with FASD. Here are some things I learnt along the way…

Establishing a relationship of trust is very important and *nothing else will get done without it*. While this is important with any client, people with FASD tend to be more sensitive to being liked and valued, and feel it acutely when professional relationships change or come to an end. Relationships of trust are built by being warm, nurturing, reliable, having a sense of humour, taking time to get to know them and *bringing food* to meetings!

Having food is important. It plays many roles - practical and emotional. When clients are poor as many of ours are, they may not have eaten. Having a hot coffee and muffin available goes a long way to adding comfort to our meetings. It helps the person concentrate. Our clinic has a small flexible budget for food. Sharing a tasty and nutritious lunch is a bonus for everyone on clinic day!

It is important to visit my clinic clients at home rather than office visits. This practice helps to avoid no shows and allows the assessment team a chance to gain a sense of their home environment. At times, clients prefer to meet at a coffee shop. *It is important to give them the choice.*

Be proactive to avoid difficulties: know that people with FASD often have problems with memory. I phone or text them the day before (or the morning of) appointments to remind them. And for clinic day, because it is crucial they attend, I request that a support worker brings the client and accompanies them for the day. At times we have even paid for cell phone minutes the week leading up to clinic to ensure we can contact them when we need to!

When talking with clients, I try to keep my language simple and uncluttered. I repeat key information and check back on what they have heard. I often use visuals such as drawings to illustrate a key point such as the probable consequences of a particular action or decision.

It is very important for people to have a chance to offload emotional upsets. Otherwise, stresses take control of their attention and prevent them being able to concentrate on anything else. One of our clients, for example, was so anxious about picking up her welfare cheque the day of her psychological testing, that she could not pay attention to the tests until the reason for her worry was resolved.

While I'm not a smoker, I have come to appreciate the importance of smoking as a coping strategy for any of our clients with FASD who are smokers. Having access to a cigarette at a crucial time of upset can be a huge comfort and helps them regain a sense of calm and control. I confess I have occasionally bought a pack of cigarettes to help a client through a crisis. It was worth it!

People with FASD are often extra sensitive to busy, noisy, bright environments, which are overwhelming. I try to choose coffee shops that are not too busy, and to schedule more frequent breaks during meetings.

It can be a tricky balance to make necessary accommodations for the needs of clients with FASD, but not so they feel patronized. One client for example needed frequent reassurance from me that she wasn't 'a retard' (her words). She was aware she had difficulties, but also needed to feel competent and respected.

At the end of the day people with FASD need all the same ingredients in a professional relationship that anyone else needs: respect, attention, compassion, care and trust. They just need it expressed *more clearly*, and by people who genuinely want to understand them. Professionals must be willing to think flexibly and make accommodations for their client's differences in ability and function. As one person said, *"FASD is what I have, not who I am."*

7. **Ron Jorgenson**, M. Ed; RCC, Port Alberni, B.C. Educator, Counselor, Community Developer

These are my observations as an educator, counselor and community developer:

There are many things that in hindsight, I wished I had known at the "beginning" of my journey with FASD. I am better for the journey. I was forced to decide how to deal with difficult situations and struggles. My responses to the challenges of FASD vary from being in denial - acknowledging and doing nothing - to attempting *to do it all*, which can be exhausting! It is exciting to be part of a movement, part of a team of support for people with FASD, and part of a growing field of awareness and action.

The three most significant learnings over time have been:

1) The significance of **attachment and sensory** issues. Intuitively, I knew the central importance of relationships. But I did not appreciate how dramatically *Leaving situations* (separations from those they were attached to such as a beloved teacher) could affect those with FASD. Separations exacerbate their difficulties with attachment, whether shifting teachers, homes or schools. Linked to that has been the compromised sensory systems of youth with FASD. Tragically, for years, society has failed to understand how accommodations within the environment allow greater success.

Working with students who have FASD requires understanding the long-term impact of alcohol-induced neurochemical and biophysiological changes. What are alcohol's effects on the fetal brain…and how does that damaged brain develop over time? How does understanding the brain help us mitigate ongoing difficulties children experience? We failed to offer adequate sensory accommodations for a group of young people who did field trips into nature. Overall, the field trips were successful but we should have done more planning for kids' sensory needs. The children were either over or under sensitive to new or novel sensations from the environment - they became overwhelmed. Regrettably, what we hoped would be entirely positive ended up, partially, as a negative experience. Failure to accommodate their sensory needs created increased detachment for a time.

2) The importance of **being part of a community** of awareness and action. As an individual struggling with my own issues in education and attempting to assist others whom I perceived as marginalized within the education system, I attempted to make a difference on my own. I could not do it alone. Now I know that *a community* of individuals can make a difference as they work together in partnerships, sharing the journey and sharing the "paddling." Working together helps us avoid falling

into the trap of despair, frustration and grief. It has also meant that the triumphs and the successes have been a shared celebration and that "together we can."

Building a compassionate, dedicated community takes time. Additionally, a shift from knowing about the need to creative action is necessary. It *means stepping outside of the box*, a characteristic we have been carefully coached through education and training *not* to do! Even in large institutions passionate individuals can make a difference. They can hold the door a little wider; they can shift policies and structures to be more accommodating. They can allow the needs of individuals with FASD to be influential factors.

I have seen classrooms change, curriculum adapted and schools emerge that are friendlier, more accommodating with teachers who understand the specific needs of their students with FASD. When Educational Assistants (E.A.'s) have embraced the sensory and adaptive needs and support the students the most amazing progress happens. Often teachers pick up on the E.A.'s sensory accommodations. A spirit of compassionate awareness about the child's struggles enters the class. I have seen a Ministry of Education recognize the struggle of students with FASD and a Provincial Outreach Program for FASD emerge that did not exist 5 years ago. We still have a long way to go. Changing the direction of a dinosaur is no small task!

3) The **duration and life long nature of FASD.**

FASD places relentless and persistent stress on individuals, families and communities. People start to learn about FASD from many different starting places. For some it is as a foster or adoptive parent working with preschoolers, others encounter FASD in students they work with. For others it is in the adolescent as he/she struggles to belong. For others it is within the adult population of encounters with independent living, employability, encounters with law, or social struggle. It is a characteristic of FASD that it will not manifest in the same way at each stage in an individual's life.

We must respond flexibly and compassionately to the unique and ever changing difficulties FASD presents to those we care for. Rigid formulaic approaches - "this is how we do this programme - take it or leave it" - don't work. We must shift to being conscious of process…good approaches grow from flexible responses to deep understanding. In this evolving format of change, the links and transitions between phases in an individual's lifetime become critical moments of support.

8. **Larry Keats**, Music Therapist

"There are so many paths up the mountain but the view from the top is still the same" ***--- Little River Band circa 1978***

Or... Things I learned from children with FAS

My 16 years of private Music Therapy practice in Salmon Arm has given me an opportunity to share "music time" with children and adults with a diverse range of behavioral disorders, learning disabilities and developmental disabilities, including FASD.

Essentially, I have learned that each person under the umbrella of FASD presents a unique mountain. Challenging behaviors, learning or motor skills deficits, when treated in the playful metaphorical musical world, can be redefined... sometimes for profound musical effect and, more importantly, life affect.

Each individual's musical journey follows a unique pathway of exploration. Sometimes it is an expressway; sometimes it is windy with many curves and barriers. My role as a therapist is to provide a safe, non-confrontational environment assisting the individual discover their own "self" as reflected in their musical activity. Musical activity provides the energy to travel the road, meeting challenging behaviours and deficits, which are redirected, reduced, rerouted during the interaction in the music room. My hope is the following short anecdotes can illustrate how some common behaviours associated with FASD have seen positive change in purpose as the person travels the music journey to self-awareness and ultimately self-control.

Hyperactivity, for example, became a lesson taught in the form of an 8 yr old child, "Abel," who arrived at my music studio for what was to be his first guitar lesson. He raced into the music room, ignoring the waiting guitar, to begin an intense playing of literally every instrument hanging on the walls, including the wall itself at one point. Next, he proceeded to the percussion cupboard, exploring each instrument for sound, touch and even taste. He went around, over and under the drum set, then on to the bookshelf, leafing through a few books before spotting the computer..., which was quickly abandoned when it took too long to boot up.

After a brief period of adjusting the brightness on the computer monitor he discovered the keyboard synthesizer, which he began playing with one hand while with the other hand, rapidly pushing a myriad of buttons, changing the sound from string orchestra to garbage can lids followed by lyrical flutes, on to fog horns and crashing drums in a blur. After all of this he then zoomed out of the studio as fast as he arrived, ultimately leaving the guitar untouched. This child had participated in thirty separate musical activities in a span of twenty minutes!

Through musical interaction in subsequent sessions, the child continued this musical grazing. It was refined into a series of mini - lessons on specific instruments, growing with more purpose and intent through musical interaction in his preferred activities. The quantity of activities was effectively traded for quality of musical activity. His attention span to task increased to the point that he was able to develop some basic skills on drum set, keyboard, computer music sequencing, multi–track recording, and guitar (yes, he did eventually have his guitar lesson). Session time soon expanded from 20 minutes to one full hour. During one of these hour sessions he was able to showcase his skills by producing his own Blues demo-tune in order to feature his current favourite instrument, the harmonica. Using a "Band in a Box" program as a starting point, he built his own band from the ground up, layering recordings of his own playing on drum set, keyboard and guitar to create a background or bed track. After creating the accompanying music mix, he performed layers of solo harmonica to create a wall of sound, which was then all mixed down to a finished product. This was quite a complex process and his ability to achieve his goal in one hour was amazing. His hyperactivity was under control. His self-image was effectively redefined to become an "eight year old harmonica playing recording wizard."

Another lesson in challenging behaviour was in working with a young man who displayed obsessive compulsions. These compulsions transpired in the music room to randomly pushing buttons on the keyboard synthesizer. Initially, all his activity was random and self-indulgent leaving no space for any musical interventions by the therapist. He would often ask me to stop intervening musically. He resisted offers of assistance when his button pushing was not getting the effect he expected. He pushed more buttons with more intensity. Gradually, he began playing the keyboard for approximately two seconds between each button push. This resulted in a short musical snippet on each sound. This became a connecting point when a story using the young man's sounds as thematic material for the narrative engaged his attention. Soon a highly interactive and humourous outer space adventure was created. Sessions became increasingly interactive from then on, each one getting more sophisticated, requiring further precision to his button pushing. One of his favourite activities involved short solos of his favourite sounds with musical accompaniment. These explorations took on the title "Short Snappy Synthonies" (making word play mixing the words symphonies and synthesizer).

During this process he:

» learned to count to 100 forwards and backwards (the number of different sounds in each section)

» learned to identify many instruments by sound characteristics (strings, brass etc.)

» learned musical terms such a pitch, melody, harmony.

» became acquainted with basic recording functions.

» was introduced to the physics of sound design. He created his own sounds by adjusting keyboard parameters

His compulsions were under control. They were redefined as a musical style. His dexterity and his multi-digit ability were among the most adept. Another positive outcome for this young man was that his increased ability in self-control furthered success in managing academic demands. He was able to show more attention to tasks in classroom social situations.

A powerful aspect of music is that much of the therapeutic process happens without any words or explanation. During my musical travels I had a music program with the school district's Early Intervention Programs where I met a ten-year-old boy (let's call him Rory). Rory has a variety of learning and behavioural challenges associated with FASD. He seemed to live in his own world. He was unable to focus on the current task at hand during classroom time. He would often drift off on his own agenda. He was oblivious to how his behaviour often disrupted the classroom environment. His peers viewed him as a bit eccentric. For example, he wore a blue suede leisure suit to school complete with too-short pant legs. His "cooler" classmates ridiculed him until the teachers took them to task. In general, Rory marched to the beat of his own drummer in a world understood only by him. This resulted in ostracism and teasing by his peers at school.

Rory experienced the tragedy of losing both his natural mother and his stepmother in the same car accident. Staff at the program indicated that Rory seemed outwardly unaffected. He carried on with no sign of grieving. At a music session Rory told me he had written a song that he wanted to play. He started his song by randomly playing all notes utilizing four fingers of each hand. I started to accompany him on the guitar thinking this was all there was to his song. All of sudden he started singing with this emotionally charged angelic voice. His song was entitled "The Heart of Death." Out came such a heartfelt mournful delivery that it was all I could do to hide my own tears as he shared his grief with me ending with a sustained high intense note complete with quivering vibrato. He chose to share this song at the year- end concert. This was his first performance in front of an audience. He introduced his song, informing all that he wrote it for "My mom who died, and for all the other people who have died, even those who died in the war and stuff." Within the audience there was a collective awareness that Rory was about to share an emotional experience that most who worked with him thought improbable, given his denial behaviour during the months since his mothers' death. He proceeded to deliver his song "The Heart of Death." It truly came from his heart. It was the only time he had acknowledged the tragedy or his relation to it. His message came across loud and clear.

Despite the diverse paths of these young people they all achieved a measure of success in seeing "the view from the top." They had an enhanced awareness of themselves as humans. They transcended their labels.

In witnessing the journey I have learned patience and humour are major assets. One can never have enough ways of adapting music activity...keep going until success happens! Fortunately, music has the flexibility to embrace such challenges.

9. **Mary Culshaw**, Occupational Therapist

What I'd like primary care teams to know about FASD, from an Occupational Therapist's point of view

Sensory Processing Problems

At all times people take in sensory input from their environment. They process it, organize it and then act upon it. Problems with sensory processing can be in the areas of modulation (the ability to maintain an appropriate level of arousal or alertness); discrimination (detecting differences within the sensory input); praxis (planning and executing individual movements or series of movements). People with FASD frequently have problems processing sensory input. They may be sensitive to noise or touch. They may not perceive differences between sounds. They have problems planning their movements in response to input. All areas of their lives are impacted and greatly contribute to their frustration levels and behaviour.

Sensory processing problems have been well researched in the general population. However, it is just starting with the FASD population. Many resources for FASD include suggestions to decrease sensory overload and organize the environment.

Modulation is the ability to maintain *an appropriate* level of arousal. When a person has problems in this area they can become overwhelmed with input or conversely not even register input. "You're not listening!" or "calm down!" can frequently be heard. Modulation problems can put a person on "high alert" so any small problem "puts them over the edge." Changes to brain function and structure make it more difficult for these individuals to modulate. The neurological framework may not be there. People who have experienced trauma and long-term stress also have problems regulating or modulating themselves. Thus, if a person has trauma *and* FASD it is even more difficult for them to maintain an appropriate level of alertness. Recent research has shown those with FASD have sensory modulation problems.

Other research has shown people with FASD have problems with the vestibular or movement system. This affects their balance, and gross motor skills. These issues can be very frustrating. They may have problems with proprioception, (the awareness of their body in space). Visual processing can be impaired, leading to problems with visual motor actions and perception of the environment. They have problems in discerning auditory input. They cannot "listen" to instructions and follow the instructions at the same time. This gets them into trouble. It can be overwhelming for anyone to be bombarded by sensory input or not be able to process it quickly enough. They get into trouble, but they don't know why they are trouble…and they can't control the processes that could get them out of trouble. People with FASD may not be able to problem solve or think objectively through their frustrations because of their cognitive impairments. This leads to increased aggression, noncompliance and resistance to new situations.

Sensory processing problems play a significant part in the daily life of a person with FASD. They are unable to respond appropriately to sensory input during a situation; which can get them into trouble and/or increase their level of frustration/ anger. A person with FASD needs the support of a team to analyze situations and provide the appropriate strategies. A behaviour approach alone *will not work*.

OT

Access to Occupational Therapy

Occupational therapy works with people on their daily activities - skills for the job of living. These can be the crucial skills needed for paid or unpaid work, school, leisure activities and personal care. Often we see children and adults with FASD struggle in all aspects of their lives. Other authors within this book have spoken at length of the far- reaching implications of this disorder. A person's trouble in a specific situation can be from problems with social interaction, cognition, motor skills and/ or communication. With all these possible problems, it is hard for caregivers or the FASD-affected individuals themselves to know what is making a situation so difficult.

An occupational therapist (OT) can analyze the activity and can help determine what is at the root of the trouble. While the health, social and education systems may understand the role of an OT; they do not always access this resource. Many families can report working with an OT when their child was young. However they do not have access to an OT at later ages even though their youth/adult continues to "get into trouble."

When a child is young, an OT can help with personal care, developing specific motor skills, improving the child's ability to participate in school and address sensory issues. These provide a framework for a child as he grows. When he's older these strategies must change. Now he needs to take a bus to school, complete chores, go to the local store to buy milk, rent a video, socialize with friends or work. Very often funding allows an OT to consult to the school/home for a couple of visits but this does little to help the individual or the family. With regular and meaning intervention, the OT can work with both family and school/work to set the person up for success. The OT can link the family with other professionals and resources when the source of the trouble is found.

What is the solution? Include occupational therapy in a written care or a treatment plan, or prescription. This helps families to negotiate funding for their family member. Tell families about occupational therapy if they do not know. Many families with younger children can access an OT through the school, health or social services funding. When talking with policy makers, inform them of the role of occupational therapy and the importance of funding. Many occupational therapy colleges are more than happy to talk to policy makers and work with stakeholders. You can link with an OT in your neighbourhood or health centre to refer clients. Many health jurisdictions are developing primary care teams, which an OT can be part of. The primary care OT can assess your patient. They can make appropriate recommendations for intervention and organization of further referrals.

Mary Culshaw is an occupational therapist with 17 years experience specializing in sensory processing and FASD. She has been a member of FASD assessment teams and provides services in a large geographical area of Northeast Alberta. She recently presented a workshop on sensory processing problems of FASD to the 2010 American Association of Occupational Therapists Annual Convention.

Physicians/Medical Office Reception

10. **Renata Johnson**, Medical Office Receptionist

The golden rule: Do unto others as you would have them do unto you.

This rule is one that I have applied from very early in life and one that my parents instilled in me. I grew up in a missionary home and lived on and off reserve for many years. When I started working at the Urban Native Health Centre, I knew I would be drawing on what I thought was a wealth of knowledge.

I was in for a big surprise. For the first year, Karen (nurse practitioner) and I would constantly say, "I just learned more than I wanted to." The population seen in our office stretches from First Nations to the homeless, the drug addicted and the alcoholic and a bit of everything in between. The common threads we have discovered for most who come through our doors are – undiagnosed FASD, traumatic brain injury (TBI), and posttraumatic stress disorder (PTSD). Most have lived unbelievable horrors in their lives because of the conditions into which they were born. They did not and would not *choose* to grow up in the situations they were born into. Their escape from reality is what we all frown upon, but is the only coping mechanism they know.

I have learned to have great amounts of patience for each of our patients who do not do well in mainstream medical offices. Many of our patients have been let go by their doctor's office because they have missed 3 appointments or more. Right from the start, I did not want our patients to feel the sting of shame when they missed an appointment and today most patients remember their appointments. Many of our patients cannot remember what they are doing from one moment to the next...expecting them to remember an appointment is wishful thinking. Developing a collaborative effort with some of the different agencies in our neighbourhood and with the help of our street nurses we can track down most of our patients and get them in to the office even when others can't find them.

I have learned to provide a quiet, calm atmosphere for patients to come and wait for their appointments. They are willing to wait longer than most because they know they will be treated with honour and dignity. They will be given the time to tell their story. Most importantly, I have learned their names and their voices. When they come to the office they are greeted like they are coming home. I have many patients who just come in and sit or nap because it is the only quiet, safe, warm place they know.

The very best thing I have learned while working in the Urban Native Health Centre is how powerful an animal can be. Daisy, my mixed breed dog has been working with us since she was just over a year old. She has taught me to greet everyone who comes through our door with unconditional kindness. Today when patients come in, they look for Daisy. She greets them like they are long lost friends. She is unafraid of anger and anxiety and she just sits herself down and put her head in their hands. She is one of the first to show our patients that she trusts them. She helps break the ice when a new patient is worried or afraid to open up. You can safely ask questions about a dog, but it opens all kinds of new doors.

If I could ask one thing of professionals who at one point in time or another come into contact with our patients, please be patient. Yes our patient will miss appointments, yes you will struggle to understand them, but if you are patient you will discover that they are real human beings who are brilliant in their own light, generous beyond measure and are capable of far more than is given credit. Be a help, not a hindrance to someone's recovery. FASD, PTSD, TBI are only diagnoses. They do not have to dictate who and what a person is to become.

Lastly, always ask yourself: is this how I want to be treated?

11. **Rod Densmore**, Primary Care Physician and Parent of a young adult who has FAS

What I wish I'd known sooner about FASD, and

What I'd like other Primary Care Physicians to know about FASD

Issue #1: Understand the high level of caregiver distress

I believe caregivers often reach a point of exhaustion before they seek help and can come across as "rigid and controlling." I have even seen an adoptive mum "diagnosed" as "Munchausen by Proxy!" A non-physician publicly declared an adoptive mum had this stigmatizing diagnosis (which means exporting your own illness on to your child for some kind of secondary gain) *during a care conference*. "Establishing" such a diagnosis (Munchausen) without the benefit of a thorough medical /psychiatric consultation and, especially, aiming your unproven, damning label at a patient in a public meeting would be grounds for launching a formal complaint against *a physician* and would prompt investigation by his/her governing body. Any care provider is unethical to attack a caregiver this way. Additionally, non-physicians are *unqualified* to make such a diagnosis. I believe the accurate diagnosis was "burned out, misunderstood and inadequately supported parent."

It would be poor medical practice to diagnose a patient with borderline personality disorder (BPD) if, at that moment, she was in the midst of ongoing domestic violence. It would be logical to try to help her extricate herself from the violent situation, offer support and then - if symptoms that fit the criteria for BPD persisted, *perhaps* that diagnosis might be accurate. In the same way, the "Munchausen" label above was equally inappropriate for this mum described above, when repeated requests for help managing out-of-control behaviours of her son were ignored.

My wife, who is a pediatric occupational therapist and I, a primary care doctor, have more educational and financial resources than the average adoptive parents yet we have been stretched to - and past - the limit of our ability to cope by ongoing behavioural crises. Additional stress resulted from the lack of being able to find understanding helpers who could tell us what to do! How do parents with limited support cope? A familiar model that could illustrate caregiver distress in FASD is the "Colicky baby." Relentless crying grinds away at parents' peace of mind. In the midst of all the crying, restorative and healthy activities for the parents: eating right, exercising, time with friends, and intimacy are "put on hold till things get resolved." Tension mounts between the parents about what strategy to try. Advice from well-meaning grammas and books often does not work. Parents blame themselves for the baby's distress or at least their not being able to effectively respond to it. This sense of inadequacy and impotence to calm distress in the child increases parental exasperation and depletion. Having dealt with both a colicky baby and an adopted child with FASD I found *caregiver depletion in FASD to be much more severe.*

Issue #2: Different types of parents face different barriers

Though I know many very caring birth parents that are successfully raising their children, in most places the majority of kids who have FASD are raised by foster or adoptive parents. Each of these three types of parents confronts slightly different barriers:

Foster parents have *all of the responsibility but often not enough authority* to act in the child's best interest. If, for example, they see that a classroom situation is toxic they have a fight on their hands (with foster care supervisors - and some of the regulations that bind what those supervisors can and cannot do) if they want to home-school the child or move her to a different school.

Birth parents, if they are in recovery from addictions, often want to be involved in their child's life. In my experience, they are *usually passionate advocates* for their kids. The burden of *mental health issues* birth mums contend with is simply staggering. Most have been abused as kids. Depression, agoraphobia, ADHD, panic, and PTSD are extremely common and very seldom diagnosed or treated. I have found traumatic brain injury, sensory processing disorder and FASD itself to be infrequently recognized, very common, and critically important to bear in mind when offering services to these women (and birth fathers too). Most have had a series of spectacularly *invalidating exchanges with authority* figures. "Tough love, 3 strikes you are out" approaches are simply ineffective. Removal of children without offering a way birth mums can be involved in their care deprives hope and leads to future alcohol-exposed pregnancies. Interest, respect and non-judgmental understanding from doctors for this group can help create the critical doctor-patient alliance that allows for:

1. treatment of mental health/ addiction issues,
2. birth control and
3. expert prenatal care.

These three services by doctors obviously are a cornerstone for any effective strategy to reduce the incidence of FASD. Being "pushed around" and harshly judged is the norm for many birth mums…if doctors or other professionals abuse them this way there is a much higher likelihood their next child will have FASD.

Infertility is a common pathway to adoption. Several years ago I learned that Harvard's Benson-Henry Institute for Mind Body Medicine, (website: http://www.mgh.harvard.edu/bhi/), had studied a cohort of infertile women. Of the many patient groups studied at the Benson Henry Institute, there was a three way tie for the most distressed - patients who scored highest on standardized tests of depression, anxiety, stress and impaired problem solving: AIDS, cancer and infertile women. Doctors must understand the high level of distress infertility often causes. We must recognize that parents who have been infertile are as fragile emotionally as patients dealing with AIDS or cancer. In addition, now that their longed-for child has arrived, parents' efforts to connect can be frustrated by the sensory issues that interfere with attachment in many FASD-affected kids. Advice from grandparents and friends who have "normal" kids often is ineffective so parents often feel inadequate because behavioural issues do not respond. Even Dr. Brazelton's and Barbara Coloroso's advice fails to help… it must be their - the adoptive parents' - fault! Tips: be gentle, patient, encouraging, expect a degree of "brittleness", rigidity and forgetfulness, and try to help treat a problem without adding undue burdens to parents who are barely coping.

Issue #3: Minimization

"He rocks," could mean that the seatbelt where he sits in the car has been worn out… twice!

"She is never still," could mean she is up from the dinner table *fifteen* times despite it being her favourite meal.

"He is distracted," could mean he is up twenty times from his chair looking at every car going down the street even though dad is attempting to read him his favourite bedtime story.

Tips: Do not minimize and dismiss such complaints. Can parents make a video displaying such behaviour to show the pediatrician or child psychiatrist? A video demonstrating extreme behavioural challenges demands solutions from the care team. Often, treatable issues of sensory overstimulation, sensory seeking and sensory discrimination difficulties underlie a portion of "misbehaviour." Get curious about these seldom-diagnosed sensory issues yourselves and encourage parents, also to learn. http://www.thespiralfoundation.org is a great place to start.

Incidentally, FAS (Fetal Alcohol Syndrome) and SPD (Sensory Processing Disorder) are in the DSM-5 planning committee's group of "Conditions Proposed by Outside Sources."

Issue #4: FASD is an invisible disability

Most children and adults with FASD look normal; yet, they have profound trouble adapting and "fitting in." They may be fluent talkers but often cannot get started on a project, know when they are "off track" or understand when they have finished. Planning, sequencing, anticipation of danger and understanding body language often are profoundly impaired. Dan Dubovsky, an adoptive dad and social worker with much experience working with FASD says affected kids are frequently mislabeled as "NURMU" (Noncompliant, Uncooperative, Resistant, Manipulative, and Unmotivated). They have brain damage. That is the reason for their issues and the only place to start from when planning intervention strategies.

12. **Dr. Jonathan Down**, Developmental Paediatrician, Victoria B.C.

Reflections on Fetal Alcohol Spectrum Disorder:

By way of introduction, I became a medical doctor in 1975; a couple of years after Smith and Jones' paper on Fetal Alcohol Syndrome was published in the Lancet. When I was at medical school in England, and during my paediatric post-graduate training in Canada, FAS was considered a rare condition. Even at the beginning of the 21st century, Nelson's

Textbook of Pediatrics contained more than 2300 pages of "gold standard" pediatric information-but only a quarter of a page about FAS.

Over the past 10 years, our understanding of the teratogenic potential of alcohol has increased significantly. We know that prenatal alcohol exposure can damage all systems and organs-not just the brain. We are beginning to comprehend the enormous public health dimensions of this disorder. For example, we know that FASD is not a rare condition and that about 1 in 100 babies are born with FASD. We know the majority of people who have FASD have not received a diagnosis of their disability. Most people with FASD are adults, and although we now have a better system in British Columbia for the diagnosis of children-there is no system in place for adult diagnosis and assessment.

We know that the majority of people with FASD look normal. Although there are measurable facial changes that can occur if prenatal alcohol exposure occurs at a critical time of embryonic life, --most people with FASD have a normal facial appearance. FASD is therefore an invisible disability. Whereas other invisible disabilities can be identified through standardized testing, people with FASD often "pass the tests but fail at life." In other words, our current tests are unable to capture the full extent of the brain injury caused by prenatal alcohol exposure. There is no behavioral phenotype for FASD, meaning that there is no standard pattern of brain impairment. FASD is a developmental disability with life-long effects.

We need to be adopting a "lifespan approach" not only in our diagnostic capacity-but also in the way we support people with this disability. In the past, it was often the paediatrician who made the diagnosis of an FASD -without the benefit of a team. We now recognize that given the complex nature of this disability paediatricians cannot function alone -they need to be part of a team. Members of the diagnostic team may include a social worker, psychologist, occupational therapist, speech language pathologist, and a psychiatrist. It is important that every effort be made to confirm –or exclude-that prenatal alcohol exposure occurred during the index pregnancy.

The social worker on the team plays a pivotal role because historically this part of the diagnostic work up has been subject to bias, and prejudice. Skepticism about the validity of an FASD diagnosis remains-even in some members of the medical profession. It is, therefore, vital that we are transparent and clear in our diagnostic process and subsequent outcomes.

My professional and scientific knowledge of FASD has been enhanced over the years by my experiential understanding of the condition. This occurred through being involved in our local FASD community support organization, volunteering at Whitecrow summer camp, and being prepared to give extra time to listen to the stories of affected people and their caregivers. It is through the individual's story that we as pediatricians can begin to truly understand what it is like to live with this disability. In fact, caregivers of people with FASD often describe the professionals in their lives as dichotomous variables-they either "get it or they don't." This relates very much to the professional's willingness to go beyond the textbook and into the kitchen, the classroom and occasionally the courtroom. The value of having access to a paediatrician-or indeed any physician-who really understands the nature of this disability is one of the key factors in the formation of resiliency. Resilient people are able to bounce back from adverse events. The lives of people with FASD are full of such setbacks.

Our understanding of the huge social impact of FASD is still in its infancy. We constantly learn more about the stress on caregivers, the frustrations of teachers, and the inadequacies of the child welfare, mental health and justice systems. This can be a source of frustration for the medical profession. Paediatricians-like most physicians are trained to "fix" things, and indeed it is the basis of the fiduciary relationship between doctor and patient. Those five key words "how can I help you?" infer that the physician will do whatever they can to cure (where possible) and to care (without exception) for their patient. However, for a condition like FASD-where there is no cure-the duty of care becomes paramount. This is where many paediatricians experience their frustration-because much of what is required for their patients and families cannot be provided through traditional medical services. Income support, adequate housing, teacher's aide support, and addiction support services for biological parents-are some of the "non medical" prescriptions required for families living with FASD.

Over the past 35 years, we have come a long way in our understanding of FASD. We still have a long way to go. The problems we readily see are only the "tip of the iceberg." I think we are only beginning to realize the extent of this hidden disability.

Chapter Seven

Interpersonal Affiliation Systems and FASD

"There is no way for the human mind to perceive the external world (directly). We perceive through relationships with objects and with others. Relationships are the stuff we are made of." ***---Ruth Feldman, Bar Ilan University, 2010***

How do we manage to perceive and interact with one another? What parts of our brain work together to allow attachment? If there are disruptions in some of these areas how might clinicians and caregivers help?

As mentioned in the introduction, this is pioneering science, advancing daily. Insights of today, 2011, might seem backward in a few years. Nevertheless, I find some of the insights from these frontiers of neuroscience and psychiatry to already be relevant for me as I try to make sense out of issues my child and patients struggle with.

Let's all "stay tuned" to new understandings in attachment/social connection neuroscience. I believe these concepts will be even more helpful for our families in the future.

Although this chapter is designed for health professionals (language in the last part of the chapter is quite technical), the general public will find the first part quite accessible.

This field already abounds in creative researchers and gifted clinicians. At this time, however, few write about FASD-induced problems specifically. Interested readers will find Daniel Goleman's *Social Intelligence: The New Science of Human Relationships* [1] and Michael Gazzaniga's *Human: The Science Behind What Makes Us Unique* [2] to be excellent general introductions to human social interaction. Jon Allen's *Mentalizing in Clinical Practice* offers health professionals wise guidance for their approach to counseling patients. Working around and even transcendence over some affiliation problems is possible. [3]

A wise place to start might be to consider the infant-mother "dance."

Baby needs lunch or a diaper change or something else so puts out a signal - sometimes a loud one - to mum. Mum does not mirror back *exactly* what baby's message is because, frankly, that message is sometimes a loud scream! Instead, Mum engages in what Peter Fonagy terms *contingency* mirroring - that is, she reflects back to the child what she intuits is the problem along with reassurance. [4] Perhaps she'd say, "Don't worry, little man, we'll get you changed and get you something to eat right away; it'll be ok." Having needs met empathetically and repetitions of reassurance eventually help mould the psychological core of the infant. *Baby internalizes his caregivers' representation (of himself) to form the core of his psychological self.* [4] If mum's representation of baby is, "what a great kid, a bit fussy but he's wonderful," her child will build his psychological self on a strong foundation. If dad's representation is, "This kid is driving me nuts, I cannot sleep, she howls incessantly, and nothing works," his child's psychological core and confidence may be shaky.

With nurturance, baby learns the inner working model, "if I get close, I get cared for." Baby begins to appreciate he is distinct and separate from his mum and dad. Awareness of interpersonal boundaries slowly develops. Baby also learns that he can be soothed from emotional and physical distress albeit first by connecting with mum and letting her settle him down. Later, he can "graduate" to using parts of his self-soothing apparatus to calm down all by himself. [4] The fruit of secure, nurturing early attachments includes:

» *a sense of self as distinct from mum or others*

» *knowledge that distress <u>can</u> be soothed*

» *the potential to eventually be able to engage one's own self-soothing apparatus*

» *confidence that "getting close leads to getting helped"*

» *relief from the restless pursuit of connection; nurturing attachment, once provided, allows baby to relax (at least until the next dirty diaper!) and even start to explore his world, learn and imagine.*

"That's my baby!"
(Endearment-part one)

Peter Fonagy says," The attachment system is a striatal area that is activated, for example, by a mum or dad seeing her/his *own* baby as opposed to a baby belonging to someone else." [4] Seeing her *own happy* baby caused much more activation of mothers' dorsal putamen and sustantia nigra (striatal) areas versus seeing someone else's happy child. Their own baby, with a *neutral* expression, caused slight increase in activation of striatal areas compared to viewing another's neutral child. If baby was *sad*, whether she was mum's own or someone else's, mums displayed very little activation of the dorsal putamen or substantia nigra. "For mums to have that special connection feeling, their baby'd better smile," suggests Dr. Fonagy. [4]

Later, we will return to the topic of endearment as we discuss Ruth Feldman's concepts of *synchrony* and some of Dr. Fonagy's most recent work.

How might FASD disrupt the development of the infant-parent dance?

Preoccupied parents beset, for example, by sleep deprivation from a dangerous living situation, mental health issues such as post-partum depression and/or substance abuse issues will *not be as emotionally available* to their infant. Contingency mirroring, essential for the infant to sense empathetic connection, might be replaced by reactive thoughts that the baby is "making me (the parent) mad." Not sensing empathetic connection, the infant might cry even more vigorously, but this act might further overwhelm and alienate exhausted parents, already at their wits' end.

Children with FASD can be born with their stress sensitivity already set to "Hyper-reactive" (over-reactivity of the hypothalamic-pituitary-adrenal [HPA] axis). Reduction in cortisol receptors is just one of the differences prenatal alcohol often induces. Less activity at cortisol receptors effectively limits the child's ability to settle down from upsets. Cortisol receptors, effectively, function as "off switch" for the stress system so less activity at these receptors means emotional upset happens with less provocation and lasts longer. [5]

Disrupted sleep affects not just the child, but also his whole family. Unfortunately, circadian rhythm problems (which can contribute to feeding and sleep problems) are common in FASD. [6] Prenatal alcohol may harm a child's ability to make melatonin in response to dim light. This surge of melatonin contributes to sleep onset and maintenance. [7] I encourage readers to review Jim Jan's group's excellent review article on sleep problems in FASD [6] and make use of the patient information resources it contains. Prenatal alcohol exposure may also be a risk factor for enough sleep apnea or restless leg movement to disrupt sleep. Disrupted sleep reduces coping abilities of kids and parents; conflicts erupt more easily and attachments can be disrupted. Assessment and treatment of sleep problems is a central goal of preventive health care of families raising FASD-affected children.

Sensory processing difficulties in FASD

Of course, to fully appreciate a parent's nurturance, baby must accurately perceive caregiver's overtures. What if a child cannot see accurately or finds touch to be *irritating* instead of relaxing? Many patients with FASD I work with have profound sensory processing issues; we will review several of them shortly. An introductory Power Point session entitled Come to your Senses: *An Introduction to Sensory Processing Issues That Affect People Who Have FASD* appears earlier in this book. In this chapter, we will expand on how certain sensory perception problems complicate attachment.

Let's look at some patients' struggles:

J.S. Life must be so frustrating for J.S. because each time she simply shakes her head "no" she gets an immediate headache followed by two to three minutes of having her eyes flit back and forth (excessive horizontal nystagmus). J.S. has a balance (vestibular sense) problem.

R.J. This little fellow, in grade three, was "normal" on an *audiologist's hearing test* yet has no clue what to pay attention to in class because the teacher's voice is "drowned out " by the truck going by, the noisy fan, the buzz of the lights (auditory figure-ground discrimination problem). His itchy wool sox and his shirt's "scratchy" tag also distract him (touch oversensitivity). What R.J. requires is an assessment of *auditory figure-ground discrimination - a listening test!* We need to know if he can hear the teacher's voice when it is only 20 decibels louder than background noise...if not, he needs a way of amplifying the teacher's voice.

J.L. This little girl vomits anytime she is on a swing or trampoline (vestibular oversensitivity).

A.N. This boy, in grade one, craves touch so much he "invades the personal space" of his classmates by touching their hair or their soft new coat (touch seeking).

All these kids have no clue their experiences are unusual - *they have never felt things differently!*

Unless **J.S.'s** parents understood her sensitivity to head movement they might try to soothe her by rocking and be mystified why they were unable to settle her. After all, rocking helped their other kids! Unless R.J.'s teacher amplifies her voice she might interpret his distractibility as willful "fooling around" and her connection with R.J. might be at risk. J.L., as a young child, would probably become *more* distressed if placed in a "Jolly Jumper" because of her balance system's oversensitivity. If parents' attempts to calm her increased her distress, her mum and dad might feel incompetent and become demoralized. J.L.'s warm, emotional connection to her parents might be at risk. Their sense of effectiveness as parents *would* be at risk. If A.N. (the "Touch *seeker*") had a dad who was *irritated* by touch (Tactile defensive) the two would need to connect using strategies other than "hugs and cuddles" or risk alienating each other.

The eight sensory systems include smell, touch, vision, hearing, taste, position of joints/muscles (proprioception), gravity/balance (vestibular sense), and perceptions from body organs (interoception). Individuals with FASD (or autism, prematurity, head injuries and other conditions) can be *over*-sensitive or *under*-sensitive to sensory input to any of these systems. Prenatal alcohol can also cause some individuals to seek sensory input and can *impair processing* of sensory messages. In this chapter, our focus is attachment, so - for brevity - details of alcohol-related impairment in all sensory systems won't be discussed. However, we will look at details of sensory processing in the *visual system* so readers can appreciate how far-reaching some of the sensory struggles are. In my experience, extensive problems also affect the vestibular, interoceptive, touch, and hearing systems in FASD. Choosing to look at details of vision is not based on that sense being more impaired than other systems. The intention is simply to use vision *as an example* to demonstrate how profoundly altered sensory processing can be in FASD.

Visual system problems in FASD

Let's consider the steps of visual processing required for Jesse, a grade two student, to complete a "simple" visual task - copying the words: "Today's lesson" from the whiteboard.

1) The image of "Today's lesson" must first be registered by retinal rods and cones and converted into an electrical signal. In order see the whiteboard Jesse had to be sitting up which is accomplished by vestibular, touch and proprioceptive senses coordinating to help each other "tell the posture muscles what to do." Also, a system of *horizontal cells and bipolar cells* in the retina help to create nice "sharp edges" to the objects we see (good contrast sensitivity).

Drs. Stomland and Hellstrom found problems at the level of the retina in a study of 25 children who have FASD. Half had visual impairment; acuity was drastically impaired (less than 20/100) in 10 out of 50 eyes! Half had a loss of neurons in the optic nerve (optic nerve hypoplasia) and half has an increase in the number of blood vessels in the retina (increased tortuosity of retinal arteries). Half had eye movement difficulties (strabismus). [8] Strabismus (which is a motor planning and coordination of motor commands issue) could affect control of Jesse's eye movement across the page while reading and finding his "place" when going to the next line to read in a book or on the whiteboard.

Dr. Darren Sass, a developmental optometrist, has introduced me to the concept of *synchrony* of eye movements and accommodation, which is the lens' ability to change so one can focus on close work or distant objects. To read up close, the eyes must converge (go slightly cross-eyed) and the lens must become rounder to focus. To then look up at a distant whiteboard and still see clearly, eyes must move to a "straight" (not cross-eyed) position and the lens must be pulled into a more oblong shape so it can focus on distant objects. [9] For the most part, these eye movement and lens focus activities occur automatically but if they are not well coordinated the speed of processing visual information is impaired. Anecdotally, I can report many of the patients I see who have FASD have been found to have accommodation, acuity, and eye movement problems and eye exercises and strategies from developmental optometrists have been helpful. Contact information for developmental optometrists is listed in the appendix.

Overwhelmed working memory areas impair learning

Recently, Dr. Brock Eide alerted me to an overarching learning problem that kids affected by FASD must deal with. Practicing *compensatory strategies* for slow visual processing, impaired memory, distractibility (or numerous other challenges) is possible - and helps - but the act of keeping these compensatory strategies in mind *fills up (already compromised) working memory areas* thus leaving less "space" available in working memory for new learning. [10] Thus, success with vision therapy and many other treatments is better if kids are "not trying to do everything all at once." Don't undermine potentially effective treatments by overloading working memory capacity. I have not seen recent studies linking impaired social ability to an overwhelmed working memory system but I believe such associations are likely.

2) After "Today's lesson" is imprinted on Jesse's retina, the electrical "image" is sent down nerves that stop at a big sensory relay station called the thalamus. It is early days for specialized MRI (DTI or Diffusion Tensor Imaging) but Catherine Lebel and colleagues have shown the left thalamus has less intact or less developed microstructure in a recent study of kids who have FASD. She found decreased "fractional anistropy" in the left thalamus - this just means the little organelles inside this part of thalamus' nerve cells are not as organized as they should be so this area of the brain cannot work optimally. [11] In the thalamus, visual information gets analyzed by one area (the magnetocellular layer) for *movement of the image* and *coarse details* of the object. Another area of the thalamus (the parvocellular layer) analyses *colour* and *finer details* of objects. If Jesse was catching a ball his magnetocellular layer would be more important at first - to help him see the moving ball and his parvocellular layer would be more important later, as he reached out to snap his baseball mitt shut at the correct moment. Visual information also arrives at the superior colliculus of the midbrain and there, it is mixed with auditory and touch cues to produce a "map" of the space around us - this is one area of *multisensory* "spatial perception." [12] Before you say, "who the heck cares about the superior colliculus?" consider this: from this structure messages are sent to the brainstem to help control eye movements and through a large fast nerve tract (tectopontine) to the cerebellum where fine-tuning eye-hand control is controlled. Jesse would drop the ball or never get close to catching it without his superior colliculus! Prenatal alcohol reduces the speed of nerve conduction along fast tracts because it reduces production of myelin, the nerve "insulator" chemical that permits fast transmission of electrical impulses along nerve cell appendages (certain axons but not dendrites). [13]

3) Next "stop" for visual information is the primary visual cortex in the occipital lobes. This is the area where Alex Medina and his colleagues found "blurry, fuzzy" central processing in their 2006 study. Visual images form electrical "imprints" which are circuits of occipital cortex neurons. The more such circuits are "worked" - the more one looks at something - the more likely the image forms a *cortical functional map*. Prenatal alcohol results in excessive activity of an enzyme (called Phosphodiesterase type 1) and this impairs the brain's ability to construct a nice, crisp visual "map" because there is less ability to *perceive where the corners and borders of the image* are. In other words, prenatal alcohol exposure can result in "un-crisp, fuzzy" image production via excessive activation of a common enzyme. A "drug" that helped decrease activity of the enzyme (Vinpocetine - this is just an extract of the periwinkle plant available at most health food stores) seemed to *help crispness of the image* (read: the brain *learned* better!) in this animal study. [14]

4) In the occipital visual cortex, electrical impulses from the retina start to form an image but it is not until visual information is sent down a busy superhighway (called the inferior longitudinal fasciculus) to the temporal lobes that Jesse can understand the image on the whiteboard is actually a couple of words. Profound abnormalities of large tracts including the inferior longitudinal fasciculus are seen in FASD. [13] At minimum, visual information takes longer to reach the temporal lobe. Some visual information might not even make it as far as the temporal lobe because of damage to these big connecting tracts.

5) Visual information is first analyzed in a part of the temporal lobes called *Wernicke's area*; processing here allows Jesse to know that the images: "Today's" and "lesson" are *words*.

6) Wernicke's then sends the "word" information to adjacent temporal lobe *memory* areas that allow Jesse to put the words *into context and understand their meaning*. Now maybe he'll recall (with the amygdala's help) that he forgot to do "Today's lesson" yesterday! Yipes!

Temporal lobe impairments including decreased memory center (hippocampus) activity have been demonstrated following prenatal alcohol exposure. [13] [15]

7) *To write* what he now recognizes as words Jesse's Wernicke's area sends a message down the next "big superhighway connection tract" (the arcuate fasciculus) all the way around to…

8) Broca's area in the frontal lobe. There, plans for the muscle movements required to "say" "Today's lesson" (either aloud or "in your head") are formulated and then pushed "next door" to…

9) Motor cortex areas of the parietal lobe. This is where nerves that actually "tell" Jesse's muscles of his face, tongue and voice box to "say" a specific word or his hand to write the word originate. Prenatal alcohol exposure often impairs parietal lobe function. [13] [16]

Forcing eye contact can *sabotage* discipline

Ability to engage in eye contact can be important to establishing close emotional connection. Some kids affected by FASD feel "invaded and overwhelmed" by being forced to maintain eye contact (they are oversensitive to eye contact or "gaze averse"). Insisting on eye contact can push some kids into "fight/flight or freeze." This situation may result: "forced" eye contact ➔ child withdraws ➔ less connection with parent ➔➔ conflict!

When do caregivers most often *demand* eye contact? When their child did something wrong and they are trying to teach the kid a lesson. Insisting a child that is oversensitive to eye contact look at you as you are trying to discipline him/her almost guarantees the child will be so overwhelmed that they will not be able to "learn their lesson."

Facial recognition

Brain systems to recognize a face are critical to developing a sense of what is "*you*" versus what is the "other" person. Recognizing your parents' faces is a foundation for initial stages of attachment. Three brain regions are critically damaged in *Wilson's Syndrome*: 1) Fusiform Gyrus - an area that tells us "is *it a face or not*", 2) Superior Temporal Gyrus and Sulcus - areas that tell us "*is that face mean or happy*" i.e. is it safe to approach or not, and 3) Amygdala and prefrontal cortex - these areas help us decide if we *want* to approach or avoid that face. Patients with Wilson's Syndrome are often "indiscriminately hypersocial." Likely, these same brain areas are affected to some degree in some of our kids who have FASD. [13]

Activated by motion, the superior temporal sulcus integrates visual information and connects to social understanding areas. These circuits allow us to perceive *intentions* of others and are important in predicting the next move in a sequence. [17] Quite profound delays in the transfer speed of visual information to the temporal lobe exist in FASD making "real-time" predictions of others' intentions slow and awkward at best. [11]

Social Safety depends on recognition of danger

A practical problem parents struggle with is impairment of their daughter's ability to discern who is a "safe" boy to go out with versus who is "dangerous?" Individuals that have some damage to their "Facial recognition hardware and software" (fusiform gyrus, superior temporal gyrus, amygdala and prefronatal cortex) may need to abide by rehearsed rules (I will only go to a party if I am accompanied by a sober, trusted friend) or practice specific habits (I will always call one of three friends to discuss whether it is a good idea to go on a date with a specific girl or boy) in order to be safe. Those not familiar with FASD may believe such measures are restrictive to a young person's freedom but I believe such safety plans actually allow people affected by FASD to avoid some anticipatable dangers and achieve optimal success.

As a physician, I witness countless examples of when such safety plans are not practiced. From my perspective, working with patients who have been molested and abused, *lack* of such safety plans is dangerous. Those who believe individuals with FASD have no impairment of facial recognition systems would find it difficult to explain a young man's art therapy project. He drew all members of his grade ten class and all members of his family the same size and with very similar facial expressions. He did not know who the class bullies were and who was dependable. Possibly he could form a picture in his brain of individual differences (i.e. who was safe and who was dangerous) and simply had a drawing (expressive output) problem. Possibly he had the same brain problems as Wilson's patients do. More research might eventually clarify this question but, in the meanwhile, his family and friends must help him develop strategies to avoid danger. He has already been sexually molested and has posttraumatic stress symptoms.

Conclusions regarding impaired visual perceptions:

Jesse's "simple" visual task of reading the whiteboard and copying down the words "Today's Lesson" illustrates how hard everyday tasks can be for kids who have FASD because of their difficulties with visual sensory processing. Multiple areas can be harmed by prenatal alcohol exposure: the retina (fuzzy image), eye muscle coordination (double vision, difficulties "finding the beginning of the line of print"), the thalamus (where some filtering of irrelevant info happens), the visual cortex (crisp "corners and borders" of images), the big communication tract that takes visual information from the visual cortex to the temporal lobe, and the memory banks of the temporal lobes where we make sense of what the word means are all affected. Beyond this, processing speed is impaired by many mechanisms including damage to myelin (the sheath which makes nerve conduction quick).

Suitable accommodations for Jesse follow these understandings:

- Do not "overload" him with *volume* of work - a few less words on the spelling list or a few less paragraphs to read would be suitable

- Give time to allow for slower processing speed

- Help him sit where he is not distracted (not too many things up on the walls; ensure Jesse has a well organized work space)

- Let him practice at least some things "till he gets it." "*A habit*" is much easier to remember than something new.

- It is hard work being Jesse in class! - allow breaks and rests, let him know in some way that does not single him out (perhaps a "secret code") when it is his turn to answer a question…then try to set up a "no way you can lose" helping strategy till he understands the answer. (See, "Non shaming solutions," figure 2 in *Chapter One, FASD 101: Fetal Alcohol Spectrum Disorder For A General Audience* in this book.)

- He will be tired at the end of the school day - does he really have to go home at the end of the day and struggle with homework? Point: allow for the slower processing speed.

- If Jesse shares my older patient's impairments in facial recognition he may not know who is safe to be with and who might abuse him - practicing safety rules might prevent a dangerous situation.

How could Jesse's visual issues affect his social interactions?

Imprecise visual processing could lead to impaired interpretation of vital information such as interpreting facial expressions correctly. Muddled visual processing might result in poor movement planning. Jesse might misjudge where objects are in space and get hit by a soccer ball or be in danger trying to cross the road because estimation of how fast cars are approaching is impaired. Clumsiness might lead to ridicule. Sensory overload or preoccupation with compensatory strategies might overwhelm Jesse enough that he misses others' visual cues ("non-verbal communication" and gestures).

The amygdala directs the visual system

The amygdala acts as an "editor" in the social brain. The amygdala directs the visual system to attend others' eyes (searching for emotional information there such as a tear, a frown or a smile). The amygdala then assigns emotional significance to others' signals thus helping us answer: is he dangerous? or is she trustworthy?

Numbing

Recently, Martin Bohus has discussed states of emotional upset at the American Psychiatric Association Meeting. Dr. Bohus explains that in overwhelming stress, when fight and flight cannot help us overcome adversity, an ancient system of *numbing* becomes activated. Numbing actually *shuts-down* the overactivated amygdala. *Learning anything* that has emotional significance involves the amygdala. Difficulties always have emotional significance! Thus, if in a state of numbing, one cannot think about feelings or learn ways to overcome difficulties. [18]

Patients with FASD, born with hyperactivation of their stress systems [5], often are overwhelmed and appear to be numbed out, especially if they have been abused. When numbed out, their amygdala - the area that assigns emotional significance to behaviour - is "off line." Abilities to determine if others are safe (and can be approached) or dangerous (so must be avoided) are blocked until the amygdala recovers at least some function. Attempts to learn and remember strategies that can "keep you safe" will also be less successful until the amygdala regains some activity. This neurobiology explains a component of the inertia seen in the presence of terror such as when a person cannot leave an abusive relationship. Lack of willpower to effect change is not an accurate assessment of such situations. Rather, terrified individuals are derailed by shut down of their ability to process emotional information mediated by the ancient process of numbing. Obviously, the only humane or effective approach is to provide safety and reassurance so that terrified people can calm down enough to restart their emotional processing abilities.

Inconsolable crying: how *caregiver* auditory oversensitivity can disrupt attachment

Consider newborns...all infants in all cultures have an "inconsolable crying curve" which shows that inconsolable crying tends to "peak" in the second month after birth and decrease by the forth month. Inconsolable crying might be caused, in part, by oversensitivity of infants to certain touch sensations, certain movements, food textures, etc. [19] Prolonged inconsolable crying is a source of frustration and anger for parents and other caregivers. How difficult prolonged crying might be for parents will, in part, be predicted by *parental* sensitivity to loud noise. Tragically, frustration can build to a point of shaking the children.

The peak incidence of shaken baby syndrome follows a similar pattern to that of inconsolable crying (but with a "lag" of 4-6 weeks). However, shaking can occur as early as the second week of age. [19] Thus, effective intervention strategies (support people assisting new mums and their families, and provision of welcoming 24/7 "phone coaching" NOT just handing parents printed literature) must be offered to at-risk families *very soon after birth and continue until the sleep patterns are properly established and " inconsolable crying" is resolving*. Male relatives of the babies must be included in interventions also. I think it is important to anticipate that caregivers who have over-sensitivity to loud, unexpected noise (acoustic startle), especially if they do not have good supports readily at hand, may be especially vulnerable to frustration when their child is crying inconsolably and unremittingly.

Other parts of the social brain

Disclaimer: Since sensory processing is a central preoccupation of at least the back two-thirds of the brain, and most cognitive functions involve "whole brain" (very widespread) circuits, separating other brain activities from sensory processing is somewhat artificial.

Temporal lobes

The front part of both temporal lobes (anterior poles) mixes sensory information with limbic system signals.

The left side is particularly active when language processing is involved with social understanding.

Temporal lobes recognize if a social situation deviates from expectations (Yikes! I did not know *everyone* was going to get dressed up for this birthday party), and then pass on the problem to the *theory of mind system* to solve (they are all good friends, I'll just ask Jill if I can borrow a sweater). [17] (Theory of mind is the ability to separate what is on your mind from what you think is going on in another's mind.)

Unfortunately, temporal lobe changes are seen in FASD. Reductions of grey and white matter volumes were seen in the occipital-temporal regions of young adults with FASD. [20] Temporal lobe connections across the midline and with parietal lobes also appear to be reduced in FASD. [21] Furthermore, temporal poles (and the base of the prefronatal cortex) are the most likely areas to be damaged in traumatic brain injuries. [22] Regrettably, especially if living in unsafe situations, head trauma is so common it is almost *the norm* in patients with FASD that I see clinically.

Daniel Amen suggests that damage to temporal lobes may result in temper problems, a short fuse, unstable or unpredictable moods, misinterpreting comments as negative when they are not intended to be, déjà vu, or out-of-the-blue aggression. [23] In my experience, mood-stabilizing medications such as valproic acid or lamotrigen often improve concentration, performance of tasks and mood, sometimes to the extent patients with temporal lobe injuries can regain lost function. Literature supports the effectiveness of valproic acid on destructive and aggressive behaviours [24] and lamotrigine for aggression and agitation [25] in patients with traumatic brain injuries. I recall one interesting lady who reported to me, somewhat incredulously, that she'd *written a letter* to her (bleep bleep) landlord. In her constant battle with her callous landlord she frequently resorted to yelling, punching walls, etc. However, since starting lamotrigine, she sat down and wrote a letter of complaint - she won the dispute too! Later, we changed her medication to valproic acid, not because we were unhappy with lamotrigine's effect, but because she was quite forgetful and each time she forgot to take the med for several days she'd need to start at a very low dose and then gradually increase it (lamotrigine must be very gradually increased because a highish dose to start would have a bigger chance of inducing a

Meds

very severe rash). Valproic acid was more practical because when she forgot it, this med was easier to restart.

Discussing her son, a mother told me, "He seems pushed around by whatever the emotional event of the day is."

Dr. Larry Siever says that the temporo-parietal junction works in concert with midline deep frontal lobe structures (the anterior and pregenual cingulate). By combined action of the cingulate dampening down or attenuating signals of alarm and the temporo-parietal junction deliberatively "tuning in" or "tuning out" specific sensory signals, people are able to *direct their attention*. Less activity in the cingulate/temporo-parietal attentional control system means that emotions (the limbic system) direct attention. [26] We know the lower part of the parietal lobe (an area right next to or involving the temporo-parietal junction) is often harmed by prenatal alcohol. [27] Impaired function of the anterior cingulate in individuals with heavy prenatal alcohol exposure has also been demonstrated. [28]

Dr. Siever goes on to say the top part of the temporal lobe (superior temporal gyrus) is an area of self-referential processing of emotional data - the "it's all about me" or "reactive processing" center. Dr. Siever found *increased* activity in the superior temporal gyrus in patients with borderline personality disorder versus the *middle* temporal gyrus which an area of *conscious deliberative evaluation*. [26] Decreased function (decreased fractional anisotropy on diffusion tensor MRI images), especially on the right side, has been reported in temporal lobes of individuals with FASD. [28]

Mirror Neurons

Each of us has circuits of neurons that resonate with *observed* actions, sensations and emotions *in others*! It does not matter if we see another's leg *being touched* or if our own leg is touched. Activation of our somatosensory cortex occurs in either situation. If we observe another's *action* the same areas of the premotor cortex that planned that muscle action in the other person also are activated in us. The same area of neuronal activation occurs whether we observe an action or perform it. Mirror neurons help us understand another's actions and imitate them. Mirror neurons are also active when the final part of another's actions are hidden and must be inferred. [17]

Observed *action* mirror neurons

1) The superior temporal sulcus provides an initial description of an action to...

2) Parietal mirror neurons, which add somatosensory information and send the message to...

3) Frontal lobes where the action is encoded. For example: If listening to speech, activation of the speech production center (ventral premotor cortex) occurs. [17]

Significant volume reduction of parietal lobes was seen in adolescents after heavy prenatal alcohol exposure. [27]

Observed *disgust* mirror neurons

If we smell or see another exposed to a disgusting smell our anterior insula is activated - this area regulates visceral and autonomic responses to smell and taste sensory input, plus it receives input from the superior temporal sulcus and the facial recognition area. [4]

Observed *pain* mirror neurons

Empathy towards those we see in pain results from activation of our somatosensory mirror neurons *plus* two areas (anterior cingulate and anterior insula) that process the emotional affective component of pain. But empathy is deeper than just resonating in these three areas with the other person. Empathy requires you to *set aside your perspective* occasionally so you can estimate what the other person's take is of their situation. [29]

I am not aware of studies of mirror neurons in individuals with FASD. Thus, my conclusions are speculative. I believe motor mirror neurons (which allow imitation of actions) are unharmed, for the most part, by prenatal alcohol. Kids I see are often great imitators! However, appreciation of others' pain, disgust and emotional states is often severely compromised. Anterior cingulate and anterior insula damage may cause part of these deficits.

The anterior cingulate (and adjacent areas of the medial prefrontal cortex) are activated if you examine thoughts, experiences *or emotions* of yourself or another. [29] Functional problems were identified in tracts connecting to the prefronatal cortex in individuals with FASD. [30]

When you "put yourself in the shoes" of another person

This task is not simple. Coordination of these areas is required:

The lower (ventral) part of the medial prefrontal cortex considers emotions, example: will that help him feel better?

The upper (dorsal) part of the medial prefrontal cortex considers cognitions, example: how will he think about this?

The temporo-parietal junction helps to focus in on the others' perspectives and signals.

The inferior parietal cortex (an area possessing rich interconnections with the prefrontal cortex) becomes activated when one tries to take the perspective of another.

Endearment part two

Ruth Feldman has devoted much of her recent work life to the study of selective (I love you *more than others*) long lasting attachment. Chemical/hormonal, mental, brain, epigenetic and genetic factors mediate the biologic systems of attachment, but attachment is much more than just activating these different systems. *Synchrony* between all these biological and behavioural attachment systems in two different people is key.

Gazing at their infant's face, talking in a high-pitched singsong manner ("motherese"), expressing emotional warmth and affectionately touching (not just wiping food off the mouth!) are optimal ways *mothers* can connect with their infants. But they can overdo a good thing by continuing their motherese, touch, etc. when the infant is trying to respond - "standing back" enough to give the infant some time and space to respond helps to set up the synchronous dance of back and forth energy. Components of the dance are:

1) Gaze synchrony: looking at each other in a natural pattern of maintaining eye contact for a few moments, then looking away, then looking at each other again. Sensory over-sensitivities such as gaze aversion in autism can disrupt gaze synchrony.

2) Touch synchrony: a comfortable exchange of touch that develops a little later than gaze synchrony.

3) Vocal synchrony: typically develops by three to six months. Interestingly, *at first,* vocal synchrony starts with mum and baby talking *together*; only later do they "take turns." [31]

Fathers also have a number of robust biologic and behavioural systems of attachment. In fact, Dr. Feldman reported that involved fathers had similar levels of oxytocin to mothers! More on oxytocin just below, but before we leave fathers - Dr. Feldman points out dads' optimal ways of engaging socially with their kids are *slightly different from mothers' methods! Fathers usually carry kids facing away from them - out towards the world.* Interaction with dad usually involves high-energy stimulating touch. Interaction with mums tends to involve soothing touch. Fathers are more likely to stimulate their infants, carry them in space ("playing airplanes"), and encourage exploration. Neither sex is "right or wrong" in how they interact with infants and small children, they are just different. [31]

Are Ruth Feldman's descriptions of optimal ways mothers and fathers can interact with their babies the human equivalence of Michael Meaney's "high licking and grooming" rats?

Michael Meaney's research group at McGill University in Montreal have shown that *attentive nurturing* (mothers that display high amounts of licking/grooming and arched-back nursing behaviour) can actually "grow" cortisol receptors in their offspring; nurturing alcohol-exposed rat pups resulted in *acetylation* of their already methylated DNA areas which code for cortisol receptors. Acetylation allowed mRNA to transcribe enough of the DNA areas that code for cortisol receptors that at least some of this protein (the cortisol receptor) could be synthesized. [32] Dr. Feldman stated that the parent-child synchronous interaction patterns described above - slightly different for mums and dads - are the human equivalent of high licking/grooming nurturance in animal models. [31] Dr. Meaney says: "*Attentive parenting can influence prenatal alcohol-mediated damage to the glucocorticoid receptors.*" [32] To review further details of Dr. Meaney's work access **The Importance of Epigenetic Influences** in this book's chapter eight: Genetics and FASD.

Oxytocin

Oxytocin is an environmentally dependent neuropeptide with complex actions. In mothers, oxytocin stimulates milk let-down and uterine contractions. Increased by touch in a nurturing relationship, oxytocin primes bonding, trust and social affiliation (with each other and the infant) *for both mums and dads.* Oxytocin helps one to engage with another person in vocal, touch and gaze synchrony. Both oxytocin level and oxytocin receptor gene activity have been correlated to duration of gaze synchrony. [31] Curiously, if oxytocin levels are too low *or too high* relationships are less rewarding.

Synchrony results in a natural attunement of a mum her child and vice versa. Each can now pay attention to and respond to subtle signals from the other.

Functional MRI (fMRI) studies of parent-infant dyads

fMRI studies of 45 sets of mothers and fathers viewing videos of parent-infant interactions when their children were 2 weeks and 3 months postpartum show:

- *own* baby cry causes activation of areas that regulate emotion and empathy (frontal, basal ganglia, cingulate, thalamus and brainstem circuits) in a pattern similar to that observed in obsessive compulsive disorder (OCD) - this pattern, which fits with post-partum habits, worries (about the infant), and preoccupation (with the infant) is seen in male and female parents but is stronger in mothers, especially first time mothers

-later, by 3 months, new areas become activated to *own* baby cry including striatum, hypothalamus, and anterior cingulate - these areas are associated with reward and hormonal regulation.

Thus, fathers and mothers show earlier post-partum activation of OCD-like brain circuitry patterns that correlate with checking behaviours, worries and obsessions; later, parenting activates reward circuitry. [33] (Comment: don't worry - it is very helpful - from your baby's point of view - to have mum and dad obsessed about her!)

Previously (in: *endearment part one*) we learned Peter Fonagy had seen the largest activation of mothers' striatal attachment areas (dorsal putamen and substantia nigra) when they saw their own happy infant (versus their own sad infant or another person's infant). Summarizing more recent work, he says that attachment security is, to a degree, transgenerational. If you are a mum or a dad with secure attachments you are more likely to have a child with secure attachment patterns. Dr. Fonagy says that several biologic factors underpin secure attachment:

1) Oxytocin release in secure mums during play with infants was far higher than oxytocin release in insecure mums. This release of oxytocin is correlated with activation of the hypothalamic-pituitary region.

2) Secure mums showed a larger activation of the medial prefrontal cortex in addition to the dorsal putamen and substantia nigra (striatal attachment areas) on seeing

their infant's smiling face - but more importantly...

3) *When baby is sad*, attachment-secure mums *still have some striatal attachment circuit activation* (so still have the special, " this is my baby" feeling) whereas insecure mothers do not.

4) Instead (of striatal attachment center activation) insecure mums show activation of their *insula* when seeing their sad infant. Insula activation is usually associated with an experience of *negative* affect including memories of negative experiences. Insular activation also primes activation of autobiographical memory systems. [4] (Have you ever been flooded by recollections of every little [and big] disappointment and failure in your life when you were scared and upset? This was your insula "on overdrive.")

In FASD, due in part to sensory issues, infants can be so irritable and fussy they can sometimes be diagnosed as having a *regulation disorder of sensory processing.* [34]

This degree of fussiness and irritability could challenge the bonding abilities and patience of Mother Thersa. Mere mortal parents such as I need a network of helpers to "keep body and soul" intact raising such an infant. Parents unlucky enough to have a personal history of attachment insecurity may find that insula-mediated flooding of negative thoughts distract their attention and undermine confidence when caring for sad or fussy infants.

Recently studies have shown prenatal alcohol exposure can reduce function in the right putamen and thalamus. [9] Thus, those with FASD may struggle more to have the special feeling of affection mediated by this area. Readers may wonder if I am suggesting that people with FASD are not loving? Of course not! Most people with FASD that I know are very loving. Dr. Fonagy's insights simply suggest one part of the attachment brain may not work as efficiently in some people. Catherine Lebel's neuroimaging work has identified damage in parts of this circuitry in individuals exposed to alcohol prenatally.

Given that most people with FASD that I know are loving and friendly... have they figured out a "work around" for the putamen/thalamus component of attachment system damage? Maybe - or perhaps different structures are more critical for attachment when the brain has been damaged by prenatal alcohol. Sorry to repeat an overused cliché - but we do need more research.

Serotonin and emotional dysregulation ("Spazz!")

In the fetus, serotonin neurons arising from brainstem nuclei project forward to forebrain areas. In animal models, there is a critical window of time for serotinergic projections to arrive in the forebrain. With cooperation of glial cells, forebrain serotinergic (5-HT 1A) receptor activity facilitates maturation, migration and differentiation of neurons. Decreased serotinergic activity, seen in animal models of FASD, results in "cascading deficiencies of forebrain development." [35]

Reduced serotonin activity contributes to decreased control of emotions. Dr. Glen Gabbard says: "The prefrontal cortex is the place of self-directed regulation of emotional response - *our goal is to extend its influence!* Serotonin is the brake fluid for the brakes in emotion control systems. In borderline personality disorder, there is less serotonin-mediated orbital prefrontal cortex inhibition of over-reactivity in the amygdala." [36] Whether similar reductions in serotonin activity undermine emotional control in FASD is not known at this time. I have not come across studies of serotinergic activity or serotinergic 1A receptor density in FASD in recent medical literature.

Opioid Receptor tone and emotional distress

I don't know if depleted opioid receptor tone results from prenatal alcohol, but recent studies have pointed to this mechanism underlying some of the most distressing symptoms encountered by my patients - self-harm activities (cutting) and drug seeking.

Opioids (such as the body's own endorphins and encephalins) mediate physical pain but also *mediate social pain* such as the distress of social isolation, exclusion or separation. Opioids mediate, in a positive way, self-soothing and suppression of stress-induced negative affects. In other words, adequate opioid tone helps people cope with upset and not be overwhelmed by stress. Conversely, low opioid tone reduces the ability to calm down and results in a situation of "being pushed around by negative feelings." [26]

Buprenorphine is a narcotic medication often used in place of methadone for people recovering from opioid abuse. Buprenorphine, unlike methadone, maintains a steadier "baseline tone" of stimulation of opioid receptors - this baseline tone helps patients avoid a sensation of "raw achy" craving that often leads to drug seeking. At higher doses, buprenorphine tends to block opioid receptors, which in turn reduces stimulation of brain reward centers. With less drug-induced activation of the reward center, patients find it easier to think about topics other than drugs. For some years now, in Seattle, buprenorphine has been used successfully for patients recovering from heroin and other opioid addictions. [37] At present, it is not covered by government pharmaceutical coverage for indigent populations in British Columbia.

Self-injury such as cutting actually increases opioid tone at opioid (mu) receptors because the injury releases the body's own opioids - endorphins and encephalins - into the circulation. Recent studies confirm high rates of self-harm behaviours in those seeking buprenorphine treatment. [38] Hopefully, we will soon learn if partial blockade of the opioid mu receptor by buprenorphine can help reduce self-injury as well as drug seeking. I have a number of patients in my practice whose lives are profoundly limited by drug seeking - I would like to be able to use meds such as buprenorphine for them. If research confirms buprenorphine reduces self-harm - I would like to be able to use it for that indication also.

Conclusions: Parent-child relationships are a synchronous dance, controlled by many social and biologic factors

Effective parenting is a dance; a dance that involves at least two partners. *Either* partner has the potential to make or break an interaction. Infants activate parents' basal forebrain regions, which regulate nurturing and caregiving responses. Handling emotions (about the infant), setting aside personal concerns so attention can be focused on the infant, empathy and maintaining motivation despite sleep disruptions are all crucial to successful parenting. [39] FASD, whether in parents or children, causes changes to some of the key structures and circuits of interpersonal affiliation. James Swain states: "We argue that an integrated understanding of the brain basis of parenting has profound implications for mental health." [39]

Problems in social interaction affect FASD. Foster care or adoption breakdowns, marital conflict, child neglect and abuse, ostracism at school, and poor self esteem are all, at least in part, the result of relationship breakdown. These destructive heartbreaks tear families apart.

Conversely, interpersonal success builds confidence. Let's use what we can of recent understandings to build resilient, empowering relationships.

References:

[1] Goleman D. 2006. Social Intelligence: The New Science of Human Relationships. New York: Bantam Books.

[2] Gazzaniga MS. 2008. Human: The Science Behind What Makes Us Unique. New York: HarperCollins Publishers

[3] Allen JG, Fonagy P, Bateman AW. 2008. Mentalizing in Clinical Practice. Washington, DC: American Psychiatric Publishing, Inc.

[4] Fonagy P. 2009. (Conference presentation) Advances in Personality Disorders: Attachment and borderline personality disorder: a mentilization – based approach. American Psychiatric Association Meeting, San Francisco, May 16-21, 2009.

[5] Uban KA, Bodnar T, Butts K, et al. 2010. Direct and Indirect Mechanisms of Alcohol Teratogenesis: Implications for Understanding Alterations in Brain and Behavior in FASD. In: Riley EP, Clarren S, Weinberg J, Jonsson E, editors. Fetal Alcohol Spectrum Disorder: Management and Policy Perspectives of FASD, First Edition. Weinheim, Germany: Wiley-VCH Verlag GmbH & Co. KGaA. doi: 10.1002/9783527632510.ch6. p 109-126.

[6] Jan JE, Asante KO, Conry JL, et al. 2010. Sleep health issues for children with FASD: Clinical considerations. International Journal of Pediatrics. Published online July 14, 2010. Accessed at: http://www.ncbi.nlm.nih.gov/pmc/articles/PMC2913852/ November 28, 2010.

[7] Goril S, Shapiro CM. 2010. The prevalence and patterns of sleep disorders and circadian rhythm disruptions in children with Fetal Alcohol Spectrum Disorders (FASD). Poster presentation at 2010 Fetal Alcohol Canadian Expertise (FACE) research roundtable meeting published as: 2010 FACE Poster Competition Abstracts Supplement. Journal of Population Therapeutics and Clinical Pharmacology 17(2) Summer 2010: e284-e301.

[8] Stomland K, Hellstrom A. 1996. Fetal Alcohol Syndrome: an opthalmological and socioeducational prospective study. Pediatrics 97(6): 845-849

[9] Sass D. 2010. Personal communication.

[10] Eide B, Eide F. 2010. Common Learning Challenges in Sensory Processing Disorder. (Conference presentation) at: Sensory Processing Disorder Foundation 11th International Symposium and Pre-Conference Institute, Bellevue, Washington, November 12, 2010.

[11] Lebel C, Rasmussen C, Wyper K, et al. 2008. Brain Diffusion Abnormalities in Children With Fetal Alcohol Spectrum Disorder. Alcoholism: Clinical and Experimental Research, 32: 1732–1740. doi: 10.1111/j.1530-0277.2008.00750.

[12] Barthel K. 2004. Evidence and Art: Merging Forces in Pediatric Therapy. Victoria, BC: Labyrith Therapies. Available from: www.labyrthjourneys.com p 34.

[13] Norman AL, Crocker N, Mattson SN, et al. 2009. Neuroimaging and Fetal alcohol Spectrum Disorders. Developmental Disabilities Research Reviews 15: 209-217

[14] Medina AE, Krahe TE, Romoa AS. 2006. Restoration of neuronal plasticity by a phosphodiesterase type 1 inhibitor in a model of fetal alcohol exposure. Journal of Neuroscience 26(3): 1057-1060

[15] Sutherland, RJ. 2003. Prenatal alcohol exposure neuropathology and cognition: integrating behavioral and neural approaches in rats and humans. (Conference presentation) Fetal Alcohol Canadian Expertise (FACE) 2003 Research Roundtable. (available webcast at:

http://www.knowledgenetwork.ca/fasii/index.html)

[16] Powrozek TA, Zhou FC. 2005. Effects of prenatal alcohol exposure on the development of vibrissal somatosensory cortical barrel network. Brain Research Developmental Brain Research 155(2): 135-146

[17] Allen JG, Fonagy P, Bateman AW. 2008. Mentalizing in Clinical Practice. Washington, DC: American Psychiatric Publishing, Inc. p 118.

[18] Bohus M. 2009. (Conference presentation) Pain processing in BPD: functional and genetic approach. American Psychiatric Association Meeting, San Francisco, May 16-21, 2009.

[19] Barr RG, Barr M, Fujiwara T, et al. 2009. Do educational materials change knowledge and behaviour about crying and shaken baby syndrome? A randomized controlled study. Canadian Medical Association Journal 180(7): 727-733

[20] Li Z, Ma X, Peltier S, et al. 2008. Occipital-temporal reduction and sustained visual attention deficit in prenatal alcohol exposed adults. Brain Imaging and Behavior 2: 39-48

[21] Sowell ER, Mattson SN, Thompson PM. 2001. Mapping callosal morphology and cognitive correlates: effects of heavy prenatal alcohol exposure. Neurology 57: 235-244

[22] Phan N, Hemphill JC, Aminoff MJ, et al. 2010. Traumatic brain injury: Epidemiology, classification, and pathophysiology. UpToDate Desktop 18.2 CD-ROM Medical Reference

[23] Amen DG. 2010. Change your brain change your body. New York: Harmony Books. p 316.

[24] Wrolewki BA, Joseph AB, Kupfer J, et al. 1997. Effectiveness of valproic acid on destructive and aggressive behaviours in patients with acquired brain injury. Brain Injury 11(1): 37-47

[25] Pachet A, Friesen S, Winkelaar D, et al. 2003. Beneficial effects of lamotrigen in traumatic brain injury. Brain Injury 17(8): 715-722

[26] Siever L. 2009. (Conference presentation) Neurobiology of Personality Disorders. American Psychiatric Association Meeting, San Francisco, May 16-21, 2009.

[27] Sowell ER, Thompson PM, Mattson SN, et al. 2002. Regional brain shape abnormalities persist into adolescence after heavy prenatal alcohol exposure. Cerebral Cortex 12: 856-865

[28] Sowell ER, Mattson SN, Kan E, et al. 2008. Abnormal cortical thickness and brain behavior correlation patterns in individuals with heavy prenatal alcohol exposure. Cerebral Cortex 18: 136-144

[29] Allen JG, Fonagy P, Bateman AW. 2008. Mentalizing in Clinical Practice. Washington, DC: American Psychiatric Publishing, Inc. p 122.

[30] Fryer SL, Schweinsburg BC, Bjorkquist OA, et al. 2009. Characterization of white matter microstructure in fetal alcohol spectrum disorders. Alcoholism: Clinical and Experimental Research 33: 514-521

[31] Feldman R. 2010. (Conference presentation) The biologic basis for parent-infant bonding. Third biennial UBC conference on: Brain Development and Learning: Making Sense of the Science. Vancouver, BC. July 16-20, 2010.

[32] Meaney M. 2010. (Conference presentation) Maternal Care and Gene-environment Interactions Defining Development. Third biennial UBC conference on: Brain Development and Learning: Making Sense of the Science. Vancouver, BC. July 16-20, 2010.

[33] Swain JE, Leckman JF, Mayes LC, et al. 2008. Functional Brain Imaging of Parents: Associations with thoughts, timing, experience, delivery and dyadic experience. (Poster presentation) Canadian Academy of Child and Adolescent Psychiatrists Annual Meeting. September, 2008.

[34] O'Malley KD. 2007. Infant, toddler and young child systems of care for patients with Fetal Alcohol Spectrum Disorders (FASD) and their families. In: O'Malley KD. Editor. ADHD and Fetal Alcohol Spectrum Disorders (FASD). New York: Nova Science Publishers.

[35] Zhou FC, West JR, Blake CA, et al. 2005. General discussion at the Fetal Alcohol Syndrome Symposium. Experimental Biology and Medicine 230: 407-412

[36] Gabbard G. How neurobiology informs psychotherapy in personality disorders. (Conference presentation) American Psychiatric Association Meeting, San Francisco, May 16-21, 2009.

[37] Yuodelis-Flores C. (addictions psychiatrist). 2010. Personal communication.

[38] Sansone RA, Whitecar P, Weiderman MW. 2010. Self-harm behaviors among buprenorphine-treated patients. Primary Care Companion, Journal of Clinical Psychiatry 12(2): PCC.09100813. doi: 10.4088/PCC.09100813ecr.

[39] Swain JE, Lorberbaum JP, Kose S, et al. 2007. Brain basis of early parent-infant interactions: psychology, physiology, and in vivo functional neuroimaging studies. Journal of Child Psychology and Psychiatry 48(3-4): 262-287

Chapter Eight

Genetics and FASD: Heritability information gives us a deeper perspective on "Secondary Disabilities"

This chapter reviews some of the details of genes, identified to date, that increase the risk of developing alcoholism and other conditions which co-exist with and even relate to the development of FASD - impulsivity, sensory processing problems, externalizing behaviours, emotional volatility, attachment problems, and other mental health issues. If we can understand elements of this emerging field we can develop effective, targeted, public health preventative plans, and learn how to interact more effectively with all kids, but especially those who have FASD.

Although this chapter's focus is those genetics relevant to traits found in FASD-affected individuals and their birth parents, I cannot stop myself from discussing clinically relevant ideas because I am a primary care doctor. Thus, I will share a few "pearls" that Montreal psychiatrist Dr. Joel Paris finds practical and effective when dealing with volatile, impulsive patients.

As a parent of a child with Fetal Alcohol Spectrum Disorder (FASD) and a physician who cares for patients who have FASD, I have known the emptiness that comes from my own failures - many times over! At times, symptoms from the scary list of "Secondary Disabilities" that Ann Streissguth's 1996 study [1] highlights overwhelm my ability to cope. Yet Diane Malbin has given caregivers a helpful template [2]: if we can lessen the gap between environmental expectations and our child's abilities, less frustration and less secondary disabilities will result. Despite our best efforts, sometimes "crisis mode" seemed to last forever in my family! Our children's negativity and volatile emotions led to impulsive and dangerous behaviour and were honestly the bane of my existence for several years. Try as I might, I could do little to improve the situation. Like all caregivers I sought advice from whomever I could access. Often, the ideas I gathered were ineffective. Once in a long while, however, when I was reading something "unrelated," I would sit up in bed with a "Eureka" moment! One of these moments involved Joel Paris.

Dr. Paris, a Montreal-based psychiatrist, wrote an interesting (and brief) book in 2003, entitled *Personality Disorders Over Time*: Precursors, Course and Outcome. Joel has provided mental health care for, and closely followed, a large group of patients who have been diagnosed with Borderline Personality Disorder (and other types of personality disorder) for *over 30 years.* Arguably, this group of patients may have suffered and/or do suffer from some of the most problematical cases of impulsivity and volatile, labile emotional patterns of any patient group. Dr. Paris' wisdom and experience have provided himself, and consequently others, with many useful ideas with which to positively influence the outcomes of people who suffer from extreme and dysregulated emotions. If the personality traits of *impulsivity and emotional lability* were further "wound up" by stressful or abusive environments, borderline or antisocial symptoms could result. I thought I could perhaps "borrow" some of Dr Paris' "pearls" because many of the people with FASD that I was (rather ineffectively) working with were caught in crises, which had, in part, been triggered, by impulsive actions and very volatile, unregulated emotions.

What really struck me, though, was how *heritable* the personality traits of impulsivity and emotional lability/ volatility/ dysregulation were. In other words, notwithstanding the brain damage caused by prenatal alcohol, kids who have FASD are likely to carry a considerable genetic *predisposition* to many other mental health issues. Furthermore, a child's FASD - i.e. pattern of brain damage caused by prenatal alcohol exposure - certainly will not protect him or her from genetic risk. In order to understand our children and their pattern of alcohol-induced brain damage we need to ask ourselves what genetic factors, good and bad, did they inherit from their birthparents?

Some "pearls" from Dr. Paris' book, *Personality Disorders over Time,* regarding how to work with those who have extreme emotional volatility and/ or impulsivity: -recognize that suicidal ideas, self-harm and other crises are "a cry for help"... *and offer that help*; be sure that attention to (albeit necessary) details at a time of crisis, for instance documenting the degree of suicidal intent, planning, access to means, etc., does not distract you from your *most* critical responsibility: attending to that "cry for help" -remember that the *foundation* of any work that deals with volatile or distressed people is *the security and strength of your relationship with them*... maintaining that respectful relationship is a primary goal, for without it "helpers" can do nothing-(as a doctor) NEVER "fire" a patient (even if provoked by the patient's behaviour: i.e. not showing up to appointments, not taking meds as prescribed, or other "no-no's") because often the precipitant for another crisis (self-harm or similar) is the patient's *perception of being abandoned by a social attachment.* Maintaining reasonable boundaries is encouraged, yet should the patient disregard these boundaries the penalty must never result in the severing of the relationship; that therapeutic bond is the foundation on which any intervention is built.

Dr. Paris explains that the trait of impulsivity has a heritability of well over 50%; emotional lability, though less precisely studied, is thought to have a heritability of close to 50% [3]. As I was reading Dr. Paris' book and "filtering" his ideas through "the lens" of my FASD-affected child's turmoil, I also kept thinking about a 14-year-old patient with FASD that I had been seeing in my clinic. We were all wracking our brains trying to figure out what more could be done for him. He was often in crisis; something had to change. I had no idea how his environment could be improved. He had a good Individualized Education Plan (IEP), warm and caring parents, a counselor at school that took great interest in him, and concerned, empathetic friends and teachers. Yet despite this support, the boy was suicidal, volatile, and explosive. He became entangled in substance abuse and stealing, and was almost "impossible" for his parents to talk to on account of his defiance and negativity. I, his parents, the school, everyone: we were scared and overwhelmed. I knew that this fellow suffered from FASD (i.e. alcohol-induced brain damage) but I also could not help but wonder... *what traits had he inherited*? His symptoms appeared to be impulsivity, "externalizing" behaviours (anti-social traits and substance abuse) and emotional lability "squared." Could he have inherited these traits from his birthparents? The answer is yes. Personality and behavioural traits have a significant heritability; the most interesting part was, however, the ways in which we could all help him *not express these genetic predispositions.* I have observed that the preservation of caring relationships with concerned adults and the reception of age-appropriate interventions that have been tailored to the child's specific patterns of sensory and medical needs can yield positive results.

How can genetics information be effectively used?

Genetics researcher Dr. Marc Schuckit not only helps us understand some of the genes that lead to problem drinking, but he also suggests how we should approach and evaluate genetic information: "…the more we understand about *risk factors*, the *genes* associated with them, and the *mechanisms* through which those genes work - for *any* health concern be it alcohol problems, diabetes, cancer, coronary heart disease, depression, schizophrenia or other - the better we should be able to provide *early identification* and *prevention* of any of these disorders." [4]

Birth Mums and Birth Dads

I feel reluctant to accept the theory of *Assortative Mating*, a term which scientists use to refer to a human being's tendency to choose a mate who possesses similar traits to his or her own, despite the positive or negative implications of these traits. Perhaps a hopeless optimist, I nevertheless cling to my "positive illusion" that wonder, love, romance, destiny and divine forces bring couples together. Schuckit, et al. have decided, however, that assortative mating is "a complex effect that has been shown to occur in families with alcohol dependence."[5,6] This statement implies that birth dads of children who have FASD are likely to add to the birth mum's already significant contribution of genetic risk factors for alcohol dependence.

Birth Dads

With the exception of recent data from epidemiologist Susan Astley and her group from the Fetal Alcohol Syndrome Diagnostic and Prevention Network (FASDPN) Clinic at the University of Washington, Seattle, I have not seen statistical data about birth dads. [7]

Statistics regarding the birth dads of 1400 patients seen at FASDPN for assessment and diagnosis of FASD:

Only 8 % of the birth dads accompanied their child to the diagnostic evaluation (vs. 20% of patient's birth mothers). On average, birth dads were 32 years old at the birth of their FASD child (birth mums were 3-4 yrs younger). 39% did not finish high school; 50% reportedly had learning disabilities.

The names of 765 of the birth dads and 955 of the birth mums were known.

I asked different birth mums (seen as patients in my medical practice) about the birth dads of their children. This is not a scientifically rigorous method of studying the demographics of this group. Nevertheless, the following are *real* examples of birth dads:

(Birth dad #1): "Don't know where he is, he left as soon as he knew I was pregnant, I honestly don't remember much about him - that was a time of a lot of partying in my life." (Birth dad #1 probably carries genes that predispose his children to substance abuse, impulsivity and reduced social attachment)

(Birth dad #2) "Quick-to-anger fellow, now in jail for assault, "out-of-control" drinker, has not contacted me (birth mother) for several years, had learning problems especially with math, "bored" with school, "jumpy," quit in grade 9." (Birth dad #2 probably carries genes that are predispose his children to learning disorders, impulsivity, ADHD, sensory processing issues, difficulty regulating emotions and externalizing symptoms such as conduct disorder and substance use disorders)

(Birth dad #3): "Drinking buddy with me (birth mum), often wanted me to drink with him, could be abusive when drunk but a really nice guy when sober, have not seen him for 10 years, his brother and sister died of cirrhosis." (Birth dad #3 probably carries genes that are predispose his children to substance abuse, cirrhosis and emotional dysregulation)

(Birth dad #4): "Caring, nurturing, attentive dad, Masters of Science Degree, married me (birth mum) when I was in medical school. (Birth mum is a physician but is now unable to work in this capacity). He thought my drinking was a "partying phase" and that I'd be able to reduce it later; now he looks after our son, who has FAS, full time - at this point I cannot stop drinking, I've lost my job. I don't live with my husband or my son. My husband had to give up his job advancement plans as the care of our son is so consuming." (Birth dad #4 seems to be studious and "steady" - he may well have been attracted to his wife because she was exciting and flamboyant - it is tragic that she could not reduce her level of drinking)

I suppose nothing is straightforward; birth dads are composed of a varied group of individuals. When someone with more resources than I possess gets around to studying this diverse group I expect my observations will be proven. Fathers' genetic contributions to their children matter as much as mothers' genetic contributions!

Understanding both birthparents' inheritable traits can help caregivers plan preventative medicine interventions for their children.

As a physician, knowing the birth family history of these conditions would help in the planning of preventive medicine interventions:

Experiences, Heritable Symptoms and Traits Relevant to Mental Health Outcomes:

Do *either* of the birth parents or their families have, or have they experienced:

» Major Depression, "Subthreshold" depression such as dysthymia?

» Abuse of alcohol and other substances including: tobacco, marijuana, cocaine, methamphetamine, phencyclidine (PCP), heroin or other opioids, prescription drugs, or inhalants?

» Bipolar Disorder?

» Anxiety disorders including posttraumatic stress disorder (PTSD), phobias, panic disorder, or generalized anxiety disorder?

» Schizophrenia?

» Abuse or neglect?

» The effects of *witnessing* violence?

» Foster care (number of placements, duration of each placement) and the effect of early family dynamics?

» Adoptions, early family dynamics?

» Autism Spectrum Disorder?

» Learning disorders, educational difficulties?

» ADHD, ADD?

» Obsessions, compulsions?

» Sensory processing problems (over or undersensitivity or craving certain sensations), especially touch oversensitivity, auditory oversensitivity ("acoustic startle"), and difficulty perceiving "bitter" tastes?

» Personality disorders?

» Personality traits of impulsivity, emotional lability/ dysregulation, metacognition issues such as alexithymia, poor selfconcept, difficulty appreciating others' points of view and diminished sense of social worth?

» "Externalizing symptoms," e.g. the combination of conduct disorder, substance abuse or dependence, antisocial personality disorder, or the traits associated with these conditions?

The above is a current but incomplete list of conditions that we know have significant heritability and/or influence on mental health. Furthermore, issues such as impulsivity, emotional dysregulation, depression, anxiety, PTSD, bipolar symptoms, externalizing traits, ADHD, and substance abuse can lead to trouble with the law, disrupted school experience, confinement in jail or in patient facilities for treatment of mental health issues, inappropriate sexual behaviour, difficulties living independently, and problems with employment. These are the issues Dr. Ann Streissguth and her researchers, from the University of Washington, Seattle, refer to as "Secondary Disabilities"[1]; regardless of whether you are a parent, professional, person who has FASD or a general community member these negative outcomes are expensive heartbreaks we must *all strive to prevent*.

Birth Mother study

In 2000, a group from the University of Washington, Seattle, published *A Comprehensive Profile of 80 Birth Mothers of Children with FAS*. [8] Susan Astley and her team studied 257 birth mothers whose child(ren) had been assessed at the University of Washington FAS Diagnostic Clinic. Details of the selection of 80 birth mums from this group can be reviewed in this article: Astley et al., 2000 [9] To be eligible for the study, birth mums had to be locatable, live in Washington State and have given birth to at least one child who was diagnosed as having FAS or *static encephalopathy* (a pattern of behavioural and cognitive problems similar to that seen in FAS but without the growth restriction and facial anomalies required to make the FAS diagnosis). *107 of the 257 mums could not be found* at the time of this study, which was, on average, 11 years after the birth of their child and 3 years after the FAS or static encephalopathy diagnosis was established for their child. 58 out of the 257 mums were ineligible for the study because they had moved out of state or *died*. A quarter of the women had either died or disappeared within just three years of their child's diagnosis. This is a *devastating* level of mortality - I know of no type of cancer with this level of mortality in 30-year-old women! 92 of 257 mums fit the eligibility requirements for the study and 80 women were enrolled. The children whose mothers were enrolled in the study had an average age of 7.8 years at the time of diagnosis; over half no longer lived with their birth mum when they were diagnosed. Each birth mum participated in a *4-hour* structured interview answering *2044 questions* - to complete this number of responses demonstrates "heart for your kids" and interest in their best welfare. Helping to keep birth mums, many of whom had serious mental health issues, "on-task" enough to complete these detailed interviews is also a testament to the flexibility, approachability and supportiveness of the interviewers.

Birth mums averaged 27 years of age when they gave birth to their child who was diagnosed with FASD. 39% had completed high school; 25% had some college education. Average maternal I.Q was 90. 59% had annual household incomes of less than $10,000 at the time of the study; most lived in poverty at the time of the index child's birth. An astonishing 95% had been physically or sexually abused during their lifetime. The mental health burden of birth mums was *overwhelming*: 96% had psychiatric diagnoses. The average number of psychiatric diagnoses per birth mum was 4.7. Two thirds of the women were not receiving mental health treatment at the time of the interview. Policy makers must start by understanding and addressing these last two sentences - the *average* number of psychiatric diagnoses is 4.7 and 2/3 are not receiving *any* mental health treatment! *Not one of us* could function effectively (and not seek maladaptive coping strategies) while coping with this level of burden of untreated psychiatric illness.

Most common diagnoses affecting birth mothers included tobacco smoking (95%), alcohol abuse (86%), posttraumatic stress disorder (PTSD) - which 77% of birth mums had at the time of the interview or in the past, followed by depression (60%), simple phobias (44%), social phobias (43%), antisocial personality (39%), agoraphobia (34%)/ mania/ bipolar (21%), panic disorder (20%), bulimia (13%) and schizophrenia/ schizophreniform (7%). Hindsight is always 20:20, but I did not see that ADHD, borderline personality disorder (BPD), traumatic brain injury (TBI) or sensory processing disorder (SPD) were assessed. Perhaps these issues are more easily recognized clinically only more recently; I have observed them often in birth mums I see in clinic. I bring up these four diagnoses because they are often overlooked, which is a pity, because each of these conditions is common, can lead to very significant impairments of function, and can be effectively treated.

A possible bias in the study is that the women who went missing or died between the time of their child's diagnosis and the interview a few years later were not interviewed. This (missing or deceased) group of mothers likely had to contend with an even more severe burden of mental health issues than the 80 women who were enrolled in the study. Also, as noted above, I do not think the study assessed prevalence of ADHD, TBI, BPD or SPD in birth mothers. Thus, the "average" inventory of mental health conditions for birth mothers is likely to be *even more severe* than what the study concluded. As a primary care physician, I am familiar with the devastating legacy these conditions can inflict on an individual and his/her family; I recall my own reactions to these data when I first read them about a decade ago. Firstly, the notion that "FASD is 100% Preventable" (which we all get told at conferences by well-meaning but poorly-informed speakers) is nonsense! My response: 1) This statement ignores the important contributions of birth fathers to genetics and outcome, and 2) Society could reduce FASD prevalence by *diagnosing and effectively treating* the crushing burden of mental health disorders birth mothers contend with. Until barrier-free diagnosis and treatments are available the statement: "FASD is 100% preventable" is simply empty rhetoric.

It is beyond the scope of this genetics chapter to detail the prevalence of co-morbid alcohol and drug abuse combined with each of the above mental health diagnoses. However, two very relevant considerations must be noted: 1) People with PTSD, depression, eating disorders, ADHD, traumatic brain injury or bipolar disorder have a high incidence of co-morbid alcohol abuse, and 2) Frequently, especially for women, the mental health issue (e.g. depression or PTSD) pre-dates and precipitates the alcohol abuse. [10] Let us be clear: firstly - accessible, validating, accepting, non-stigmatizing mental health care must be made available for marginalized women - and *then* we can hope to see the legacy of untreated addictions (including the prevalence of FASD) decrease. This is "get-in-there-and–get-your–hands-dirty" work with some of society's least advantaged folks. An additional barrier - some birth parents are more than a little suspicious of the professionals that work in clinics and family support because most have had rough experiences in their brushes with "authority figures" in the past. I don't blame them; if I had experienced a fraction of the trauma many of my patients report I believe I'd be much less "intact" than they are.

In 2011 we have evidence-based drug and psychotherapeutic [11,12] methods which are proven to be effective in the treatment of even the most severe of these issues (e.g. PTSD). To not have these strategies readily available where we encounter traumatized women (e.g. victims services, women's shelters, outreach clinics) is a public health disgrace. As mentioned above, I believe we'd find the incidence of borderline personality disorder symptoms, traumatic brain injury, sensory processing disorder and ADHD symptoms to be quite high in birth mums if the Seattle Study had assessed those conditions - treatment must be made available for these issues also. That means funding occupational therapists to assess and treat sensory processing disorder. We now understand that those suffering from domestic abuse often have symptoms that look like borderline or other personality disorders, and that these symptoms often abate when the abuse is stopped. The more that we, as a society, recognize and treat the mental health and safety issues of birth parents, especially those of the birth mums, the more we can hope to reduce the crushing levels of emotional distress which lead to self-medicating by means of drugs and alcohol. Non-stigmatizing, accessible mental health care and psychiatric rehabilitation will reduce the incidence of FASD because birth parents will then have better tools than alcohol with which to cope.

Resiliency factors??

Returning briefly to Dr. Astley's *2010* presentation, [7], Susan questioned what is going on with the 9.3% of the 1400 children assessed in her clinics that were exposed to alcohol but do not have measurable deficits. Did they have less exposure to alcohol than their peers who were diagnosed with having an FASD? No. They were more likely to be females - maybe estrogen is, to some extent, neuroprotective, partially diminishing the toxic effects of alcohol on the fetus. They were *more* likely to be younger and *less* likely to be affected by adverse postnatal events such as multiple placements, sexual or physical abuse, chaotic, unpredictable homes, etc. Though not measured as deficient, "blunting" will have occurred i.e. loss of genetic potential. Susan Astley said no genetic studies have yet been done on this relatively resilient group; I wonder whether they have two "long" (ll) alleles of the serotonin transporter gene (as opposed to long/short [ls], or short/short [ss].) Please see reference 28 for more details, re: serotonin transporter genes.

More recently, geneticist Albert Chudley estimated approximately half the alcohol-exposed children he had seen clinically "show no substantial neurocognitive impairments or birth defects." [13] Dr. Chudley's observations clearly support Dr. Astley's contentions that resiliency factors exist; an opportunity to decrease prevalence of FASD might result from further study of resiliency factor mechanisms.

Heritability of mental health problems can be high.

Mental health and other health problems can be caused by prenatal alcohol exposure - but also, risk for developing these conditions can be inherited. For instance: you have a lifetime risk of developing *bipolar disorder* (BD) of 40-70% if your identical twin has it. You have a 5-10% lifetime risk of developing BD if you have a brother, sister, mum or dad (first degree relative) with it. [14] 69% of the variance for expression of symptoms of *borderline personality disorder* is accounted for by genetic influences. [3] The lifetime risk of developing *depression* if your identical twin has it is 37%. [15] Heritability of *ADHD* may be as high as 76%. [16] *Alcohol dependence* has 50-60% heritability. [17] *Externalizing behaviour* such as conduct disorder or antisocial personality disorder associated with substance abuse can have a heritability of 80%. [18]

Children born to parents who have mental health and addiction issues will inherit a genetic susceptibility to those issues. The extent of this genetic predisposition varies with each mental health diagnosis; some conditions can have a moderate heritability (30-50%) but others can have higher levels of heritability (60-80%).

Consider, also, an additional effect: the *direct* effect of alcohol on genes and the proteins that are made by those genes. LeStrat, et al. have reported that, in addition to causing direct damage to developing fetal tissues, alcohol can harm an individual by *changing gene expression* in genes that control neurogenesis (new nerve cell growth), cell adhesion (the "glue" between cells), apoptosis (controlled cell death), myelination (an essential part of helping nerve cells communicate quickly), ubiquitination* (a process of protein modification), cell survival, energy metabolism, * and manufacture of mitochondrial proteins.* Alcohol also has a direct disruptive effect *on the proteins* which are made by the transcription of genes responsible for the processes which are marked * - that is mitochondrial, ubiquination, and energy metabolism proteins. [19] Recently, Albert Chudley adds that alcohol can cause detrimental effects on gene regulation, transcription

Genetic Issues

and translation, molecular transport, and secretion and various enzyme systems. [13]

Genes that increase the risk of developing substance abuse

At this time, genes that increase the risk of developing substance use problems are better understood than genetic mechanisms underlying other serious mental health issues. The National Institute on Alcohol Abuse and Alcoholism in the USA has funded the Collaborative Studies on the Genetics of Alcoholism (COGA) since 1989, with the goal of identifying the specific genes underlying this vulnerability. Alcohol-use disorders have 50-60% heritability and the genes that explain about half of this heritable risk have been identified thus far. [17]

Amanda Kalaydjian and Kathleen Merikangas say, "aggregate twin study data are remarkably consistent in demonstrating that genetic factors play a far greater role in the etiology of *more severe* patterns of substance use, particularly abuse or dependence, as compared to initial use or *early* stages of addictive substance use which appear to be more strongly determined by environmental influences."[20]

If the *sequence of DNA bases* (Adenine, Thymine, Guanine, Cytosine) is changed then gene expression from that area of the DNA will change.If factors such as the development of chemical bonds (methylation) between parts of the DNA prevent the chromosome from "unwrapping" (thus not letting messenger RNA [mRNA] get "close enough" to "learn" the sequence pattern required to manufacture proteins) then *genetic expression is altered without changing the DNA sequence* - an *Epi* (on top of) *genetic* event has occurred. To form a protein, RNA bases must gain intimate proximity to DNA; this close access is denied if DNA bases remain tightly coiled up. The process of DNA, acting as a template for an appropriately assembled messenger RNA, is called *transcription*. mRNA then proceeds to code for the appropriate amino acid sequence that will create a specific protein - assembling a protein according to the mRNA code is called *translation*.

Epigenetic processes involve inaccessibility of DNA base sequence templates to RNA because methyl bonds (between different DNA bases) or tight bonds to *histones* (small proteins that DNA chains are wrapped around) have prevented the unfolding of DNA strands. Recent work on epigenetics implicates birth dads in adverse consequences for their offspring *whether the birth mum used alcohol or not!* [21] I like to explain epigenetics using the "cheesy" metaphor of a reluctant father sizing up his daughter's boyfriend. (Sometimes it is easier to remember things that are presented in a "silly" story!)

Epigenetics, DeeNA and ReNAldo - A Love Story

(This "Cheesy love story" is a metaphor for just how inaccessible DNA can be)As mentioned above, DNA strands are tightly wound around histones. Then, histone-bound DNA is tightly *coiled*. Such "bound up" DNA is inaccessible to RNA. DNA coils and folds must open up and tight bonds to histones must release in order for RNA to get close enough to DNA to allow transcription. Methyl bonds make it hard for DNA to "open up" - thus, transcription is reduced and the amount of a specific protein that can be made by that mRNA is reduced.

"Cheesy" Metaphor: It is Friday night and this rather scraggly boy (the mRNA - let's call him ReNAldo) shows up at your front door wanting to take out your teenage daughter (the DNA - let's call her DeeNA). You, the dad, are the methyl bonds which bind DeeNA's *chromatin* layers together so they cannot unfold (you told her there is no way she can go out in that skimpy red dress!) thus she is "inaccessible" to ReNAldo's wishes for intimacy! (Chromatin is the combination of DNA, histone and other proteins that make up chromosomes.) Ah - if it were only that simple! Alas, ReNAldo is smarter than he looks and so arranges for DeeNA to have some of her base pairs *acetylated* which is a way of him gaining intimate access to her base sequences "through the back door." The methyl bonds are still there, keeping DeeNA from being fully open to transcription, but acetylation has allowed ReNAldo a pathway for transcription - after which he can go on to make the specific protein DeeNA has programmed his bases to produce. Score: one for Mother Nature, zero for Dad. Damn!

The importance of Epigenetic Influences

Now the "punch line": maternal *stress, emotional trauma*, and *prenatal alcohol* can cause methylation of parts of children's DNA that codes for *proteins* called *cortisol receptors* Cortisol receptors act as "off switches" for the stress (fight/ flight/ freeze/ hypothalamic pituitary adrenal [HPA] axis) system. Without an "off" switch the child cannot "turn off" his/her hormonally driven stress system.

Successes for mum or dad in their efforts to "calm you down", or being able to "self-soothe," are elusive. Such a baby might be diagnosed as having "*Regulatory Disorder of Infancy*" - there is limited capacity to settle distress because the "off switches" for the stress system, the cortisol receptors, are in short supply.

Michael Meaney's research group at McGill University in Montreal has shown that *attentive nurturing* can actually "grow" cortisol receptors; nurturing alcohol-exposed rat pups results in *acetylation* of their already methylated DNA areas that code for cortisol receptors. Acetylation allows RNA to transcribe enough of the DNA that codes for cortisol receptors that at least some of this protein (the cortisol receptor) can be manufactured. [22]

Keen students of Michael Meany's paradigm might ask, "did all that high LG mother-kindness so empower her pups that they became foolish and overconfident - thus exposing themselves to excessive danger?" *Maybe*, but I think close attachment would make rat pups (or human toddlers) far more likely to "listen" to their mum's directions for staying out of trouble. Furthermore, according to Dr. Gordon Neufeld (see reference 23) poorly attached kids often become "guarded or armored", not letting others see their vulnerabilities. Dr. Neufeld further suggests that such "distancing" from feelings of vulnerability may result in emotional desensitization and eventually a "craving" for at least feeling the "adrenaline high" of potent (sensory) stimulation. Dr. Neufeld thinks this drive for an adrenaline high may partly explain risk-taking behaviour such as engaging in "extreme sports".

Avril Levigne, the Canadian songstress, in her "rebellious teen" stage had a song *"Anything but Ordinary"* which exemplifies adolescent risk craving.

Her song's lyrics, "sometimes I drive so fast, just to feel the danger..." and "I wanna scream... it makes me feel alive" express teenage seeking of risky or edgy physical activities. Most parents, recalling their own teenage angst, could endorse Avril's wishes to scream but would have problems with her wanting to drive fast "just to feel the danger." However, parents shouldn't throw Avril's CD into the trash because in verse three Lavine tells her audience to let down their defences, appreciate the beauty in the world around them and savour, don't waste away their time.

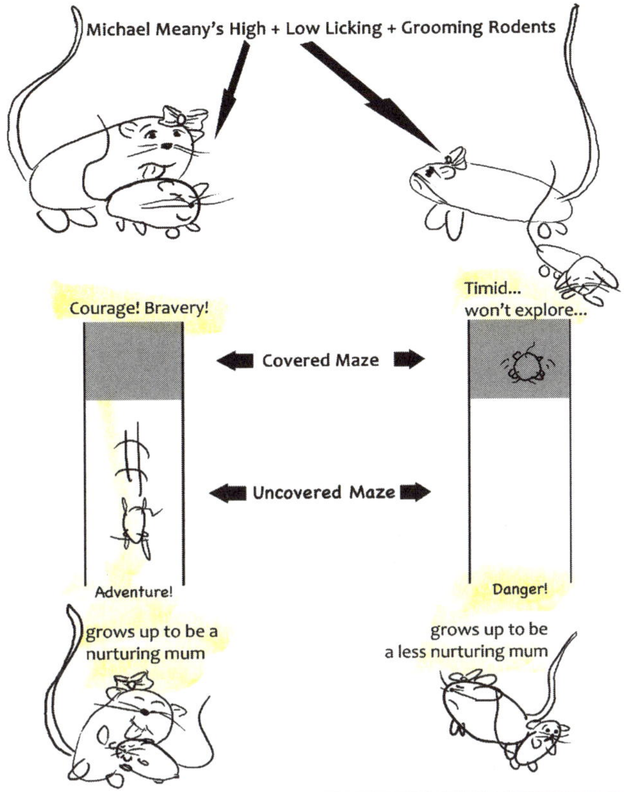

Graphic adapted from: Higgins ES. 2007. [reference 16]

Above, we see a "high licking and grooming" (high LG) mum and her contented pup on the left and a "low licking and grooming" (low LG) mum and her "tuned out" pup on the right. Unfortunately the sequelae of disinterested parenting include timidity in the pups - in rat experiments low LG pups were not risk-taking enough to bravely venture out on the "exposed" limb of the rat maze...and when they grew up they were "low LG" mums to their pups. (Gordon Neufeld's concept of "emergent play" wherein children, *once they became confident of a secure connection with their parents*, are energized to curiously explore and learn [23] appears to me to be a human equivalent of bravery and curious exploration shown by the high LG rat pups.)

Obviously if the low LG pups so craved sensory input (or adrenaline) that they took reckless risks "in order to feel alive" then this could be a great danger for them.

The next level of research Michael Meaney undertook (not pictured in the figure above) was to *foster* low LG pups to high LG mums - attentive early nurturing allowed those pups to become brave (able to explore the uncovered limb of the rat maze) and grow up to be nurturing parents. Fostering high LG pups to low LG mums had the opposite effect - those pups grew up to be timid, non-nurturing parents. The low and high LG rats had the same genes but attentive nurturing had thus been proven as a way to alter genetic *expression*. The high LG rats could express the part of their DNA that codes for cortisol receptors - thus they could grow more "off" switches for their stress systems. The low LG rats *had the same DNA as the High LG rats* to code for cortisol receptors but *could not express that DNA* (because the DNA was methylated and the attentive nurturing [which allows for *acetylation*] had not occurred).

Warm, attentive nurturing (i.e. empathetic attachment) has the power to effect positive epigenetic changes on control mechanisms of the hypothalamic-pituitary-adrenal (HPA) stress axis. This conclusion, which follows from Michael Meaney's research, gives hope to parents of kids who were exposed to prenatal *alcohol, trauma, broken attachments* or any combination of these hardships. (Psychiatrist, Bruce Perry calls these three factors "the triple threat.") Joanne Weinberg, Ph.D., says that prenatal alcohol exposure causes enduring increases in fetal HPA tone (hyper-reactivity of the hypothalamic-pituitary-adrenal stress axis) which cause over-reaction to stressful events in children. This "difficulty in calming down" likely contributes to the development of some symptoms we call secondary disabilities [24], for example, anxiety disorders. Dr. Meaney's studies suggest that attentive nurturing of alcohol-exposed children has the potential to effect epigenetic changes that improve stress sensitivity; "We live by hope!" said an adoptive Dad recently at a parenting course I was facilitating.

How can nurturing attachment actually heal over-active stress circuits in the brain? What is the neurobiology that underlies this powerful force of attachment? How might we help restore vital attachments in those parent-infant "dyads" who are "at risk" because of infant (FASD, prematurity, sensory hyper or hyporesponsivity) or parent factors (post-partum depression or mental illness or addiction issues)? Detailed analysis of these factors is beyond the scope of this chapter but I believe this is such an important factor for optimal outcome for children with FASD that I'd like to share some introductory information.

Attachment

Attachment of children to their parents and vice versa has been studied using neuroimaging techniques. Early on in the parent-infant relationship there is increased activation in dopamine-rich areas of the *"reward pathway"* (cell bodies in the ventral tegmental area which project to the nucleus accumbens). Parents fall *in love* with their infant! Later, *"obsession"* areas in the (dopamine-rich) caudate show most of the activation. Parents become *obsessed* with their infant! Oxytocin receptor activation (in the nucleus accumbens) in an estrogen, progesterone and prolactin-primed brain facilitates attachment for new mums. Vasopressin receptor activation (in the ventral pallidum) facilitates dad's attachments. [25]

Front-line professionals and parents already know how important attachment is, and that healthy "working relationships" are the foundations required for *being able to offer families and kids any programme or care*. The only problem is that sometimes those kids don't want to have a relationship; maybe they even sabotage social connections. How to stay connected to kids who are experts at distancing themselves from parents is the gist of Psychologist Gordon Neufeld's DVD Series and book. I like Gordon's ideas enough to have taken extra training in the facilitation of his video courses. I think they are the most accessible and empowering "attachment-focused" materials for parents and teachers that I have found. Interested readers could obtain the book: Neufeld G, Mate' G. 2004. Hold on to Your Kids: Why Parents Need to Matter More Than Peers. Toronto (Canada): Vintage Books of Random House Canada, Inc. The book is really practical and has excellent suggestions but I find the DVD series called "The Vital Connection" even more helpful. To obtain the DVD access Dr Neufeld's website at: http://www.gordonneufeld.com/

Fathers' Roles

Animal studies have shown offspring of alcohol-exposed *fathers* to have a lowered birth weight, hyperactivity, lowered cognitive ability, reduced length, lower serum testosterone, smaller seminal vesicles, lower beta endorphin levels in the hypothalamus, more malformations, smaller eye globe size, increased incidence of microcephalus, more problems with muscle coordination and a higher likelihood of hydronephrosis. This list of findings is similar to what physicians find when they diagnose children severely affected with FASD. Philip Haycock, working with the Department of Public Health and Primary Care, Strangeways Research Laboratory, University of Cambridge, thinks that the mechanism of these changes is "likely to involve alcohol-induced epigenetic changes" and that "environmentally acquired epigenetic states (*will be transmitted) between generations* in animals and humans." [21] Fathers' alcohol intake harming their children brings to mind poor old James Bond. In 2011, we now appreciate that James has a dilemma; he must choose to either trade his "shaken not stirred" martini for a tasty mocktail, ensure "Goddess number 12" (or whatever her number is) has effective birth control, or apply a condom. Given the incidence of chlamydia (5-28%) my advice would be for him to use a condom whatever option he chooses! [26] Given James' philandering past, Goddess number 12 would be wise to insist on a condom plus a complete STD screen in any event!

Epigenetic influences from *both birth mums and birth dads* result in a significant part of the pattern of prenatal injury we call FASD. Clearly, *neither* dad nor mum should drink alcohol when conceiving a child. If anyone can read Philip Haycock's review [21] and not come to the conclusion that conceiving a child and parental consumption of booze (whether it be maternal or paternal) do not mix, I would be interested in their "logic!" In the interest of public health awareness the journal publishing Dr. Haycock's study, Biology of Reproduction, took the unusual step of making article [21] available as a free download. Our friend James Bond is likely to say, "Philip Haycock's ideas that dads must not drink describe studies done on animals so they don't apply to me"; sorry James, it isn't so! Recent work by Lillian Ouko and her group at The Division of Human Genetics, University of the Witwatersrand, Johannesburg, South Africa, shows how alcohol influences human sperm by effecting epigenetic changes to DNA methylation patterns and that such changes are likely to be passed on to the next generation. [27]

Gene by Environment Interaction

One gene can affect several different types of mental health issues. Different forms (called the short [s] allele and the long [l] allele) of the promoter part of the serotonin transporter gene **(5-HTT)** predispose to different mental health outcomes *in the presence of stressful or negative life events*. One or two copies of the short allele of 5-HTT not only increase the incidence of and severity of depression, but also decrease depression's responsiveness to treatment. If a patient has one or two short alleles of 5-HTT, he/she is at increased risk of developing depression or posttraumatic stress disorder (PTSD) *if exposed to stressful life events*. This increased risk is compounded if the patient has *low levels of social support*. [28]

Furthermore, *various age* groups with the short allele show different adverse effects - for instance, college students exposed to negative life events show increased drinking and drug use. Also, maltreated small children who have a short allele went on to start drinking alcohol at an earlier age and at an increased amount compared to their peers. [29]

Mary Schneider and her team at the University of Wisconsin-Madison have performed some elegant studies with these same gene polymorphisms (l and s alleles of the serotonin transporter) in monkeys. Offspring that carry the *short* allele of 5-HTT, when exposed to alcohol prenatally, are much more likely to have increased activation of their HPA stress axis and to display irritability compared with their peers who carry *long* 5-HTT alleles (even if those "long allele" peers were exposed to alcohol). [28] In other words, the short allele conferred increased irritability to the offspring of monkeys who (prenatally) consumed moderate amounts of alcohol. *This short allele is common in humans, with prevalence rates depending on racial ancestry of the sample group. (25% [African] to 80% [Asian])*

Monkey babies from Mary Schneider's lab *that carried the short allele* of 5-HTT *and were exposed to prenatal alcohol* displayed behaviour very similar to what is described as "Regulation Disorders of Sensory Processing".[30] Irish pediatric psychiatrist, Kieran O'Malley says: "Infants and young children with FASD commonly demonstrate Regulation Disorders of Sensory Processing which are characterized by difficulties in tolerating environmental stimuli, co-coordinating basic motor movements or in approaching and interacting with others in their immediate environment." The difficulties that alcohol-exposed babies have with feeding, irritability, sleep regulation, and fussiness could be consistent with Type A: Hypersensitive Regulation Disorders of Sensory Processing (Fearful/ Cautious subtype). [31]

I do not know of studies to assess the prevalence of the short allele of 5-HTT in human infants that fit the diagnostic criteria for Regulation Disorder of Sensory Processing and who have been exposed to alcohol prenatally. Let's just imagine, however, that we have this information. Mary Schneider's studies would predict a high likelihood of enduring fussiness, difficulties with feeding, problems with self-regulation and trouble falling sleep. It would be entirely appropriate to organize intensive support for *any* parents trying to take care of such an infant. If parents were single, and/or have other risk factors such as isolation, depression, substance use issues, PTSD, low income, or lack of support from grandparents and other family members, then trying to care for such a difficult-to-settle infant could be a "perfect storm" of stress. Anyone who thinks I am over-dramatic in insisting that this combination of unsupported parents and difficult-to-settle infants creates the "perfect storm" for risk of shaken baby syndrome does not appreciate current understanding about pediatric abuse and would be wise to view: http://www.PURPLECrying.info/. The practical implication is that high risk situations need intensive interventions early because "inconsolable crying" and sleep dysregulation, key triggers for shaken baby syndrome, are very common in newborn infants with regulation disorders. A public health nurse visiting at 6 weeks is *far too late* to be able to recognize and help at-risk parent-infant dyads.

Genetics Basics - What Does DNA Do?

We each have 46 chromosomes - ½ from our mum and ½ from our dad - in each of our cells (except eggs and sperm which have 23 chromosomes each). These 46 chromosomes are arranged in 23 pairs. Each of us has 25,000 genes - scientists now know where and on which chromosomes these genes are located.

Perhaps the key question is "what turns these genes on and off?" Most genes are inactive, for instance women have two X chromosomes in each cell but one typically stays "dormant" while the other "does all the work" of making the individual female. Cells carry DNA that codes for any body activity, but, for instance, if a spleen cell used its genetic codes to make unnecessary proteins (for a spleen) such as nerve growth factors that would be a waste of cellular resources and could eventually cause disease. Spleen cells must inhibit or turn off genes that do not have to do with optimal spleen function. *To a large extent the question is not whether a person has a specific gene but whether that gene is expressed or unexpressed - i.e. can he/she "turn a specific gene on or off?"*

Genes control many aspects of our most fundamental body processes. For example, genes can influence traits of touch and auditory oversensitivity, the learning of new facts (episodic learning difficulties), impulsivity and aggression.

In a study of toddler-aged twins, auditory and especially tactile defensiveness had moderate heritability and, importantly, was associated with anxiety and the possession of a fearful temperament. [32] Touch and auditory oversensitivity is a "sensory profile" which other clinicians (and I) have found to be common in kids affected by FASD. [33] Sensory overresponsivity (SOR) likely involves dopamine 2 receptor (D2R) binding in the striatum (caudate, putamen and globus pallidus). Genetic modulation of D2R and dopamine transporter proteins would affect expression of SOR. [34]

DNA's activity is central to learning a new fact. For example, the first time you learned 2+2=4 glutamate was released into a synapse ➔ then glutamate bound to NMDA receptors ➔ which changed the structure of the NMDA receptors in such a way as to allow a "secondary messenger", calcium, to enter the post-synaptic cell ➔ calcium then signaled DNA in the post-synaptic cell to synthesize a number of proteins (including more NMDA receptors)! Thus, the strength of transmission for the next similar glutamate release is increased. *Long-term potentiation* (LTP) is the term for long-lasting enhancement in signal transmission between two neurons and is caused, in part, by new protein synthesis. Long-term potentiation is considered to be basic to memory and learning. [35] Individuals who have FASD are often found to have impaired episodic learning (of "new" facts) [36] but I am not aware of studies that confirm alterations of LTP in this group.

"Impulsivity" includes terms such as sensation seeking, risk-taking, novelty seeking, boredom susceptibility and unreliability - impulsivity has been associated with risky behaviours including sexual risk taking and drug use. [37] Impulsivity has at least 50% heritability. [3] Impulsivity may relate to FASD in that it seems to be associated with engaging in unprotected sex while under the influence of alcohol. In a study of "sexual debut age 16 or younger" it was found genetics influenced disinhibitory traits such as sensation seeking, impulsivity and non-conformity; 20-25% of the youth had been drinking when they had sex, and if youth showed more conduct disorder traits or drug use there was an increased chance of having *unprotected* sex and/or sex *in exchange* for drugs or money. [38]

"Externalizing" disorders such as conduct disorder, antisocial personality disorder or substance abuse disorders appear to have a high heritability and are strongly associated with alcohol abuse. [39]

Genes ARE NOT DESTINY

Caregivers and environments **do influence outcomes**; that is why I am writing this chapter! Kids of alcoholics have a two to four times increased risk of becoming alcoholic themselves - but less than half become alcoholics. [17] Nevertheless, four lines of evidence: adoption studies, twin studies, animal models and human genetics all say there is a significant genetic component to alcohol use disorders. [17] If we can understand mechanisms that allow expression of potentially harmful genes we can target interventions to people at high risk. Those who carry high-risk genes *do not necessarily* develop even highly heritable diseases (e.g. even if your identical twin has Bipolar Disease you have at least a 30 % chance of *not* developing it).

Reduce exposure/access to addictive substances. You may have a large genetic predisposition (lots of family members with addictions) but if you are not exposed to a substance of abuse you will NOT develop an addiction to it. **One way to avoid expressing a high-risk gene for alcoholism is not to drink.** Reducing access to substances of abuse by is an essential public health policy. A liquor store on every corner is ludicrous. Society needs to very carefully decide the best approaches to drug access decisions. Providing "free" injectable drugs to addicts reduces harm from contaminated drugs, unintentional overdose and dirty needles but will increase the amount of drug consumed. When access to alcohol is increased by opening more liquor stores, allowing longer opening times at drinking establishments or lowering drink costs, the public health burden from more drinking (cirrhosis, alcohol-related road traffic accidents and alcohol-related violence) increases. [40] Prof. Griffith Edwards, considering the link between increased availability, increased consumption and increased drinking problems in Eastern Europe in the 1990's says, " Where controls on price and access (to alcohol) already exist they should not be removed for political, ideological or trade reasons, with their public health significance ignored."[40]

While genetics are a central factor in pathogenesis of drug addictions, Howard Edenberg helpfully points out, "If someone self-administers enough of any substance (of abuse) he/she will 'swamp' the effects of any genetic tendencies!"[41]

Nicotine dependence has 50-60% heritability and some genetic locations associated with nicotine addiction (a cluster of nicotine receptor genes on chromosome 15) also contribute an increased chance of *alcohol use problems*. [41] Other nicotine receptor genes on chromosomes 9 and 11 are "candidate" genes that might predispose to *impulsivity, cocaine dependence and nicotine dependence* - one cannot separate the effect of one factor on another i.e. the cocaine dependence might result from the impulsivity effect. [17]

Not all that is familial is genetic; e.g. choices and habits, "the way we do it in this family," play a role in whether risk-taking behaviour will occur.

What Actual Genes Appear to Increase the Risk of Developing Alcohol Abuse?

"Genes we already know predict a bit less than 50% of drug dependence so lots is unknown at this point," says Howard Edenberg. [41] Especially in complex conditions (such as personality traits, alcohol addiction, diabetes or hypertension) *many* genes influence an outcome - any single gene accounts for just a *small part* of an eventual outcome. Each gene may also affect some other important characteristics - and these might directly or indirectly affect addictions. For example if you have the **GABRA2** gene the odds ratio for you to develop alcoholism is 1.2 (an increased risk of 20%); if you have this same GABRA2 gene the odds ratio of you *not* being married is 2.2 (an increased risk of *120%)*! [41] Clearly, GABRA2 carries genetic codes that influence skills needed to maintain long-term relationships such as reciprocity, control of anger, volatility, and impulse control.

Alcohol Metabolism (simplified)

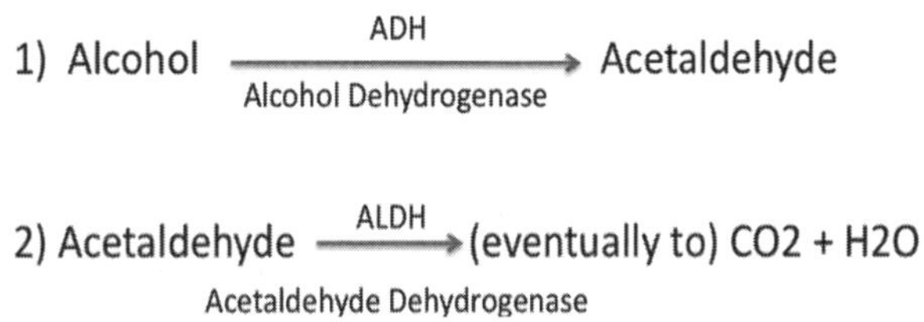

Step 2) of alcohol metabolism, above, actually involves three separate reactions: acetaldehyde to acetic acid, acetic acid to acetyl-CoA and then acetyl-CoA to water and carbon dioxide.

Some genes influence enzymes that break down alcohol. For example, ALDH2 is a gene that codes for *Acetaldehyde Dehydrogenase* - an enzyme that breaks down acetaldehyde. Acetaldehyde is a toxic breakdown product of alcohol. If acetaldehyde accumulates it causes flushing, nausea, lightheadedness and a fast heart rate (sometimes called "the flushing reaction"). If an individual carries the gene for the *inactive form of acetaldehyde dehyrogenase* he or she will develop this flushing reaction after drink. Booze "isn't worth it!" Individuals are at virtually no risk for alcohol dependence if they are *homozygous* for this gene (i.e. if they inherit the gene for the inactive form of aldehyde dehydrogenase from both their mum and their dad). [40]

ADH1B*2 (also called ADH2*2) is a variation of the gene that codes for a more active form of the *alcohol dehydrogenase* enzyme. Mothers with ADH1B*2 have a lower risk of producing children with FASD because they break down alcohol into acetaldehyde more quickly. Thus, they tend to have higher acetaldehyde blood levels, which may, in turn, reduce drinking (due to the flushing reaction). [42]

Another way that alcohol is broken down in the liver involves the *microsomal ethanol-oxidizing system (MEOS)*, which is located in the *smooth endoplasmic reticulum (SER)*. MEOS depends on *cytochrome P450 enzyme* systems which are also located in the SER. Chronic alcohol intake can induce a form of P450 called *CYP2E1* that leads to an increase in the rate of metabolic break down of alcohol, increased *alcohol tolerance* (which means a higher dose of alcohol is needed to achieve intoxication), increased production of *toxic breakdown products* from alcohol or other drugs (such as acetaminophen [Tylenol]) which, together with *increased reactive radicals,* increases liver damage. [40] Genes govern activity of the MEOS system but I have not seen any mention of these genes as risk factors for FASD or alcoholism in my review of medical literature.

Little alcohol is broken down outside the liver but some alcohol metabolism occurs is the stomach. A form of the *alcohol dehydrogenase* (ADH) enzyme called *class IV or "sigma" ADH* is present in the stomach. Caucasian women and many Japanese people have reduced activity of this enzyme so there is less alcohol breakdown in their stomach and more alcohol is absorbed into the bloodstream, which results in higher blood alcohol levels. Women also have a smaller amount of body water so for any given alcohol intake they will have higher blood alcohol concentrations than males. Higher blood alcohol concentrations lead to more organ damage for a given "dose" of alcohol. [40] Genes govern sigma ADH activity but I have not seen any information about this enzyme system in alcohol abuse literature.

I recommend interested readers review Dr. Albert Chudley's recent genetics chapter in *Fetal Alcohol Spectrum Disorder-Management and Policy Perspectives of FASD*. It contains a succinct and precise review of genetic factors that affect alcohol metabolism enzyme activity. Dr. Chudley notes that the genes which code for faster breakdown of alcohol into acetaldehyde **(ADH1B*3)** or for slower breakdown of acetaldehyde into acetate **(ALDH2*2)** will elevate acetaldehyde levels, cause a flushing reaction and reduce alcohol drinking. [13]

The Collaborative Study on Genetics of Alcoholism

The Collaborative Study on Genetics of Alcoholism (COGA) is on a quest to find variations of genes that increase the risk of alcoholism. COGA has studied the genes of 14,000 family members of alcoholics in treatment. That is a lot of genome mapping! A single nucleotide polymorphism (SNP) is one structural change in an area of a gene. COGA looks at the entire genome of family members of alcoholics to see where there is increased incidence of certain SNP's that increase the risk of developing alcoholism. Thus far, the following areas appear to contain genes that increase risk of developing alcoholism:

GABA GENES: The GABA A receptor is inhibitory - it mediates anxiolysis, sedation, drug tolerance and drug dependence. As mentioned above, genes for the GABA A receptor, especially **GABRA2** increase the risk of alcoholism. These "high risk" GABA A receptor genes include many SNPs on chromosome 11 (the 3' end of the gene not the 5' end) which are more common in relatives of alcoholics. If SNPs from adjacent or very close areas are grouped together these "clusters" are called "halplotypes." High risk haplotypes predict areas of the genome associated with alcoholism more accurately than high risk SNPs.

GABRA2 does not act by changing the order or arrangement of DNA's bases (adenine, cytosine, guanine and thymine). Instead, GABRA2 changes *how promoters and splicing variants work.* GABRA2 is seen in populations with *profound* addiction issues. Individuals with the "phenotype" (pattern of observable traits and behaviours) associated with GABRA2 have *drug* as well as alcohol dependence, a lower age of onset of heavy drinking, a higher number of maximum drinks per episode of drinking (i.e. larger binges) and more extreme withdrawal symptoms. People with GABRA2 are also more likely to have co-morbid antisocial personality disorder, conduct disorder, major depressive disorder and "novelty seeking" traits. [17] As mentioned above, GABRA2 increases the risk of alcoholism by 20% but increases the chance of not being married by 120% (compared to "control" populations that do not have this gene). [17] Study of such extreme phenotypes might *not* help us understand addictions in the majority because different genes might play a more influential role for those who drink more moderately.

Below, we see that expression of GABRA2 is associated with conduct disorder symptoms in younger people and a severe pattern of alcohol abuse in older people. These tendencies are more profound for people who have more than one copy of the gene (homozygotes).

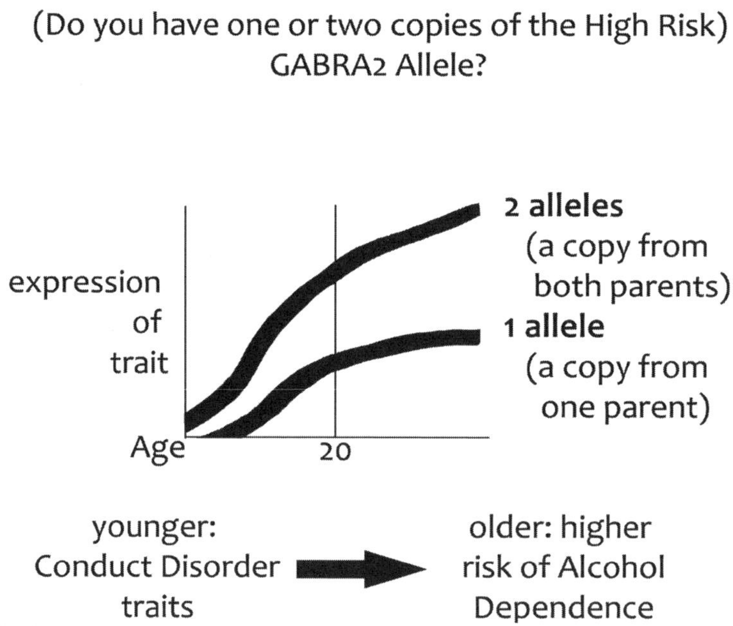

Adapted from: Gelernter J. 2009. [17]

Clinical Comment: Members of families affected by GABRA2 are at very significant risk. If a family you are working with fits the profile (kids with conduct disorder, antisocial tendencies in the adults, early-onset of very heavy drinking, large binges, extreme withdrawal symptoms, marked "risk-taking" and comorbid depression) please consider the possibility they could be dealing with GABRA2 or similar severe genotype. Would you ask parents from such a family to take on more duties or special-needs interventions for their kids? Sometimes "Discharge Planning Meetings" for at-risk kids whose families also have high levels of mental health issues are "a set-up for failure." I have seen a single mum (from a family that fits the GABRA2 behavioural phenotype) told to do 24/7 supervision of her "sneaking-out, fire-setting, and suicidal" 16 year-old daughter at the same time as trying to look after her new baby. Put yourself in this mum's shoes. I don't know how I could do this level of supervision, even with friends' and my wife's help. 24/7 supervision might be *required* - my point is that services need to be provided to help caregivers achieve this level of observation. If issues involve younger kids, maybe ideas like "therapeutic daycare" *with transportation provided* might be more likely to succeed. If a family has GABRA2 or similar genes, *very robust* attention to optimizing the environment is required to reduce the likelihood of "windup" of genetic predisposition into catastrophic mental health problems.

We as a society deem serious medical issues such as ovary cancer, colon cancer and breast cancer (all of which appear to have a significant heritability) worthy of well-organized genetic clinics. Such clinics counsel families and support extremely high-risk patients as they consider undertaking sometimes-drastic therapeutic options (e.g. mastectomy or oophorectomy) in a bid to reduce risk of serious disease or death. Compared with these serious cancers, uncontrolled substance abuse carries a risk of even higher levels of morbidity and death. Regrettably, compared with genetic cancer clinics, I am not aware of an equivalently comprehensive response for families at high genetic risk for substance abuse problems, including alcoholism. The lack of comprehensive intervention for families of alcoholics is, in my opinion, shortsighted and *very expensive* (due to loss of human potential, higher health care and social service costs).

Policy makers needn't "re-invent the wheel." Good models for how to approach serious diseases with genetic components are already being practiced. Consider the high risk **BRCA1** and **BRCA2** genes. These genes are rare (less than 1% of general population samples) but, if present, increase the chance of developing breast cancer from "baseline" rates of 12% of women who live to age 90 to 40-55% lifetime rates. [43] I'd like to see society move beyond shame and blame and deal with families who are unfortunate enough to have genes like GABRA2 by using the same levels of intelligence and funding we now use to support families who are unlucky enough to have BRCA genes.

In the meantime, while we wait for a GABRA2, "short" 5-HTT allele, (CRHR1, hTAS2R16, low "alcohol level of response", and Opioid OPRM1 Asp40 allele - explanation below) genetics clinic to be built, we clinicians might be dealing with a lady like Michelle who I saw last year. Michelle, a bright but exhausted thirty-eight year-old social worker, could not reduce her alcohol intake. She tried to get down to one beer a day (from four) because her liver function tests were abnormal, but she couldn't. She was discouraged. But her big worry was her son, John - 14 years old, stealing money from her purse, sneaking out, beating up his "friend" for money for pot, and recently brought home by police because he was intoxicated and "impossible to reason with." John, while drunk, tried to beat up a policeman. When I described the GABRA2 phenotype, Michelle interrupted: "Cripes, *that's my family!* My father was kicked out by Mum because he was abusive, Uncle Bob is in jail for assault, his kid, Janey, my niece is in "Juvie" (Juvenile Detention Center) for drug charges, and Bob's son, R. J., should have been caught for all his driving-under-the-influence episodes."

Both Michelle and I realized that her family's reality was pretty stark: big changes had to happen *immediately* or John would be doomed to travel down Janey's, Bob's and R.J.'s destructive pathway. John was sent to SALTS (Sail and Life Training Society) last summer because, in spite of his lament, "those preppy jerks are boring," he liked boats. Michelle's brother, Alan, ran an outboard repair business and had John help out around the shop twice a week. Alan took his Fender Stratocaster guitar to work one day and wowed John enough to get him interested in lessons. A girl from SALTS kept in touch with John and he went down to Nanaimo to see her at March Break. She doesn't like booze. Michelle's actions are designed to pre-empt (so far as possible) the expression of John's high-risk addiction genes. I hope this story has a happy ending; at this point, I can say this past year was not cheap for Michelle but was a lot better than the previous one for both her and John.

Dopamine 2 receptor genes (DRD2) are not statistically *proven* to play a role in addiction *yet*, but chances of verifying an association of dopamine activity and addiction are high. [19] Alcohol increases dopamine release in the nucleus accumbens - hence its rewarding effect. There is reduced dopamine 2 receptor activity in the striatum during alcohol withdrawal. If individuals carry the A1 allele (or variation) of the DRD2 gene the chance of them learning to *avoid the negative consequences of withdrawal* are reduced. The *active* genes for this effect (of *not* learning you have to decrease drinking in order to avoid the wicked withdrawal headaches) might be the DRD2 A1 allele itself or it's *close neighbor* genes: **ANKK1, TTC12, NCAM1**. [19]

ANKK1 acts on **TTC12** to change the risk of heavy drinking. These two genes also influence the risk of nicotine dependence. [19]

CRHR1 encodes for the corticotropin releasing hormone receptor 1 and there are two SNPs of this gene: rs242928 and rs1876831. They are associated with *binge drinking in adolescents* and *alcohol dependence* in adults. [18]

hTAS2R16 gene on chromosome 7 encodes the "bitter" taste receptor. If this gene is expressed people experience *less sensitivity* to bitter taste, drink more alcohol per 24 hours and are at increased risk for alcohol dependence. A group of Irish patients were found to have abnormalities of this taste receptor gene. I can only speculate about the frustrated novel-writing ambitions of the scientist who named the gene variation associated with alcohol dependence in this patient group: **HANGOVER / 2NF699** - if this gene variation is expressed, the risk of developing alcohol tolerance is higher. [19]

Dr. Marc Schuckit's concept of **Low Level of Response** to alcohol (a large dose is required to get you "tipsy" or you can "drink your buddies under the table") is an extremely important predictor of risk of alcoholism for all ages and with both sexes. [4] There are many "candidate" genes that are associated with a low level of response. [4] Dr. Schuckit's research has examined 40 yr-olds who are heavy drinkers and their children, particularly when those young people were in late adolescence (aged 17) and early adolescence (aged 13).

For 13 yr-olds (just beginning to experiment with alcohol): a low level of response is related to alcohol outcome, but primarily through its effect on peer's drinking behaviours. [4] Thus, to influence alcohol outcomes in young teens we must influence peers. Innovative (supervised) teaching from peers who have experienced problems from alcohol is likely to be "more real" and less likely to be sent to teen's "auto-delete files" than dry, abstinence rants from teachers and other professionals.

For 17 yr-olds, a low level of response operates *directly* and through these mediators: **expectations** (what you think will happen if you drink) and ***coping*** (if you use alcohol to cope or have poor coping mechanisms) to predict alcohol outcome. [4]

Accurate expectations: Effectively "getting the message out" to 17 yr-olds that some of their expectations about alcohol are inaccurate or at best, will not serve them well and equipping them with more effective methods for coping with stress, can be helpful. Teens should be aware that the National Center on Addiction and Substance Abuse in the USA released a study in 2003 "confirming that feelings of depression, hopelessness, sadness and suicidal ideation are a great deal more frequent in high school girls than boys and these same feelings are significantly associated with a heightened risk for not only drinking but also for other drug use." The reviewer, Dr. Monica Ziberman, goes on to say, " Substance use is often perceived by young women as a coping mechanism in dealing with shyness, anxiety, and/or depression" (Marc Schuckit's "expectations" mediator). Dr. Ziberman continues, "Prevention strategies at high school and college levels should focus on those who drink to *enhance ability to function* and self-esteem. (Rod Densmore's clinical note: I have found that drinking to *enhance ability* is often self-medication for undiagnosed ADHD or an anxiety disorder - both these mental health issues can be more effectively treated with meds and/or other strategies that have *less side-effects than alcohol.*) Dr. Ziberman adds that higher amounts of testosterone conversion in the liver of even healthy women who drink episodically "may be the basis of a variety of fertility problems such as ovulation inhibition, decreased gonadal mass, infertility and other sexual dysfunctions; women who were heavier drinkers had higher rates of difficulty reaching orgasm, vaginismus and lack of sexual interest. In men alcohol intoxication produces a transient *reduction* in testosterone levels." Ziberman discussed a 1981 survey that found a large portion of women drinkers thought alcohol lessened their sexual inhibitions and helped them feel close to others: "22% reported feeling more sexually assertive, but only 8% reported becoming less selective in partner choice. However, 60% reported having been the target of other drinkers' sexual aggression." [44] Thus, drinking for many young women is a coping mechanism - albeit not a very effective one - for stress, shyness, depression and anxiety. What better coping ideas are available?

Evidence-based coping strategies for stress in young adults include some effective (and relatively simple) school-based programs developed by the Benson-Henry Institute for Mind Body Medicine at Harvard University. After completion of classroom-based curricula that involved practicing a "relation response," students were found to have better attendance, better work habits, a higher grade point average, decreased unexcused tardiness , increased self-esteem, decreased psychological distress, but most importantly, reduction of risk of substance abuse and mental health problems. [45] Interested readers could to learn more about these school interventions by accessing the website: http://www.massgeneral.org/bhi/services/treatmentprograms.aspx?id=1274#

Like their 13 yr-old sibs, **17 yr-old** peers' attitudes about alcohol also directly predict adverse alcohol outcomes. Marc Schuckit's level of response model predicts more than three quarters of why adverse alcohol outcomes are seen in this age group! Dr. Schuckit says, "Wow - this model explains 78% of the variance of why a certain adverse alcohol outcome is seen." Schuckit goes on to say that predictions this accurate in a biological system are "too good to be true." [4] I am a Dad of a *very* self-determined 18 yr-old and muse about her response if I told her, "You are sooo predictable - I understand 78% of what makes you tick!"

For 40 yr-olds, peers *do not* have as high a degree of influence on alcohol outcomes as for their kids. However, the three factors:

1) low level of response,
2) using alcohol to cope with stress or having poor coping mechanisms and
3) expectations that somehow alcohol will make you more desirable, pro-social, etc.

predict half of the variance of why a certain alcohol outcome is seen in this 40 year-old group. [4]

OPRM1 is the genetic locus that codes for the proteins of the "mu" opioid receptor. Mu and gamma opioid receptor stimulation by alcohol adds to positive reinforcement by causing dopamine release in the nucleus accumbens. Several SNPs of the OPRM1 gene are associated with alcohol dependence. If drinkers have the *Asp*40 variation (and *not* the *Asn*40 variation) Naltrexone (an opioid receptor blocker) helps avoid relapse into heavy drinking. [18]

A SNP of OPRM1 called **A118G (rs1799971)** was seen in over 50% of adolescents that had early onset alcohol use problems but was only present in 16% of their peers who had no alcohol use issues. Naltrexone helped reduce alcohol overuse in adolescents with A118G(rs1799971) by reducing their age-related increased sensitivity to the positive reinforcing effects of drink. [46]

Variations in nicotine receptor gene clusters on chromosome 15, called **CHRNA5, CHRNA3** and **CHRNA4**, affect the risk of developing dependence to alcohol and nicotine. [17] We all minimize the effect of nicotine at our peril because tobacco kills more people than alcohol-induced illnesses do. [47] Furthermore, nicotine decreases fetal growth. Varenicline (Chantix) is a partial nicotinic receptor agonist that may also help decrease alcohol consumption. I have not used this agent with pregnant mums who are unable to stop their smoking and drinking. However, I wonder if in some very high risk situations it might be wise to consider using this medication when the risk of side effects to mother and fetus is less than the risk of continued tobacco and alcohol use. This drug's information document says: "Teratogenic effects were not observed in animal studies; however, decreased fertility, decreased fetal weight, and increased auditory startle response were observed in the offspring. There are no adequate or well-controlled studies in pregnant women." [48] Varenicline is pregnancy risk category "C" which means: "Risk cannot be ruled out. Human studies are lacking and animal studies are either positive for fetal risk or lacking as well. However, potential benefits may justify the potential risk." [48] Naltrexone is also pregnancy risk factor category C. Maybe we should be considering including these medications as part of a comprehensive strategy of support offered to high-risk pregnant women.

Are there genes of resiliency that allow drug users to *not* progress to dependence? The National Institute on Drug Abuse (NIDA) consortium has much interest in this question and research is ongoing.

COGA is a family genetic linkage study for alcoholism - are there similar genome-wide studies specifically for FASD?

Not yet, concludes Dr. Chudley in his recent review. [13] But Chudley describes work of Lomabard et al. [49] that suggests (by pooling animal and human FASD study data) *specific genes affecting three critical biologic pathways* are likely to influence the risk of developing FASD. Interested readers are again encouraged to review Dr. Chudley's chapter [13] for more details but I will briefly discuss the three biologic pathways here.

Prenatal alcohol appears to interfere with *transforming growth factor-beta* regulation of neuronal migration, growth of cerebral cortex cells, growth of axons, cell adhesion (alcohol *decreases* neuronal growth and migration but *increases* cell adhesion), neuronal apoptosis (alcohol increases apoptosis; apoptosis is controlled cell death) and regulation of the immune system. Clinically, I have observed sequellae of immune dysregulation in several patients with FASD - I understand this is anecdotal evidence, but cannot help wanting to know why breast and other cancers, multiple sclerosis, and frequent infections seem to be common issues *for patients in their twenties and thirties*. Abnormalities of neuronal migration and cortex development and reductions of axonal growth (i.e. widespread reduction of white matter myelinated tracts) are demonstrated convincingly in recent neuroimaging studies of individuals with FASD. [50]

A second critical signaling pathway affected by prenatal alcohol is the *mitogen-activated protein kinase (MAPK) system*. When alcohol dysregulates this system, changes in cell growth and migration can occur. Recently, using a mouse model of FAS, alcohol-induced impairment of cerebellar cell migration *was reversed* using caffeine to increase calcium ion secondary messenger activity and agents to increase cyclic GMP activity and decrease cyclic AMP activity. [51] Hopefully, this, and similar work will lead to strategies that could reduce prenatal alcohol's damage.

The third biologic system likely to be involved in FASD is called the *Hedgehog signaling pathway*. Alcohol reduces activity of key signaling components of the Hedgehog system (such as the Shh molecule). If Shh molecule levels are restored experimentally, alcohol-induced craniofacial anomalies are reduced because apoptosis of neural crest cells is reduced. [49]

Conclusions

Genetic influences on risk of disease involve multiple genes; there is a small effect from each - no one variation (or allele) of one gene does it all! Children with FASD have birth parents that - at least at the time of conception and early pregnancy - drank excessive amounts of alcohol. Risk of problems from alcohol overuse relate to a number of **genes** (we know about half of them thus far), **choices** and **environmental** influences.

Genes that influence activity of opioid receptors, CRH receptors, nicotinic receptors, dopamine 2 receptors, bitter taste receptors, and GABA neurotransmission have been shown to increase the risk of problem drinking.

Inherited tendencies towards impulsivity, and emotional dysregulation may affect *choices* about using an addicting substance.

Level of response to alcohol is an important heritable factor predicting risk of alcohol-related problems at all ages and with both sexes. Different factors in level of response models assume more importance for any given age group.

Supportive attachments have been shown to positively influence genetic expression of parts of the HPA stress system. To a degree, a nurturing environment can induce epigenetic activity (acetylation) that can improve the dysregulated, overreactive HPA stress axis that results from prenatal stress and/or alcohol-induced methylation of the area of DNA that codes for cortisol receptors.

While no family linkage studies have yet been done for FASD, innovative recent work suggests genes controlling three critical biologic pathways affect the risk of alcohol-exposed children developing FASD.

Some prenatally exposed children appear to be less damaged by alcohol's teratogenic effects than their peers and studying resiliency factors in this group needs to be a research priority. [7] Perhaps resilient children possess the long (not the short) variation of the promoter part of serotonin transporter genes, like the resilient monkey infants in Mary Schnieder's lab. [28]

Secondary Disabilities (background)

Readers experienced with FASD literature will be aware of Dr. Ann Streissguth's concepts of secondary disabilities but I will include this brief summary for those less familiar with her work. Current understanding suggests that *if appropriate supports are not in place* a child may develop secondary disabilities. Social worker and FASD educator Diane Malbin points out that chronic frustration results when kids with FASD are not able to meet society's (often unrealistic) expectations. [2] This frustration can result in secondary disabilities, which include:

1) Disrupted school experiences (defined as being expelled, suspended or dropping out)

2) Trouble with the law (defined as being charged or convicted of a crime, arrested or otherwise in trouble with the law)

3) Mental health problems

4) Alcohol and drug abuse or dependency

5) Inappropriate sexual behaviour (defined as inappropriate sexual advances, sexual touching or promiscuity)

6) Incarceration or confinement to inpatient psychiatric care, inpatient drug dependency programs.

Adult patients may have two additional secondary disabilities:

1) Dependent living (defined as living with family or friends, in a group home, or in some sort of assisted living facility)

2) Problems with employment (defined as requiring ongoing job training or coaching, being unable to keep a job, or being unemployed.) [52]

Secondary disabilities are a parent's, teacher's and government official's nightmare. They are costly to deal with and destroy lives.

Diane Malbin has found that it is possible to reduce these secondary disabilities by training those who are involved in a FASD-affected individual's life to ensure that environmental expectations are appropriate. [2]

Since 1996 we have known that the following are all **universal protective factors** against developing secondary disabilities:

1) Living is a stable nurturing home over 72% of life span
2) *Early* diagnosis (prior to age 6)
3) Safety (never having experienced violence against oneself)
4) Stability (staying in each living situation at least 2.8 years)
5) Experiencing a good quality home in middle childhood (age 8-12)
6) Access to supportive services designed for developmentally disabled persons
7) Paradoxically, being diagnosed with Fetal Alcohol Syndrome rather than partial Fetal Alcohol Syndrome
8) Having basic needs met for at least 13% of life span [1]

Genetic Perspectives and Secondary Disabilities

Some personality traits and mental health problems, which may be risk factors for developing secondary disabilities, have significant heritability. For example, highly heritable issues such as ADHD, conduct disorder, substance use disorder, and sensory processing disorder could play major roles in the development of "Disrupted school experiences" or "Disrupted employment." Likewise, impulsivity, a trait with over 50% heritability [3], could influence "Inappropriate sexual behaviour." Externalizing disorders which include the triad of conduct disorder, antisocial personality disorder and drug dependence share a common genetic liability with up to 80% heritability according to Joel Gelernter [18]; individuals with these genes would be at higher risk for "Troubles with the Law". In this chapter we have reviewed genes (GABRA2, "short" 5-HTT allele, CRHR1 SNP's rs242928and rs1876831, hTAS2R16, low "alcohol level of response" genes, Opioid OPRM1 Asp40 allele, and others) that, thus far, explain about half of the risk of developing "Alcohol abuse or dependency."

"Universal Protective Factors" which help *reduce* the likelihood of developing secondary disabilities are also influenced by highly heritable "Mental health problems". Streissguth, et al. have identified that the percentage of time spent in a "Stable, nurturing home environment" *is the most influential protective factor*, reducing by three- or four-fold the odds of occurrence of most secondary disabilities". [53] However, *if parents* have substance dependence, ADHD, bipolar disorder, conduct disorder or other serious mental health problems the chance of them being able to offer a stable, nurturing home over 72% of (their child's) life is likely to be diminished. Also, persistence and the ability to persevere against widespread, endlessly frustrating barriers (including long wait-lists to see specialists and high costs of diagnostic clinics) in order to achieve an "Early diagnosis (by age 6)" could be diminished if parents had significant mental health problems. Early diagnosis is a particularly helpful protective factor for "Confinement". Dr. Streissguth also notes that the risk of developing "Alcohol and drug abuse and dependencies" is reduced if children live with alcohol abusers for a shorter time (i.e. less than 30% of life).

I wonder if recently available genetics data suggest it is appropriate for those involved in FASD research and clinical work to consider updating their concept of secondary disabilities. Not to discount the importance of environmental influences, we now understand many populations have very significant heritability of personality traits and mental illnesses, including addictions. Frustrations about the poor fit between environmental expectations, and a child's actual performance can be crushing for our kids (and parents like me) - but genetics research indicate that environmental factors explain less than half of the etiology for substance use, personality and mental health issues that increase the risk of a child developing secondary disabilities.

The "poor fit of environmental expectations with achievable performance" explanation suggests that, with enough caregiver and parent energy and persistence to ensure everyone in the environment understands the child's limitations, substantial reductions in secondary disabilities are possible. As a dad and physician, I have tried very hard to "clue-in" teachers, counselors, and others that "rub shoulders" with my kid so misunderstandings could have been avoided. Sometimes these advocacy efforts pay great dividends. Often, though, poor outcomes happen *despite my wife's and my best efforts* to try to correct the "poor fit" between unrealistic expectations of stakeholders and what my child can actually do and understand. Another, possibly bigger, causative factor for the development of secondary disabilities, an "elephant in the room," is the collection of genetic risks *that our kids were born with.*

A future vision

If the FASD field could "clone" effective strategies from other health conditions that are significantly influenced by genetics then an unexplored preventative pathway would be realized. It does not matter what "hat you wear" - parent, teacher, psychologist, government official, physician - all of us strive constantly to reduce these unbelievably expensive, debilitating heartbreaks currently called secondary disabilities in the kids we love and care for. Understanding root causes of conditions we presently call secondary disabilities gives rise to the most effective ideas for preventing them. While it is not my intention to provoke controversy, if this chapter sparks debate about causes of positive and negative outcomes in FASD and innovative preventative medicine ideas that could help my child one day, I'd be delighted. As discussed, model programmes such as clinical work with families affected by high-risk cancer genes may be able to teach clinicians about effective intervention strategies in families beset by very high-risk mental health/ addiction genes.

Epigenetics

Even mainstream media has been exploring epigenetics. *Time Magazine* says, "The new field of epigenetics is showing how your environment and your choices can influence (expression of) your genetic code - and that of your kids." (Parentheses added) [54] Science writer David Shenk says epigenetics is part of a new understanding of how genes are expressed. He points out "how bankrupt the phrase 'nature versus nurture' really is." The human genome contains roughly twenty-five thousand genes, but the number of patterns of epigenetic processes (which turn those genes "off" or "on") is likely to be fifty to a hundred times larger (than 25,000) - a full epigenome map will require major advances in computing power. [54]

It seems likely that, a few years from now, we will understand much more about how genetic expression is turned on and off. My prediction is that studies will confirm the power of attentive, nurturing interpersonal attachments to cause advantageous epigenetic changes. Conversely, trauma, I believe, and drug and alcohol abuse, will be understood as amongst the most common *negative* epigenetic influences. Confronted daily with tragedy in my patients' stories of incest, other horrific interpersonal traumas, neglect, drug abuse and alcoholism, I yearn for the ability to offer more to support their healing journeys. Some answers, I hope, will emerge from this rapidly expanding field of epigenetics.

How to use genetic information

Marc Schuckit points out, " Any one gene only explains part of the risk - and anyhow

- who wants to change a gene? So, identify genes that put people at high risk and make robust changes to the environment to help decrease expression of these high risk genes." [4] Psychiatrist, Kieran O'Malley suggests there is nothing *specia*l about FASD - it should be treated with no more (**but also no less**) seriousness and respect than any other significant health issue. [55] I believe Marc Schuckit's remarks about genetics and alcoholism also pertain to FASD: "We will never reach a point where we can say we can prevent alcoholism totally but the more we understand about the **risk factors**, the **genes** associated with them, **and** the mechanisms through which they work - for depression, for schizophrenia, for cancer, for heart disease and for alcoholism (and I will add, for FASD) - the better we should be able to provide **early identification** and **prevention** of any of these disorders." [4]

References:

[1] Streissguth AP, Barr HM, Kogan J, et al. 1996. Understanding the Occurrence of Secondary Disabilities in Clients with Fetal Alcohol Syndrome (FAS) and Fetal Alcohol Effects (FAE), Final Report, August 1996, to the Centers for Disease Control and Prevention (CDC), Seattle: University of Washington, Fetal Alcohol and Drug Unit, Tech. Rep. No. 96-06

[2] Malbin D. 2002. Fetal Alcohol Spectrum Disorders: Trying Differently Rather Than Harder [online]. Portland (USA): Tectrice Inc. Available through: http://www.fascets.org/

[3] Paris J. 2003. Personality Disorders Over Time: Precursors, Course and Outcome. Washington, D.C.: American Psychiatric Publishing Inc. pp 42-44

[4] Schuckit MA. 2009. Adolf Meyer Award Lecture. How Alcoholism Develops: Identification of Genetic and Environmental Influences in a 25-year Longitudinal Study. American Psychiatric Association Meeting. San Francisco

[5] Schuckit MA, Smith TL, Eng MY, et al. 2002. Women who marry men with alcohol use disorders. Alcoholism: Clinical and Experimental Research 26(9): 1336-1343

[6] Schuchit MA, Tipp JE, Kelner E. 1994. Are daughters of alcoholics more likely to marry alcoholics? American Journal of Drug and Alcohol Abuse 20(2): 237-245.

[7] Astley S. 2010. Profiles of 1400 patients evaluated for FASD at the Washington State FAS Diagnostic and Prevention Network Clinic [WA FAS DPN] by interdisciplinary teams using the 4-digit code Presented at: 11th Annual Fetal alcohol Canadian Expertise Research Roundtable [FACE] Sept 14,2010 [available webcast at: http://www.motherisk.org/FAR/index.jsp]

[8] Astley SJ, Bailey D, Talbot C, et al. 2000. Fetal Alcohol Syndrome (FAS) Prevention Through FAS Diagnosis: Part II. Identification of High-Risk Birth Mothers Through the Diagnosis of Their Children. Alcohol & Alcoholism. 35(5): 509-519

[9] Astley SJ, Bailey D, Talbot C, et al. 2000. Fetal Alcohol Syndrome (FAS) Prevention Through FAS Diagnosis: Part I. Identification of High-Risk Birth Mothers Through the Diagnosis of Their Children. Alcohol & Alcoholism. 35(5): 499-508

[10] Pettinati HM, Plebani JG. 2009. Depression and Substance Use Disorder in Women. In: Brady KT, Back SE, Greenfield SF, editors. Women and Addiction: a Comprehensive Handbook. New York: The Guilford Press. pp 193-208.

[11] Choen JA, Mannarino AP, Deblinger E, et al. 2009. Cognitive-Behavioral Therapy for Children and Adolescents. In: Foa EB, Keane TM, Friedman MJ, Cohen JA, editors. Effective Treatments for PTSD: Practice Guidelines from the International Society for Traumatic Studies. Second edition. New York: The Guilford Press. pp 223-244

[12] Cahill SP, Rothbaum BO, Resick PA, e al. 2009. Cognitive-Behavioral Therapy for Adults. In: Effective Treatments for PTSD: Practice Guidelines from the International Society for Traumatic Studies. Second edition. Foa EB, Keane TM, Friedman MJ, Cohen JA, editors. New York: The Guilford Press. pp 139-222

[13] Chudley AE. 2010. Genetic Factors Contributing to FASD. In: Fetal Alcohol Spectrum Disorder: Management and Policy Perspectives of FASD, First Edition. Riley EP, Clarren S, Weinberg J, Jonsson E, editors. Weinheim, Germany: Wiley-VCH Verlag GmbH & Co. KGaA. doi: 10.1002/9783527632510.ch6. pp 109-126

[14] Stovall J. 2009. Bipolar Disorder: Epidemiology and Diagnosis. UpToDate Desktop 17.1, (Medical Reference CD-ROM). Feb 6, 2009

[15] Lyness JM, Schenuk TL, Sokol HN. 2009. Depression: Epidemiology and pathogenesis UpToDate Desktop 17.2, (Medical Reference CD-ROM). June 18, 2009

[16] Higgins ES, George MS. 2007. The Neuroscience of Clinical Psychiatry: The Pathophysiology of Behavior and Mental Illness. Philadelphia (USA): Lippincott, Williams and Wilkins. p 220

[17] Gelernter J. 2009. Symposium 70: Genetic Vulnerabilities for Drug Use and Co-morbid Mental Health Disorders: Approaching Co-morbidity in Addiction Genetics (conference presentation) American Psychiatric Association Annual Meeting, San Francisco

[18] Gelernter J, Kranzler HR. 2009. Genetics of alcohol dependence. Human Genetics 126: 91-99

[19] LeStrat Y, Ramoz N, Schuman G, et al. 2008. Molecular Genetics of Alcohol Dependence and Related Endotypes. Current Genomics(9): 444-457

[20] Kalaydjian A, Merikangas KR. 2009. Sex Differences in the Transmission of Substance Use Disorders. In: Brady KT, Back SE, Greenfield SF, editors. Women and Addiction: A Comprehensive Handbook. New York: The Guilford Press. pp 84-98

[21] Haycock PC. 2009. Fetal Alcohol Spectrum Disorders: The Epigenetic Perspective. Biology of Reproduction published 27 May 2009; 10.1095/biolreprod.108.074690

[22] Higgins ES, George MS. 2007. [as 16 above] p 180

[23] Neufeld G, Mate G. 2005. Hold on to Your Kids: Why Parents Need to Matter More Than Peers. Toronto (Canada); Vintage Books of Random House Canada, Inc. p 166

[24] Weinberg J. 2007. Prenatal Alcohol Exposure in an Animal Model: Fetal Programming and Implications for Vulnerability in Adulthood. Conference Presentation at: 8th Annual Fetal Alcohol Canadian Expertise (FACE) Research Roundtable, Vancouver, B.C. September 7, 2007. To View: http:www.motherisk.org/fas6/webcast/index.html

[25] Higgins ES, George MS. 2007. [as 16 above] p 186

[26] Zenilman JM. 2009. Genital Chlamydia trachomatis infection in women. UpToDate Desktop 17.2, (Medical Reference CD-ROM)

[27] Ouko LA, Shantikumar K, Knezovich J, et al. 2009. Effect of alcohol consumption on CpG Methylation in the differentially methylated regions of H19 and IG-DMR in male gametes- implications for Fetal Alcohol Spectrum Disorders. Alcoholism: Clinical and Experimental Research 33(9): 1-13

[28] Kraemer GW, Moore CF, Newman TK, et al. 2008. Moderate level fetal alcohol exposure and serotonin transporter gene promoter polymorphism affect neonatal temperament and limbic-hypothalamic-pituitary-adrenal axis regulation in monkeys. Biological Psychiatry 63: 317-324

[29] Gelernter J, Kanzler HR. 2008. Genetics of Addiction. In: Galanter M, Kleber HD, editors. Textbook of Substance Abuse Treatment, 4th edition. Washington, DC: American Psychiatric Publishing Inc. pp 17-27

[30] ZERO TO THREE. 2005. Diagnostic Classification of Mental Health and Developmental disorders of Infancy and Early childhood: Revised Edition (DC:0-3R). Washington, DC: ZERO TO THREE Press.

[31] O'Malley KD. 2007. Fetal Alcohol Spectrum Disorders: An Overview. In: O'Malley KD, editor. ADHD and Fetal Alcohol Spectrum Disorders (FASD). New York: Nova Science Publishing Inc. pp 1-24

[32] Goldsmith HH, Van Hulle CH, Arnesa CL, et al. 2006. A population-based twin study of parentally reported tactile and auditory defensiveness in young children. Journal of Abnormal Child Psychology 34(3): 378-392

[33] Jirikowic T. 2007. Sensory Integration and Sensory Processing Disorders. In: O'Malley KD, editor. ADHD and Fetal Alcohol Spectrum Disorders (FASD). New York: Nova Science Publishing Inc. pp 39-49

[34] Schneider ML, Moore CF, Gajewski LL, et al. 2008. Sensory Processing Disorder in a Primate Model: evidence from a longitudinal study of prenatal alcohol and prenatal stress effects. Child Development 79(1): 100-113

[35] Higgins ES, George MS. 2007. [as 16 above] p 58

[36] Matejko A, Lebel C, Rasmussen C, Bealieu C. 2010. Brain Imaging and Neurocognitive Functioning in Children and Twins with FASD, Conference Presentation, Promising Practices, Promising Futures, Alberta FASD Conference, Feb. 9, 2010. Calgary

[37] Reed SC, Evans SM. (2009) Research design and methodology in studies of women and addiction. In: Brady KT, Back SE, Greenfield SF, editors. Women and Addiction: A Comprehensive Handbook. New York: Guilford Press. pp 14-31.

[38] Cavazos-Rehg PA, Spitznagl EL, Bucholz KK, et al. 2008. Predictors of sexual debut at age 16 or younger. Archives of Sexual Behavior ISSN (online) 1573-2800. October 10, 2008 Retrieved, Jan.17, 2011 from: http://www.ncbi.nlm.nih.gov/pmc/articles/PMC2855761/

[39] Burckell LA, McMain S. 2009. Concurrent personality disorders and substance use disorders in women. In: Brady KT, Back SE, Greenfield SF, editors. Women and Addiction: A Comprehensive Handbook. New York (USA): The Guilford Press. pp 269-285

[40] Edwards G, Marshall EJ, Cook CCH. 2003. The Treatment of Drinking Problems: A Guide for the Helping Professions 4th Edition. Cambridge, (U.K.): Cambridge University Press. pp 18-19

[41] Edenberg H. 2009. Symposium 70: Genetic Vulnerabilities for Drug Use and Co-morbid Mental Health Disorders: Genetics of Alcoholism and other related endotypes (conference presentation) American Psychiatric Association Annual Meeting, San Francisco

[42] Viljoen D, Carr L, Foroud T, et al. 2001. Alcohol Dehydrogenase-2*2 Allele is Associated With Decreased Prevalence of Fetal Alcohol Syndrome in the Mixed-Ancestry Population of the Western Cape Province, South Africa. Alcoholism: Clinical and Experimental Research 25: 1719–1722. doi: 10.1111/j.1530-0277.2001.tb02180.x

[43] Fletcher SW. 2009. Overview of the genetics in breast and ovarian cancer. UpToDate Desktop 17.2 (Medical Reference CD-ROM)

[44] Ziberman ML. 2009. Substance Abuse across the Lifespan in Women. In: Brady KT, Back SE, Greenfield SF, editors. Women and Addiction: a Comprehensive Handbook. New York: The Guilford Press. pp 3-13

[45] Benson H, Wilcher M, Greenberg B, et al. 2000. Academic Performance Among Middle School Students After an Exposure to a Relaxation Response Curriculum. Journal of Research and Development in Education 33(3): 156-165

[46] Miranda R, Ray L, Justus A, et al. 2010. Initial evidence of association between OPRM1 and adolescent alcohol misusage. Alcoholism: Clinical and Experimental Research 34(1): 112-122

[47] Els C. 2009. Practical Strategies for Managing Tobacco Use in Psychiatric Patients. Conference Presentation, Collaborative Forums in Mental Health: Advances in Psychiatry, June 5, 2009. Vancouver, BC. Canadian Psychiatric Association CPD Institute. pp 37-42 (of Syllabus.)

[48] Varenicline- Drug Information. 2009. UpToDate Desktop 17.2 (Medical Reference CD-ROM)

[49] Lombard Z, Tiffin N, Hofmann O, et al. 2007. Computational selection and prioritization of candidate genes for Fetal Alcohol Syndrome. BMC Genomics 8, 389, http://www.biomedcentral.com/1471-2164/8/389.

[50] Norman AL, Crocker N, Mattson SN, et al. 2009. Neuroimaging and Fetal Alcohol Spectrum Disorders. Developmental Disabilities Research Reviews 15: 209-217

[51] Kamanda T, Lakshmana MK, Komoro H. 2006. Reversal of neuronal migration in a mouse model of fetal alcohol syndrome by controlling second-messenger signalings. Journal of Neuroscience 26: 742-756

[52] Streissguth AP. 1997. Fetal Alcohol Syndrome: A Guide for Families and Communities. Baltimore: Brookes Publishing

[53] Streissguth AP, Bookstein FL, Barr, HM. 2004. Risk factors for adverse life outcomes in fetal alcohol syndrome and fetal alcohol effects. Developmental Behavioral Pediatrics 25: 228-238

[54] Cloud J. Why Genes Aren't Destiny. Time. January 18, 2010. pp 49-53

[55] O'Malley K. 2009. Personal Communication.

Chapter Nine

Terminology, diagnosis, epidemiology and pathogenesis of Fetal Alcohol Spectrum Disorder (FASD) for health professionals

Introduction

Fetal Alcohol Spectrum Disorder (FASD) is an overarching term describing the various patterns of how prenatal alcohol exposure can affect people. FASD is caused by consumption of alcohol during pregnancy. Physical, learning, social and behavioural effects of prenatal alcohol last a lifetime.

Terminology

Included in FASD are:

1) Fetal Alcohol Syndrome (FAS): facial changes, growth deficiency, brain changes affecting thought, social and adaptive functions and a history of maternal intake of alcohol

2) Partial Fetal Alcohol Syndrome (PFAS): brain changes, proven maternal alcohol intake and lesser degrees of facial and growth changes

3) Alcohol-related Neurodevelopmental Disorder (ARND): brain changes and confirmed maternal alcohol intake, but no growth or facial abnormalities

4) Alcohol-related Birth Defects (ARBD): body changes due to prenatal alcohol exposure often including kidney problems, heart murmurs or heart septum problems, bone issues including small 5th fingers and toes, visual focus and eye movement problems, dental problems, and hearing impairment

5) Static Encephalopathy: this U.S. term is the same as "severe ARND" (i.e. brain(CNS) rank 3 on the 4-digit code)

6) Neurobehavioral Disorder: this U.S. term is the same as moderate ARND (i.e. CNS rank 2 on the 4-digit code)

7) Fetal Alcohol Effects (FAE): an older term (no longer commonly used) that describes

individuals with brain differences caused by prenatal alcohol but not severe enough levels of growth restriction or facial features to fit diagnostic criteria for FAS

Diagnosis

Each of four domains: growth restriction, facial features, central nervous system changes, and extent of maternal prenatal alcohol intake are assessed using a 4-digit code. Rank 1 is within norms for age, rank 4 is the most abnormal.

Different diagnostic guidelines are available - for comparison: see: Astley SJ. 2006. [1] *The 4-Digit Diagnostic Code,* developed by The University of Washington FAS Diagnostic and Prevention Network (FASDPN) clinics, forms the basis of most of the various diagnostic systems. *A simplified version* of the code is presented below. More details about the 4-digit code are explained in the FASDPN diagnostic manual. [2] Please refer to the manual [2] to see the lip/philtrum guide; clinicians hold this guide up to the patient's face to determine the most accurate lip and philtrum rank (on a 5 point scale, with 5 being the most severely affected). Palpebral fissure length is measured with a clear ruler and compared with norms for age. Palpebral fissure is a surrogate measure for eye globe size - which is reduced if alcohol exposure occurred at days 19-21 post conception. Small eye globe size is a surrogate marker for impaired frontal lobe development. Eyes *may appear* to be more widely spaced in FAS but this observation is because of the smaller sized globe. Another common misperception is that the three key facial features are not seen in babies or adults; if a patient has short palpebral fissures, a flat philtrum or a thin upper lip these features persist throughout their lives.

Table 1 (see next page): A simplified version of the 4-Digit Code (based on University of Washington FASDPN diagnostic manual)

Rank	Height and Weight	Facial Features	CNS	Prenatal Alcohol Exposure
4	Both ≤ 3rd percentile	All 3 features (see below)	Structural/neurological abnormalities e.g., head circumference ≤ -2SD or epilepsy or MRI abnormalities	Confirmed high—at least weekly early pregnancy high risk drinking
3	One ≤ 3rd percentile and other between 3rd and 10th percentile	Lesser degrees of facial features e.g., fissure length ≤-2 SD, lip rank 3 and philtrum rank 4 on the guide	Severe dysfunction i.e., 3 or more domains of brain activity which are significantly affected e.g., memory, IQ, and adaptive function are ≤-2SD on standardized tests	Confirmed moderate drinking in pregnancy-readers are invited to view exact criteria/ definitions in [2]. Also, see comments below
2	Both between 3rd and 10th percentile or one between 3rd and 10th percentile and other ≥ 10th percentile	Still lesser degrees of facial features e.g., fissure length >-2SD and ≤ -1SD, lip rank 2 and philtrum rank 3 on the guide	Moderate dysfunction-abnormalities in standardized testing of brain domains are noted but not to the level of CNS rank 3 criteria. Sometimes very young children will be rank 2 and, later, when old enough to be tested on more precise psychological tests will be rank 3	Unknown-if no direct observation of drinking in the index pregnancy have been made or if no records document prenatal drinking the rank is 2: "unknown" prenatal alcohol exposure
1	Both > 10th percentile	Fissure length no shorter than -1SD, lip and philtrum no higher than rank 3 on the guide	No current evidence of delay or dysfunction	Confirmed absence of drinking from conception to birth

DSM inclusion of FAS?

The Diagnostic and Statistical Manual of Mental Disorders (DSM) is considering inclusion of FAS (*but not FASD*) in the 2013 DSM-5. At present FAS is in the category: *Conditions Proposed by Outside Sources.* Interested readers could learn more by visiting the DSM website. [3]

Notes on diagnostic terms:

Features required to fulfill criteria for Face Rank 4:

1. Small palpebral fissure length (2 or more standard deviations below the mean)
2. Flat philtrum (rank 4 or 5 on the University of Washington Lip-Philtrum guide)
3. Thin upper lip (rank 4 or 5 on the University of Washington Lip-Philtrum guide)

CNS domains:

Planning/sequencing/working memory/ abstract reasoning/executive function,

Memory/learning/information processing,

Spatial skills and memory,

Language processing and effectiveness of using language - receptive and expressive communication skills,

Cognition (IQ),

Academic achievement,

Adaptive skills/social skills/social communication,

Motor planning/motor skills (including oral-motor and visuo-motor coordination), Hard and soft neurologic signs (including sensory-motor signs),

Brain structural changes (occipitofrontal circumference, neuroimaging findings, etc.),

Attention deficit/hyperactivity. [2], [4]

An effective assessment will determine skill levels not only in areas of reduced function but also in areas of interest/ relative gifting because engagement is optimized if caregivers work within areas of strength. Mark Ylvasaker, PhD, and researcher in rehabilitation for children with traumatic brain injury (TBI) underscores the importance of identification of strengths by his statement, "In the absence of meaningful engagement in chosen life activities, all interventions will ultimately fail." [5]

CNS Rank 4 Terms:

1. "Structural abnormalities"
   With recent improvements in brain

imaging we will see a great rise in the number of patients identified as having "structural abnormalities." In a recent neuroimaging study of children diagnosed with an FASD by the FASDPN assessment clinic, neuroradiologists found a prevalence of *MRI structural abnormalities* of 43% for children thought to be "brain rank 2" in clinical assessment, 58% for "brain rank 3" and 78% for "brain rank 4." Thus, 43% of brain rank 2 patients actually fit one of the criteria - structural abnormalities (as revealed by neuroimaging) - for brain rank 4! [6]

2. "Neurological Abnormalities" usually refers to epilepsy. Recent studies have identified a "staggering" prevalence (5.9%, which is ten times the expected rate) of epilepsy in patients diagnosed as having FASD by Edmonton and Toronto FASD clinics according to neurologist, Peter Carlen. Dr. Carlen now suggests that epilepsy is so common in people who were prenatally exposed to alcohol that screening of the FASD population for EEG abnormalities should occur. Dr. Carlen adds that screening of epilepsy clinic patients for FASD should also occur. [7]

Maternal Prenatal Drinking

"Shame and blame" destroys the health care provider-patient relationship and undermines effective care. An efficacious and respectful way to ask about alcohol use is: "*Before you knew you were pregnant, what was your smoking pattern? Any marijuana? Your drinking pattern?*

Once you became aware of your pregnancy, how did that pattern of use change - re smoking, marijuana, alcohol, other drugs?

How far along were you when you first knew you were pregnant?"

"Confirmed high" and "confirmed moderate" imply discernment of amount that is unusual in heavy drinkers. The Northern California Drink Size initiative is one helpful way to open a more accurate dialogue about amount of alcohol consumed. [8]

"Exposure unknown"

Presence of all *3 facial features* is a specific enough marker for prenatal alcohol-induced CNS damage that if growth is below the 10th percentile, and if the brain rank is 3 or 4, using the Canadian Guidelines, a diagnosis of FAS may be made *whether prenatal alcohol exposure can be confirmed or not.* [4]

Epidemiology

Prevalence

Large population studies are rare.

- Seattle: FAS and ARND: 9.1/1000 [9]
- South Africa: FAS > 4/100 [10], PFAS: 6.8-8.9/100 [11]
- Northern Canada (isolated community): FAS/FAE: 190/1000 [12]
- Northern Italy: (n=543 first grade students in several elementary schools) FAS: 3.7-7.4/1000, FASD: 2.3-4.5/100, overall FASD: 3.5/100 [13]
- "Western City," USA. (Pilot) n=128, FASD: 1.65/100 [14]
- Prison: n=106, PFAS/ARND: 10/100, "possible" prenatal alcohol damage but unable to prove prenatal alcohol exposure: 18/100 [15]
- "Juvie" (youth jail): n=287, FASD: 23/100 [16]

I think the *details* of May, et al.'s 2006 study in Northern Italy [13] are especially compelling. May's group recruited children from a number of elementary schools near Milan. Following informed consent protocols, parents were asked if they would allow their children to be assessed for clinical evidence of prenatal alcohol exposure. *Half* the parents consented for their children to be examined. Depending on which school, between 2.3 and 4.5 of 100 children were found to fit criteria for FASD. Believing the *other half - the children from families that did not consent to allow their children to be assessed* - would plausibly have an even higher prevalence of FASD is speculation, but tenable. Even at a prevalence of 3.5 per 100 - Dr. May's study's average - FASD's prevalence is 3.85 times more common than the highest Autism Spectrum Disorder prevalence figures I am aware of (1 in 110). [17]

Differential Diagnosis

Susan Astley reports 1.3% of the patients referred to the Washington State FAS Diagnostic and Prevention Network had a diagnosis other than an FASD. [6]

Prevalence of other syndromes (1.3%) among 1400 patients assessed at FASDPN clinics (entrance criteria for assessment included know prenatal alcohol exposure):

Other syndromes/malformations	N
Sticklers	4
Hemifacial microsomnia	2
Williams	2
Marfan	1
Moebius sequence	2
Binder	1
Kabuki Makeup	1
Kleinfelters	1
Neurofibromatosis	1
Amniotic Band Sequence	1
Down	1

Geneticist and FASD expert, Dr. Albert Chudley reports in Winnipeg his FASD clinic physicians have diagnosed a higher number (than 1.3%) of other syndromes/ malformations in patients referred for assessment. [18]

The Canadian Guidelines for FASD diagnosis contain a list of "syndromes with features that overlap with those of FAS" - and ways to differentiate each from FAS. Listed conditions include: Aarskog syndrome, Cornelia deLange syndrome, Dubowitz syndrome, Fetal hydantoin syndrome, Fetal valproate syndrome, Phenylketonuria, Noonan syndrome, Williams syndrome, Toluene embryopathy and other chromosome alteration syndromes (such as Fragile X.) [4]

Associated conditions

95% of children exposed prenatally to alcohol had **ADHD** (compared to a 30% prevalence of ADHD in control children exposed prenatally to similar levels of nicotine, THC, and maternal nutrition). [21]

In a retrospective chart review (n=425 children with FASD) almost 18% had *some form of seizures* and 5.9% *were diagnosed with epilepsy* - a "staggering" result ten times the expected prevalence according to Dr. Peter Carlen. [22] Likelihood of seizure activity increased with the male sex (60/40 ratio), with a heavier pattern of alcohol intake in the pregnancy, with maternal use of multiple substances and with unnatural birthing such as cesarean section because of hypoxia.

Dr. Carlen's group queried whether seizures could be a manifestation of underlying hyperexcitable brain circuitry in FASD - affecting even those without a history of clinically observable seizures - which could predispose to ADD and other psychopathologies. [22]

Dr. Carlen notes that seizures appear to be caused by an unusual pattern of brain hyperexcitability related to enhanced GAP junctional mechanisms, *not* due to neurotransmitter/synaptic anomalies. [23]

Anecdotally, Dr. Jonathan Down, Developmental Pediatrician at the Queen Alexandra Health Center for Children in Victoria, B.C., felt that very few children found to have FASD by his assessment team did not also have *sensory processing abnormalities.* [24] Both Sensory Processing Disorder (SPD) and FAS currently hold the status, "Conditions proposed by outside sources," with the 2013 Diagnostics and Statistics Manual (DSM-5) Committee. [3] Dr. Down's experience is supported by recent work on SPD in FASD from the Seattle assessment clinic at University of Washington FASDPN. [25]

I have two young patients affected by prenatal alcohol (women in their early 30's) with breast cancer (one bilateral.) Anecdotally, I wonder if *immune system impairment* could be associated with FASD, though I have not seen much discussion about this possibility in medical literature. Polanco, et al. found alcohol exposure in utero increased susceptibility to mammary tumors in adulthood; alcohol-induced changes in activity of Insulin-like Growth Factor (IGF) and estradiol systems may play a role in underlying mechanisms of tumorigenesis. [26] Dendritic cells are the predominant class of antigen presenting cells; they are highly active in processing and presenting antigen to T cells. [27] Although they did not specifically study individuals with FASD, Babu, et al, found consumption of alcohol elevated cyclic AMP in dendritic cells. The cyclic AMP changes altered serotonin activity by altering activity of monoamine oxidase-A (MAO-A) and serotonin transporter. Changes in serotonin affect both its role as a neurotransmitter and immune regulator. [28]

A Diagnosis for (at least) two

Diagnosing a child with FASD ought to lead clinicians to locating *birth mothers*; diagnosing and treating birth mother mental health issues is sound pubic health policy that would reduce FASD rates. Improving access to contraception would also reduce FASD rates.

In a large Washington State study, *birth mothers* of children with FAS had, on average, more than 4 DSM-4 psychiatric diagnoses. Seldom, were these serious issues diagnosed or treated to a standard of care consistent with current clinical practice guidelines. Most birth mothers lived in poverty. 95% had been sexually and/or physically abused. Many lived in social isolation. Most common mental health problems were alcohol abuse (86%), posttraumatic stress (77%), depression (60%), simple phobia (44%), social phobia (43%), antisocial personality (39%), agoraphobia (37%) and generalized anxiety disorder (34%). Bipolar (21%) and panic disorder (20%) were also common. [19] I don't believe borderline personality disorder, traumatic brain injury, attention deficit hyperactivity disorder or sensory processing disorder were specifically assessed in Astley's study [19]; in my clinical work, anecdotally, all are under-recognized, common in birth mothers, and readily treatable.

Removing barriers for at-risk women to access effective birth control is a sensible approach to helping reduce the number of alcohol-exposed pregnancies. Because of *discontinuation*, effective contraceptives like "the birth control pill" have poor "first year failure rates" in real-world use...8% for typical users! (I wonder if "failure rates" would be closer to 10 or 15% for women contending with distractibility from ADHD or an unsafe living situation, memory issues from depression, or focus issues caused by insomnia.) Real world first year pregnancy rates for Depo-provera are 3%, 0.8% for copper IUD (NovaT) and 0.1% for progestin IUD (Mirena). [20]

Statistics regarding *birth fathers* of 1400 patients seen at FASDPN (University of Washington clinic) for assessment and diagnosis of FASD are as follows: Only 8% of the birth fathers accompanied their child to the diagnostic evaluation (vs. 20% of patients' birth mothers). On average, birth dads were 32 years old at birth of their child with FASD (birth mums were 3-4 yrs younger). 39% did not finish high school; 50% reportedly had learning disabilities and the names of 765 of birth dads and 955 of birth mums were known. [6]

Alcohol–Related Birth Defects (ARBD)

The two criteria for ARBD are confirmed prenatal alcohol exposure and one or more congenital defects including malformations and dysplasias of the heart, skeletal system, kidney, visual and hearing systems. [29]

Cardiac problems associated with prenatal alcohol exposure include atrial and

Cardiac problems associated with prenatal alcohol exposure include atrial and ventricular septal defects, teratology of Fallot, transposition of the great arteries. Ethanol can produce related changes in zebrafish heart - this animal is a possible model for understanding mechanisms of cardiac prenatal alcohol toxicity [30]

I have observed the following malformations/symptoms in my clinical experience with patients who have FASD:

Cardiac: conduction delays, long QT intervals, atrial and ventricular septal defects

Skeletal: hypoplastic nails, shortened fifth digits, abnormal dentition, pectus excavatum and carinatum, scoliosis, cleft palate

Renal: duplex ureters, horseshoe kidney, hydronephrosis, decreased awareness of the sensation to urinate (interoceptive hypo-responsivity)

Ocular: strabismus, refractive problems secondary to small globes, retinal vascular abnormalities, optic nerve hypoplasia, difficulties in maintaining conjugate gaze, visual discrimination problems (cannot determine what to look at in a cluttered environment)

Auditory: conductive and neurosensory hearing loss, auditory figure-ground discrimination problems (cannot decipher information if distracting background noise is present)

The neural crest develops embryonically into the midface, heart septae and eyes, thus, a prenatal insult to neural crest tissues by alcohol or another teratogen could cause hypoplasia of the optic nerve, smaller eye globe size, ventricular and atrial septal defects, Tetralogy of Fallot, cleft lip/palate, malformed teeth, abnormally weak dental enamel, eustachian tube problems that can lead to hearing loss and hypotonic pharyngeal muscles which can cause sleep disordered breathing. [31]

"Secondary Disabilities"

When individuals with FASD are inadequately supported, Secondary Disabilities result. These include:

1. Disrupted school experiences (defined as being expelled, suspended or dropping out)
2. Trouble with the law (defined as ever being charged, convicted, arrested or otherwise in trouble with the law)
3. Mental health problems

4. Alcohol and drug abuse or dependency
5. Inappropriate sexual behaviour (defined as inappropriate sexual advances, sexual touching or promiscuity)
6. "Confinement" to inpatient psychiatric care, inpatient drug dependency programs or incarcerated.

Adult patients have two additional secondary disabilities:

1. Dependent living (living with family or friends, group home or in some sort of assisted living)
2. Problems with employment (defined as requiring ongoing job training or coaching, not being able to keep a job, or unemployment.) [32]

Since 1996 we have known that the following are all *"universal protective factors"* against developing secondary disabilities:

1. Living is a stable nurturing home over 72% of life
2. Early diagnosis (prior to age 6)
3. Safety (never having experienced violence against oneself)
4. Stability (staying in each living situation at least 2.8 years)
5. Experiencing a "good quality home" in middle childhood (age 8-12)
6. Getting access to supportive services designed for developmentally disabled persons
7. Paradoxically, being diagnosed with Fetal Alcohol Syndrome rather than partial Fetal Alcohol Syndrome
8. Having "basic needs" met for at least 13% of life [32]

Streissguth et al. have identified that the percentage of time spent in a stable, nurturing home environment is *the most influential protective factor*, reducing by three- or four fold the odds of occurrence of most secondary disabilities. [33]

Siblings born *prior* to children diagnosed with FAS were found to also have FAS signs that - if recognized - could have predicted the next child was at risk for FAS. Siblings born *after* their brother or sister was diagnosed had less risk of FAS signs. Less maternal alcohol consumption in "after diagnosis" pregnancies was noted [34] confirming that diagnosing her child may help a mother reduce her risk of having another child with FASD.

Pathogenesis

Biological pathophysiology

Prenatal alcohol exposure causes toxicity to the fetus by a number of mechanisms:

Directly acting on the fetus, alcohol decreases cell division of both neurons and glial cells; inhibits synthesis of proteins, RNA, and DNA; reduces cell division of stem cells; and increases cell death. Alcohol reduces the number of neurons, especially in the hippocampus, cerebellum and amygdala. [35]

Indirect fetal damage occurs from alcohol-induced interference with zinc, folate and vitamin A metabolism; disrupted cell adhesion - blocking alcohol's impairment of cell adhesion by treating animal models with glial proteins SALLPSIPA (SAL) and NAPVSIPQ (NAP) is neuroprotective; interference with growth factors; oxidative stress/free radical damage - NAP has been used to reduce oxidative damage in an animal model; and disrupted endocrine balance including alterations in estrogen, testosterone, growth hormone, prolactin, vasopressin, ACTH and gonadotropins. Alcohol alters fetal programming of the hypothalamic-pituitary-adrenal (HPA) stress axis which causes prenatally exposed fetuses to have a larger and less modulated (less controllable) response to stress compared to non-exposed peers. [35] Alcohol-induced damage to the serotonergic system reduces serotinergic neurotrophic effects (reducing neural proliferation in the frontal lobes and reducing serotonin 1A receptor activity in brainstem chemoceptors). [36] [37]

Also, alcohol-induced changes to serotinergic signaling are involved in programming fetal HPA axis hyper-responsiveness to stress. [35]

Placental factors

Ethanol consumption during pregnancy causes oxidative stress, DNA damage and intrauterine growth restriction, and increases the risk spontaneous abortion. Alcohol-mediated inhibition of insulin and insulin growth factor signaling impairs placentation. In a rodent model for FASD, alcohol was also associated with increased trophoblast apoptosis, mitochondrial injury and prolactin dysregulation. [35]

Impaired Vitamin A metabolism

Prenatal alcohol interferes with activation of retinoic acid receptors. Retinoic acid, an active metabolite of Vitamin A synthesized in the cerebellum, is needed for neuronal development. [38]

Oxidative Stress

Oxidative stress can impair growth and damage the CNS. Recently, antioxidants have been shown to reduce oxidative stress markers and growth retardation in animal models of FASD. [39]

I recommend interested readers review Uban, et al.'s recent chapter [35] and Joanne Weinberg's 2007 lecture [40] for recent comprehensive reviews of FASD pathophysiology.

Comorbid traumatic brain injury

Clinically, many adults I see who have FASD also have a devastating comorbidity: traumatic brain injuries (TBI) from accidents, assaults, etc. Brain damage caused by trauma or ischemia is made worse by alcohol-induced changes to NAD(P)H oxidase and superoxides. [41]

Neurobiology of FASD's symptoms and signs

Memory

Prenatal alcohol is more likely to impair (both verbal and nonverbal) memory by compromising *encoding* (initial laying down of memories) as opposed to impairing *retrieval.* [42] Impaired hippocamal learning has been demonstrated in individuals exposed prenatally to alcohol. [43] Drs. Brock and Fernette Eide suggest that even more important memory problems many children with FASD or similar conditions contend with are cerebellar-mediated *procedural* learning deficits. Drs. Eide note that many - if not most - basic academic skills (writing, spelling, etc.) are learned in procedural memory circuits. When procedures are less clearly understood, children attempt compensatory strategies (for instance, "sounding the word's syllables out"). However, keeping these compensatory strategies in mind *fills up the (already compromised) working memory areas* thus leaving less "space" available in working memory for new learning. [44]

Sensory processing and adaptive function

As the severity level of 4-digit diagnosis increases (for example from "ARND" to "FAS") more problems with sensory processing are seen. Reduced scores in a test of sensory processing (the Short Sensory Profile) - but not lower IQ - correlate with lower scores of *adaptive behaviour.* This fact confirms the association between sensory processing difficulties and impaired adaptability.

Satisfactory adaptive function predicts self-care, social and academic success. [45]

Math

For all populations, the left parietal area is important for math skills. However, this area is particularly damaged by prenatal alcohol exposure (compared to other brain areas). [46]

A diffusion tensor imaging (DTI) investigation of math skills in children with FASD revealed changes in white matter tracts, internal capsule, and the middle cerebellar peduncle are associated with reduced math scores. [47]

Children prenatally exposed to alcohol must recruit more brain regions to perform simple number processing tasks. Activation of the right and left angular gyrus and the posterior cingulate/precuneus may correlate with increased "self-talk" as the children attempt to problem solve. Activation of the cerebellar vermis and cortex that would only occur for control subjects when they were trying to solve a particularly challenging math problem was seen in alcohol exposed subjects engaged in relatively simple calculations. [48]

Do children with FASD "fit" a cognitive/behavioural phenotype?

Compared to other CNS functions, measures of executive function and spatial processing are especially sensitive to prenatal alcohol exposure. [49]

Disinhibition

Circuits between the striatum and frontal lobes, thought to mediate inhibitory control, are damaged by prenatal alcohol exposure. [50]

Concept formation/ conceptual set shifting

Concept formation - "coming up with an idea," and conceptual set shifting - "moving on" to a new idea, are impaired in FASD. These difficulties impair problem solving and adaptive function. [51]

Balance

Balance depends on optimal functioning of at least two out of these three sensory systems: touch (somatosensory), vestibular and visual. [52] Exposure to prenatal alcohol impairs balance, in part, by making children more dependent on accurate visual or somatosensory information than their non-exposed peers. [53]

Structural changes

Prenatal alcohol exposure has been associated with structural MRI abnormalities including microcephaly, distortions of the corpus callosum and cerebellar vermis, and smaller volumes of basal ganglia. Smaller caudate and parietal lobes and reduced cortical white matter were also found. [54] Recently, MRI diffusion tensor imagining techniques have demonstrated abnormal microstructure in putamen, thalamus and white matter tracts including the corpus callosum and inferior longitudinal fasciculus (this would slow visual processing speed). [55]

Sleep

Animal studies show prenatal alcohol disrupts the ability to synchronize circadian rhythm to light cues. Disruptions in circadian regulation may cause disrupted sleep and feeding patterns. [56] Profound disruptions of sleep regulation can affect children with FASD. [57] Restless legs and/or obstructive sleep apnea can also contribute to non-restorative sleep. Melatonin has been used successfully. Sleep deficits further complicate cognitive and behavioural problems. Furthermore, sleep disruptions in children also disrupt caregivers' sleep. A considerable burden of family stress can result from sleep difficulties so I encourage clinicians to review Dr. Jan's group's recent study and use the resources they identify. [57]

Social cognition/social skills

Efficient executive functioning skills facilitate the development of *theory of mind skills.*

Theory of mind - the capacity to recognize that what you think may differ from what another thinks - develops around age 4 *if children have adequate maturation of executive functioning skills.* Dr. Rasmussen's group at University of Alberta has found "children with FASD have difficulty on theory of mind tasks," and this difficulty "may be related to underlying deficits in inhibition." [58]

Mentalization, a term developed by Drs. Jon Allen, Peter Fonagy and Anthony Bateman means:

1. Holding mind in mind
2. Attending to mental states in self and others
3. Understanding misunderstandings
4. Seeing yourself from the outside and others from the inside

5. Interpreting behaviour as linked to intentional mental states in self and others [59]

Drs. Allen et al. suggest *adaption* depends on mentalizing. Holding strong impulses and feelings "at bay" *while thinking of realistic pathways to satisfaction* is the essence of adaption. Dr. Allen says, "This containment process requires mentalizing as we construe it." [60]

When mentalization breaks down or does not develop individuals react to urges impulsively; introspection and insight is impaired. In FASD, often, behaviours and thoughts are *context dependent*. Parents report their children are "slimed" by the environment - kids seem unable to "think for themselves," thoughts and moods depend on "whichever direction the winds of chance blow." Anger, is "someone else's fault."

Impaired social communication is a core deficit with FASD. Resulting interpersonal difficulties cause much suffering for the patients with FASD and their families. Developing mentalization skills is a productive approach. However, some of the critical neurobiological hardware components for *interpersonal affiliation systems* and mentalization may be affected by FASD.

Interpersonal affiliation and FASD

Comprehension of social cues requires *accurate perception* of another's tone of voice or facial expression. Even at the "sensory end organ" level visual processing may be impaired by prenatal alcohol. Drs. Stomland and Hellstrom found problems at the level of the retina in a study of 25 children who have FASD. Half had visual impairment; acuity was drastically impaired (less than 20/100) in 10 out of 50 eyes! Half had a reduction in the number of neurons in the optic nerve (optic nerve hypoplasia) and half had an increase in the number of blood vessels in the retina (increased tortuosity of retinal arteries). Half had eye movement difficulties (strabismus). [61]

The *fusiform gyrus* allows identification of another's face. [62] Anecdotally, I have seen art therapy examples where patients with FAS draw "all the members of their family" or "all the members of their class" *very similarly*. Whether this is due to fusiform gyrus issues or expressive difficulties with impaired drawing skills might be speculative - but these art therapy pictures suggest visual discrimination difficulties from some source.

The *superior temporal sulcus* perceives intension in another's behaviour - is she coming to talk with me or does she just want to walk past me? The *amygdala* helps you understand if the other person is friendly, welcoming and trustworthy - or not. The *anterior temporal pole* helps place observed behaviour into a predictable script for a given situation - we are at a class party so that girl walking up to me probably wants to talk versus we are on a rush-hour train platform in Toronto so that girl probably *does not* want to talk.

Mirror neurons are activated by direct observation or imagining another's actions, sensations or emotions. Mirror neurons are found in the *prefrontal cortex, superior temporal sulcus, somatosensory cortex and parietal cortex*. Observation of pain or disgust in another person also activates affect processing in the *anterior cingulate cortex and anterior insula;* this affective processing is the *basis* for *empathy*. Yet empathy is more than just "resonating" with emotions in another; observed emotions must be processed and thought about - this work is done in the *medial prefrontal cortex and anterior cingulate*. To be able to understand "my take on what you think of your situation" (i.e., to "walk in your shoes") requires me to temporarily set aside my own perspective and focus on what is going on in your mind - this mentalizing work involves the anterior cingulate and medial prefrontal cortex. [63]

Recent neuroimaging studies reveal that, compared to controls, individuals exposed to prenatal alcohol demonstrate: [64]

1. Specific reduction in size of the parietal lobe even after controlling for reduced overall brain volume.
2. Reduced white/grey matter ratio especially in the occipital-temporal region
3. Reduced white matter integrity (as demonstrated by altered fractional anisotropy on Diffusion Tensor Imaging [DTI] MRI scans) of the cingulate, right temporal lobes, and occipital-temporal myelinated tracts (that are important for efficient visual processing)
4. Magnetic resonance spectroscopy (MRS) findings of lower levels of choline compounds in frontal and parietal lobes (suggesting impaired white matter function in those areas) and abnormalities in creatine/phosocreatine in the anterior cingulate, parietal cortex and frontal cortex (suggesting abnormal glial function in those areas)

5. Positron Emission Tomography (PET) data indicating altered cerebral blood flow in the temporal lobe.

6. Single photon emission computed tomography (SPECT) data indicating altered serotonin metabolism in the medial frontal cortex (that study authors suggest may be linked with impulsivity and aggression) and altered dopamine transporter activity in the basal ganglia (that may be associated with attentional deficits)

7. Functional MRI (fMRI) data show abnormalities in function of the insula and fronto-parietal networks during spatial memory tasks; abnormal activation patterns of the left inferior parietal lobe and bilateral posterior temporal lobes in a verbal working memory task; reduced activation of medial and posterior temporal lobes (which correlates with reduced encoding) in a verbal learning task; increased activation of the occipital-temporal region (indicating subjects had "to work harder to accomplish the task") in a sustained attention task; and increased activation of the prefrontal cortex in a test of inhibition which suggests the prefrontal area had to "work harder" to make up for inefficient frontal-striatal networks.

These data from neuroimagining indicates that functions of many structures humans rely on for learning and interpersonal affiliation are harmed by prenatal alcohol. However, caregivers and children with FASD cannot engage in defeatism if they are to remain as healthy as possible. The quest is to find ways of developing optimally *in spite* of these brain differences.

Environmental influences on FASD

Social information processing was impaired in a group of alcohol-exposed children but improved following teaching of social skills. [65] Children born to *older* alcohol using mothers were more likely to have impaired attention. Maternal *binging* is the pattern of drinking that most severely impairs the ability to pay attention in alcohol-exposed children. [66] In a study of 452 children the density of alcohol problems in first and second-degree relatives *were associated with* poor inhibitory control, attention problems and conduct problems (defiance, aggression, delinquency). Parental warmth, consistency and monitoring reduced all these adverse behaviours. Poverty and maternal mental health issues increased the children's disinhibition, attention and conduct problems. [67]

Calgary-based clinical social worker Liz Lawryk says that prenatal alcohol can damage so many different body and brain areas at so many different stages of gestation that generalizations about specific patterns of impaired function are impossible - but 100% of the people with FASD she works with have one crippling problem: *low self-esteem*. Resilience against further wounding experiences is very limited. Efficacy - being successful at some chosen goal is a powerful factor of resilience - through coaching and mentoring young adults (see the interview with Myles Himmelreich on my website: http://fasdrelationships.ca) in areas of their interest progress can be achieved.

Gifts/interests /relative strengths

Brain injury rehabilitation researcher Dr. Mark Ylvasaker says: "*There is something that I say a lot in rehabilitation - In the absence of meaningful engagement in chosen life activities, all interventions will ultimately fail.*" [5]

Dr. Ylvasaker's comments prompt the need to know what the gifts/interests and relative strengths of each patient are, because by working in those areas optimal progress can be achieved. Dr. Kieran O'Malley and educator Francis Kapp suggest common gifts/strengths in those with FASD often include: 1) High energy, exuberance; 2) Talents at making up stories and improvising; 3) Artistic in drama, visual art, dance, and music; 4) Relating well to and a "heart" for animals or people who are younger, older or ill. [68]

Caregiver's/parent's stress and its effect on child outcome

Parental stress increases with increasing levels of child internalizing and externalizing behaviour, and decreases in child executive function and adaptive function. [69] Provision of a stable, supportive home environment is a powerful protective factor against children developing secondary disabilities such as trouble with the law, school dropout or mental health problems. [69] Epigenetics may underlie one mechanism of how nurturing home environments reduce adverse child outcomes...Michael Meany explained, "Attentive parenting can influence prenatal alcohol-mediated damage to the glucocorticoid receptors," at the recent UBC conference on: Brain Development and Learning. [70]

Unmet caregiver needs, and addressing these needs

Olson, et al. report a list of *important unmet needs* that caregivers have identified. [69] I recently facilitated Dr. Gordon Neufeld's *Vital Connection* DVD attachment-parenting course to several groups of caregivers. Topics reviewed in the course included aggression, "counterwill" (i.e. "talking back"), crisis management, reestablishing broken attachments, dealing with competing attachments (e.g. to peers), and stages of attachment. Facilitation consisted of answering participant questions about content and explaining relevant FASD brain biology differences to consider when implementing Dr. Neufeld's concepts with their children.

Parents reported significant improvements on several of the *Unmet needs* identified by Olson, et al. including improved ability to understand their child's thoughts and behaviours, a sense of being able to cope with behaviours, an ability to have realistic expectations about their child's thoughts and behaviours, and an improved sense of confidence after completing the course. [71] This psychoeducational initiative was patterned after Dr. George Singer's successful education-based parent support groups for caregivers of children affected by traumatic brain injury (TBI). [72] (TBI has a similar pattern of impairment [externalizing/ internalizing/ executive and adaptive function issues] to FASD.) [72]

Dr. Olson's review [69] also describes recent work by George Singer emphasizing improvements in *parental self-efficacy* as a goal of support interventions. To avoid depletion and burnout, parents must feel they are effective and are able to make a positive difference for their kids. I believe understanding behaviour at a brain level can lead parents to effective strategies and interventions so Chapter One - *FASD 101* - of this book contains numerous descriptions of the brain biology underlying various behavious.

Quantifying caregiver distress

Two prominent researchers in caregiver stress, Drs. Olsen and Paley, assess it using the Parenting Stress Index (PSI) tool. [69] I developed a simple questionnaire based on Dr. Betsy Robinson's (Alzheimer Disease) Caregiver Strain Questionnaire. [73] Dr. Robinson suggested a score of seven or more ("yes" answers) placed the caregiver at increased risk of developing physical illness. Anecdotally, nearly three hundred caregivers of children with FASD have an average score of ten "yes" answers. I present the adapted caregiver strain questionnaire not because it is a standardized research instrument but as a guide for clinicians wanting some ideas of relevant questions to ask when assessing the extent of caregiver distress. I suspect that clinicians may be surprised by the degree of caregiver exhaustion they discover.

Caregiver Strain Questionnaire

Answer each of the twelve questions, answered "yes" or "no"

1. Is sleep disturbed because the person you care for is in and out of bed or wanders around at night?
2. Is it inconvenient for you because helping the person you care for takes so much time?
3. Is it a physical strain because so much effort and concentration is required in looking after the person you care for?
4. Is it confining because looking after the person you care for causes such restriction of free time?
5. Have there been family adjustments because of lack of privacy or because helping the person you care for has disrupted routines?
6. Has looking after the person you care for been a reason why there were changes of personal plans such as not being able to go on a vacation, having to turn down a job, etc.?
7. Has looking after the person you care for placed other demands on your time such as attending to additional concerns of other family members?
8. Has some of the behaviour of the person you care for been upsetting - for example "taking" things, self-harm or addictions ?
9. Have there been emotional adjustments, for instance because of severe arguments?
10. Have there been work adjustments, for instance having to take time off work?
11. Has looking after the person you care for caused financial strain?
12. Have you felt completely overwhelmed because of worry about the person you care for, or how you will manage or worry about the future?

"Yes" score - is it 7 or more out of 12?

____ /12

Genetic factors

Is there a genome-wide family genetic linkage study for FASD?

Not yet, concludes Dr. Albert Chudley in his recent review. [74] But Chudley describes work of Lomabard, et al. [75] that suggests (by pooling animal and human FASD study data) *specific genes affecting three critical biologic pathways* are likely to influence the risk of developing FASD. Interested readers are again encouraged to review Dr. Chudley's chapter [74] for more details. I will briefly discuss the three biologic pathways here.

Prenatal alcohol appears to interfere with *transforming growth factor-beta* regulation of neuronal migration, growth of cerebral cortex cells, growth of axons, cell adhesion (alcohol *decreases* neuronal growth and migration but *increases* cell adhesion), neuronal apoptosis (alcohol increases apoptosis; apoptosis is controlled cell death) and regulation of the immune system. Clinically, I have observed the sequellae of immune dysregulation in several patients with FASD - I understand this is anecdotal evidence, but cannot help wanting to know why breast and other cancers, multiple sclerosis, and frequent infections seem to be relatively common issues *for patients in their twenties and thirties*. Abnormal neuronal migration, cortex development and reduced axonal growth (i.e. widespread reduction of white matter myelinated tracts) are demonstrated convincingly in recent neuroimaging studies of individuals with FASD. [76]

A second critical signaling pathway affected by prenatal alcohol is the *mitogen-activated protein kinase (MAPK) system. When alcohol dysregulates this system*, changes in cell growth and migration can occur. Recently, using a mouse model of FAS, alcohol-induced impairment of cerebellar cell migration *was reversed* using caffeine to increase calcium ion secondary messenger activity and agents to increase cyclic GMP activity and decrease cyclic AMP activity. [77] Hopefully, this, and similar work will lead to strategies that could reduce prenatal alcohol's damage.

The third biologic system likely to be involved in FASD is called the *Hedgehog signaling pathway.* Alcohol reduces activity of key signaling components of the Hedgehog system (such as the Shh molecule). If Shh molecule levels are restored experimentally, alcohol-induced craniofacial anomalies are reduced because apoptosis of neural crest cells is reduced. [75]

Heritability of components of FASD's behavioural phenotype

Clinically, traits often seen in those affected by FASD include increased impulsivity, emotional lability, increased risk-taking, externalizing behaviour, substance use and sensitivity to unanticipated touch or loud sounds. Many of these traits are highly heritable.

Sensory Processing

Traits of auditory and tactile defensiveness were found to have moderate genetic influences and be associated with an anxious, fearful temperament in a study of 394 toddler-aged twins. [78]

Alcoholism

The National Institute on Alcohol Abuse and Alcoholism in the USA has funded the Collaborative Studies on the Genetics of Alcoholism (COGA) since 1989, with the goal of identifying the specific genes underlying this vulnerability. Alcohol use disorders have a 50-60% heritability. Joel Gelernter suggested, as of 2009, that about half the genes that increase risk of developing drinking problems had been identified. [79]

Genes for the GABA A receptor, especially **GABRA2** increase the risk of alcoholism. These "high risk" GABA A receptor genes include many single nucleotide polymorphisms (SNPs) on chromosome 11 (the 3' end of the gene not the 5' end) which are more common in relatives of alcoholics. **GABRA2** acts to increase the risk of severe drug dependence outcomes *not* by being an area of the genome where altered amino acid sequences cause abnormal proteins to be synthesized. Instead, GABRA2 changes *how promoters and splicing variants work.* **GABRA2** is seen in populations with more profound addiction issues; individuals with the phenotype associated with GABRA2 have drug as well as alcohol dependence, a lower age of onset of heavy drinking, a higher number of maximum drinks per episode of drinking (i.e. larger binges) and more profound withdrawal symptoms. People with **GABRA2** are also more likely to have co-morbid antisocial personality disorder, conduct disorder, major depressive disorder and "novelty seeking" traits. [79] **GABRA2** increases the risk of alcoholism by 20% *but increases the chance of not being married by 120%* (compared to "control" populations that do not have this gene). [79] Study of such extreme phenotypes might not help us understand addictions in the majority because different genes might play a more influential role for those who drink more moderately.

If individuals carry the **A1** allele of the dopamine 2 receptor gene **(DRD2)** the chance of them learning to *avoid the negative consequences of withdrawal* are reduced. The *active* genes for this effect (of "not getting" the connection between alcohol withdrawal and one's monumental headache) might be **DRD2 A1** allele's *close neighbor* genes: **ANKK1, TTC12, NCAM1**. [80]

ANKK1 influences **TTC12** to change risk of heavy drinking. Also, both **ANKK1** and **TTC12** influence the risk of nicotine dependence. [81]

CRHR1 encodes for the corticotropin releasing hormone receptor 1 and there are two SNPs of this gene: rs242928 and rs1876831 that are associated with *binge drinking in adolescents* and *alcohol dependence* in adults [80]

hTAS2R16 gene on chromosome 7 encodes the "bitter" taste receptor. If this gene is expressed there is *less sensitivity to bitter taste*, a higher number of maximum drinks per 24 hrs and increased alcohol dependence. [81]

Dr. Marc Schuckit's concept of "Low Level of Response" to alcohol ("it takes a lot to get you tipsy") is an important predictor of risk of alcoholism for all ages and both sexes. [82] There are many "candidate" genes associated with reduced level of response. [82]

Gene by Environment Interaction

One gene can affect several different types of mental health issues. Different forms (called the short ["s"] allele and the *long* ["l"] allele) of the promoter part of the serotonin transporter gene **(5-HTT)** predispose to different mental health outcomes *in the presence of stressful or negative life events.* One or 2 copies of the short ("s") allele of 5-HTT not only increase the incidence and severity of depression, but also decrease the treatment responsiveness of depression. If a patient has one or 2 short alleles of this **5-HTT** polymorphism he/she is at increased risk of developing Major Depression or Post Traumatic Stress Disorder (PTSD) *if exposed to stressful life events.* This increased risk is compounded if the patient has *low levels of social support.* [83]

Furthermore, *various age* groups with the short allele show different adverse effects - for instance, college students exposed to negative life events show increased drinking and drug use. Maltreated small children with at least one s allele started drinking alcohol at an earlier age and at an increased amount compared to their peers. [84]

Mary Schneider and her team at the University of Wisconsin-Madison have performed some elegant studies with these same gene polymorphisms (l and s alleles of the serotonin transporter) in monkeys. If a monkey neonate carried the short allele of this **5-HTT** gene *and if that baby's mother was exposed to alcohol during her pregnancy* the baby was much more likely to show irritability, and increased activation of his/her HPA stress axis when stressed compared with controls that were not exposed to alcohol or those with long ("l") alleles *even if those* (with the long alleles) *were exposed to prenatal alcohol*. [83] In other words, the s allele conferred increased risk (of developing the behavioural phenotype of fussiness, difficulty in feeding, resistance to soothing) to offspring of monkeys who (prenatally) consumed moderate amounts of alcohol. *This s allele is common, with prevalence rates depending on racial ancestry of the sample group. (25% [African] to 80% [Asian])*

Monkey babies from Mary Schneider's lab *that carried the s allele* of 5-HTT *and were exposed to prenatal alcohol* displayed behaviour very similar to what is described as "Regulation Disorders of Sensory Processing". [85] Irish Pediatric Psychiatrist, Kieran O'Malley says, "Infants and young children with FASD commonly demonstrate Regulation Disorders of Sensory Processing which are characterized by difficulties in tolerating environmental stimuli, coordinating basic motor movements or in approaching and interacting with others in their immediate environment." The difficulties alcohol-exposed babies have with feeding, irritability, sleep dysregulation and fussiness could be consistent with "Type A: Hypersensitive Regulation Disorders of Sensory Processing (Fearful/ Cautious subtype)". [86]

I do not know of human studies to assess the prevalence of the s allele of 5-HTT in infants that fit the diagnostic criteria for Regulation Disorder of Sensory Processing who have been exposed to alcohol prenatally. Mary Schneider's studies predict fussiness, feeding difficulties, impaired self-regulation and trouble settling for sleep; caregiving for children with this phenotype would be very trying. If parents were single, isolated, depressed, prone to substance abuse, suffering from PTSD, living in poverty, or lacking support from other family members then trying to care for such a difficult-to-settle infant could be an overwhelming "perfect storm" of stress. This combination of factors could increase the risk of Shaken Baby Syndrome. [87]

Fathers' Roles

Animal studies have shown offspring of alcohol exposed *fathers* to have a lowered birth weight, hyperactivity, lowered cognitive ability, reduced length, lower serum testosterone, smaller seminal vesicles, lower beta endorphin levels in the hypothalamus, more malformations, smaller eye globe size, increased incidence of microcephalus, more problems with muscle coordination and a higher likelihood of hydronephrosis. This list of findings is similar to what physicians find when they diagnose quite severely affected children with FASD. Philip Haycock, working with the Department of Public Health and Primary Care, Strangeways Research Laboratory, University of Cambridge, thinks that the mechanism of these changes is "likely to involve alcohol-induced epigenetic changes" and that "environmentally acquired epigenetic states *(will be transmitted) between generations* in animals and humans." [88]

Recent work by Lillian Ouko and her group at The Division of Human Genetics, University of the Witwatersrand, Johannesburg, South Africa shows how alcohol influences sperm by epigenetic changes to DNA methylation patterns - and that such changes are likely to be passed on to the next generation. [89]

Resiliency factors?

Dr. Astley questioned why 9.3% of the 1400 children assessed thus far in her study do *not* have measurable deficits in spite of being exposed to alcohol prenatally. What identifies these resilient individuals? Did they have less exposure to alcohol than their peers who were diagnosed as having an FASD? No. They were more likely *female*. They were more likely to be *younger* and less likely to be affected by adverse postnatal events such as multiple placements, sexual or physical abuse, chaotic, unpredictable homes, etc. Though not measured as deficient, "blunting" will have occurred i.e. loss of genetic potential. [6] Susan Astley said no genetic studies have yet been done on this relatively resilient group; I wonder whether they might have the "two long" (ll) alleles of the serotonin transporter gene (as opposed to long/short [ls], or short/short [ss]) Please see reference [83] for more details about serotonin transporter genes.

References

[1] Astley SJ. 2006. Comparison of the 4-Digit Diagnostic Code and the Hoyme diagnostic Guidelines for Fetal Alcohol Spectrum Disorders. Pediatrics 118(4): 1532-1545

[2] Astley SJ. 2004. Diagnostic Guide for Fetal Alcohol Spectrum Disorders:

The 4-Digit Diagnostic Code, Third Edition. Seattle, Washington: Center on Human Development and Disability, School of Public Health and Community Medicine, University of Washington

[3] The part of DSM-5 website devoted to Conditions Proposed by Outside Sources: http://www.dsm5.org/ProposedRevisions/Pages/ConditionsProposedbyOutsideSources.aspx

[4] Chudley AE, Conry J, Cook JL, et al. 2005. Fetal alcohol spectrum disorder: Canadian guidelines for diagnosis. Canadian Medical Association Journal 172 (5 suppl). Doi:1503/cmaj.1040302 (can be viewed online at: http://www.cmaj.ca/cgi/content/full/172/5_suppl/S1)

[5] Durgin C, Dillon B. (spokespersons for the International Brain Injury Association) 2007. On Neurorehabilitation: a conversation with Mark Ylvisaker, PhD. (can be viewed online at: http://www.internationalbrain.org/?q=node/71)

[6] Astley SJ. 2010. Profiles of 1400 patients evaluated for FASD at the WA FAS DPN by interdisciplinary teams using the 4-digit code. Presented at: 11th Annual Fetal Alcohol Canadian Expertise (FACE) Research Roundtable. Sept 14, 2010 (available webcast at: http://www.motherisk.org/FAR/index.jsp)

[7] Bell S, Stade BS, Reynolds JN, et al. 2010. The remarkably high prevalence of epilepsy in subjects with FASD. Alcoholism: Clinical and Experimental Research 34: 1-6

[8] Armstrong MA, Kskutas LA, Witbrodt J, et al. 2009. Using drink size to talk about drinking during pregnancy: a randomized clinical trial of Early start Plus. Social Work Health Care 48(1): 90-103

[9] Sampson PD, Streissguth AP, Bookstein FL, et al. 1997. Incidence of fetal alcohol syndrome and prevalence of alcohol-related neurodevelopmental disorder. Teratology, 56: 317–326. doi: 10.1002/(SICI)1096-9926(199711)56:5<317::AID-TERA5>3.0.CO;2-

[10] May PA, Brooke L, GossageJP, et al. 2000. Epidemiology of fetal alcohol syndrome in a South African community in the Western Cape Province. American Journal of Public Health 90: 1905-1912

[11] May PA, Gossage JP, Marais AS, et al. 2007. The epidemiology of fetal alcohol syndrome and partial fetal alcohol syndrome in a South African community. Drug Alcohol Depend 88: 259-271

[12] Robinson GC, Conry JL, Conry RF. 1987. Clinical profile and prevalence of Fetal Alcohol Syndrome in an isolated community in B.C. Canadian Medical Association Journal 137: 203-207

[13] May PA, Fiorentino D, Gossage JP, et al. 2006. Epidemiology of FASD in a province in Italy: prevalence and characteristics of children in a random sample of schools. Alcoholism: Clinical and Experimental Research 30(9): 1562-1575

[14] May PA, Gossage JP, Kalberg WO, et al. 2009. Prevalence and epidemiologic characteristics of FASD from various research methods with an emphasis on recent in-school studies. Developmental Disabilities Research Reviews 15: 176-192

[15] MacPherson P, Chudley AE. 2007. FASD in a correctional population: preliminary results from an incidence study. Presented at 2007 Fetal Alcohol Canadian Expertise (FACE) Research Roundtable 2007 (Available webcast at: http://www.knowledgenetwork.ca/fasvi/webcast/index.html)

[16] Fast DK, Conry J, Loock CA, et al. (1999) Identifying fetal alcohol syndrome among youth in the Criminal Justice System. Journal of Developmental and Behavioral Pediatrics 20(5): 370-372

[17] Campbell DB. 2010. Gene-environment interactions in Autism risk. (Conference presentation) Session IL07, Canadian Psychiatric Association 60th Annual Conference. Toronto. Sept. 25, 2010.

[18] Chudley AE. 2010. Personal communication

[19] Astley SJ, Bailey D, Talbot C, et al. 2000. Fetal alcohol syndrome (FAS) primary prevention through FAS diagnosis: I. Identification of high-risk birth mothers through the diagnosis of their children. Alcohol Alcoholism 35 (5): 499-508

[20] Malleson R. 2010. Contraception: What do Women Want? (Conference Presentation) 45th Annual Post Graduate Review in Family Medicine, University of British Columbia. Vancouver, March 4, 2010.

[21] Fryer SL, Mc Gee CL, Matt GE, et al. (2007) Evaluation of psychopathological conditions in children with heavy prenatal alcohol exposure. Pediatrics 119(3): e733-e741

[22] Bell S, Stade BS, Reynolds JN, et al. 2010. The remarkably high prevalence of epilepsy in subjects with FASD. Alcoholism: Clinical and Experimental Research 34: 1-6

[23] Sutarjono B, Florez C, Brien JF, et al. Hippocampal excitability in young postnatal guinea pig following prenatal alcohol exposure. Unpublished preliminary result discussed in conference presentation: Carlen PL, 2010. Fetal ethanol exposure and postnatal brain hyperexcitability: "The tip of the neurobehavioural iceberg". 11th Annual Fetal Alcohol Canadian Expertise Research Roundtable (FACE) Sept 14, 2010 (available webcast at: http://www.motherisk.org/FAR/index.jsp)

[24] Down J. 2009. Personal communication.

[25] Franklin L, Deitz J, Jirikowic T, et al. 2008. Children with fetal alcohol spectrum disorders: problem behaviors and sensory processing. American Journal of Occupational Therapy 62: 265-273

[26] Polanco TA, Crismale-Gann C, Reuhl KR, et al. 2010. Fetal Alcohol Exposure Increases Mammary Tumor Susceptibility and Alters Tumor Phenotype in Rats. Alcoholism: Clinical and Experimental Research, no. doi: 10.1111/j.1530-0277.2010.01276.x

[27] Bonilla FA. 2010. The adaptive cellular immune response. UpToDate Desktop 18.2 Medical Reference DVD.

[28] Babu DK, Diaz A, Samikkannu T, et al. 2009. Upregulation of Serotonin Transporter by Alcohol in Human Dendritic Cells: Possible Implication in Neuroimmune Deregulation. Alcoholism: Clinical and Experimental Research, 33: 1731–1738. doi: 10.1111/j.1530-0277.2009.01010.x

[29] Warren KR, Foudin LL. 2001. Alcohol-Related Birth Defects, the Past, Present and Future. National Institute on Alcohol Abuse and Alcoholism. Retrieved Oct 14, 2010 from: http://pubs.niaaa.nih.gov/publications/arh25-3/153-158.htm

[30] Dlugos CA, Rabin RA. 2010. Structural and Functional Effects of Developmental Exposure to Ethanol on the Zebrafish Heart. Alcoholism: Clinical and Experimental Research, 34: 1013–1021. doi: 10.1111/j.1530-0277.2010.01176.x

[31] Neural Crest: Retrieved from Wikipedia October 14, 2010 as: http://en.wikipedia.org/wiki/Neural_crest

[32] Streissguth AP, Barr HM, Kogan J, et al. 1996. Understanding the Occurrence of Secondary Disabilities in Clients with Fetal Alcohol Syndrome (FAS) and Fetal Alcohol Effects (FAE), Final Report, August 1996, to the Centers for Disease Control and Prevention (CDC), Seattle: University of Washington, Fetal Alcohol and Drug Unit, Tech. Rep. No. 96-06

[33] Streissguth AP, Bookstein FL, Barr HM, et al. 2004. Risk factors for adverse life outcomes in fetal alcohol syndrome and fetal alcohol effects. Developmental Behavioral Pediatrics 25: 228-238

[34] Kvigne VL, Leonardson GR, Borzelleca, J, et al. 2009. Characteristics of Children Whose Siblings Have Fetal Alcohol Syndrome or Incomplete Fetal Alcohol Syndrome. Pediatrics 123(3): e526-e533 (doi:10.1542/peds.2008-2423)

[35] Uban KA, Bodnar T, Butts K, et al. 2010. Direct and indirect mechanisms for alcohol teratogenesis: implications for understanding alterations in brain and behaviour in FASD. In: Riley EP, Clarren S, Weinberg J, et al. Editors. Fetal Alcohol Spectrum Disorder: Management and Policy Perspectives of FASD, First Edition. Weinheim, Germany: Wiley-VCH Verlag GmbH & Co. KGaA. doi: 10.1002/9783527632510.ch6. pp 73-108.

[36] Zhou FC, West JR, Blake CA, et al. (2005) General discussion at the Fetal Alcohol Syndrome Symposium. Experimental Biology and Medicine 230: 407-412

[37] Zhou FC, Sari Y, Powrozek TA. 2005. Fetal alcohol exposure reduces serotonin innervation and compromises development of the forebrain along the serotinergic pathway. Alcoholism: Clinical and Experimental Research 29(1): 141-149

[38] Gundogan F, Elwood G, Mark P, et al. 2010. Ethanol-Induced Oxidative Stress and Mitochondrial Dysfunction in Rat Placenta: Relevance to Pregnancy Loss. Alcoholism: Clinical and Experimental Research, 34: 415–423. doi: 10.1111/j.1530-0277.2009.01106.x

[39] Kumar A, Singh CK, DiPette DD, et al. 2010. Ethanol Impairs Activation of Retinoic Acid Receptors in Cerebellar Granule Cells in a Rodent Model of Fetal Alcohol Spectrum Disorders. Alcoholism: Clinical and Experimental Research, 34: 928–937. doi: 10.1111/j.1530-0277.2010.01166.x

[40] Weinberg J. 2007. Prenatal alcohol exposure in an animal model: fetal programming and implications for vulnerability in adulthood. (Keynote Address) 8th Annual Fetal Alcohol Canadian Expertise (FACE) 2007 Meeting. (available webcast at: http://www.motherisk.org/fas6/webcast/index.html)

[41] Zhao H, Mayhan WG, Arrick DM, et al. 2010. Alcohol-Induced Exacerbation of Ischemic Brain Injury: Role of NAD(P) H Oxidase. Alcoholism: Clinical and Experimental Research, no. doi: 10.1111/j.1530-0277.2010.01284.x

[42] Coles CD, Lynch ME, Kable JA, et al. 2010. Verbal and Nonverbal Memory in Adults Prenatally Exposed to Alcohol. Alcoholism: Clinical and Experimental Research, 34: 897–906. doi: 10.1111/j.1530-0277.2010.01162.x

[43] Riley EP, Barron S, Driscoll CD, et al. 1984. Taste aversion learning in preweaning rats exposed to alcohol prenatally. Teratology 29: 325–331 doi: 10.1002/tera.1420290303

[44] Eide B, Eide F. 2010. Common Learning Challenges in Sensory Processing Disorder. (Conference presentation) at: Sensory Processing Disorder Foundation 11th International Symposium and Pre-Conference Institute. Bellevue, Washington. November 12, 2010.

[45] Carr JL, Agnihotri S, Keightley M. 2010. Sensory Processing and Adaptive Behavior Deficits of Children Across the Fetal Alcohol Spectrum Disorder Continuum. Alcoholism: Clinical and Experimental Research 34: 1022–1032. doi: 10.1111/j.1530-0277.2010.01177.x

[46] Spadoni AD, McGee CL, Fryer SL, et al. 2007. Neuroimaging and Fetal Alcohol Spectrum Disorders. Neuroscience and Neurobehavioral Review 31: 239-245

[47] Lebel C, Rasmussen C, Wyper K, et al. 2010. Brain microstructure is related to math ability in children with fetal alcohol spectrum disorder. Alcoholism: Clinical and Experimental Research, 34: 354–363. doi: 10.1111/j.1530-0277.2009.01097.x

[48] Meintjes EM, Jacobson JL, Molteno CD, et al. 2010. An fMRI Study of Number Processing in Children With Fetal Alcohol Syndrome. Alcoholism: Clinical and Experimental Research, 34: 1450–1464. doi: 10.1111/j.1530-0277.2010.01230.x

[49] Mattson SN, Roesch SC, Fagerlund Å, et al. 2010. Toward a Neurobehavioral Profile of Fetal Alcohol Spectrum Disorders. Alcoholism: Clinical and Experimental Research, 34: 1640–1650. doi: 10.1111/j.1530-0277.2010.01250.x

[50] Fryer SL, Tapert SF, Mattson SN, et al. 2007. Prenatal Alcohol Exposure Affects Frontal–Striatal BOLD Response During Inhibitory Control. Alcoholism: Clinical and Experimental Research, 31: 1415–1424. doi: 10.1111/j.1530-0277.2007.00443.x

[51] McGee CL, Schonfeld AM, Roebuck-Spencer TM, et al. 2008. Children With Heavy Prenatal Alcohol Exposure Demonstrate Deficits on Multiple Measures of Concept Formation. Alcoholism: Clinical and Experimental Research, 32: 1388–1397. doi: 10.1111/j.1530-0277.2008.00707.x

[52] Miller LJ. 2009. Personal communication.

[53] Roebuck TM, Simmons RW, Mattson SN, et al. 1998. Prenatal Exposure to Alcohol Affects the Ability to Maintain Postural Balance. Alcoholism: Clinical and Experimental Research, 22: 252–258. doi: 10.1111/j.1530-0277.1998.tb03646.x

[54] Archibald SL, Fennema-Notestine C, Gamst A, et al. 2001. Brain dysmorphology in individuals with severe prenatal alcohol exposure. Developmental Medicine & Child Neurology, 43: 148–154. doi: 10.1111/j.1469-8749.2001.tb00179.x

[55] Lebel C, Rasmussen C, Wyper K, et al. 2008. Brain diffusion abnormalities in children with fetal alcohol spectrum disorder. Alcoholism: Clinical and Experimental Research 32: 1732-1740

[56] Sakata-Haga H, Dominguez HD, Sei H, et al. 2006. Alterations in Circadian Rhythm Phase Shifting Ability in Rats Following Ethanol Exposure During the Third Trimester Brain Growth Spurt. Alcoholism: Clinical and Experimental Research, 30: 899–907. doi: 10.1111/j.1530-0277.2006.00105.x

[57] Jan JE, Asante KO, Conry JL, et al. 2010. Sleep health issues for children with FASD: Clinical considerations. International Journal of Pediatrics. Published online July 14, 2010. Accessed at: http://www.ncbi.nlm.nih.gov/pmc/articles/PMC2913852/November 28, 2010.

[58] Rasmussen C, Wyper K, Talwar V. 2009. The Relation between Theory of Mind and Executive Functions in Children with Fetal Alcohol Spectrum Disorders. Canadian Journal of Clinical Pharmacology 16(2): e370-e380

[59] Allen JG, Fonagy P, Bateman AW. 2008. Mentalizing in Clinical Practice. Washington, DC. American Psychiatric Publishing, Inc. pp 3-4.

[60] Allen JG, et al. 2008. p 9.

[61] Stromland K, Hellstrom A. 1996. Fetal Alcohol Syndrome- an opthalmological and socioeducational prospective study. Pediatrics 97(6): 845-849

[62] Allen JG, et al. 2008. p 118.

[63] Allen JG, et al. 2008. (adapted from pp 117-130.)

[64] Norman AL, Crocker N, Mattson SN, et al. 2009. Neuroimaging and Fetal alcohol Spectrum disorders. Developmental Disabilities Research Reviews 15: 209-217

[65] Keil V, Paley B, Frankel F, et al. 2010. Impact of a Social Skills Intervention on the Hostile Attributions of Children With Prenatal Alcohol Exposure. Alcoholism: Clinical and Experimental Research, 34: 231–241. doi: 10.1111/j.1530-0277.2009.01086.x

[66] Chiodo LM, Da Costa DE, Hannigan JH, et al. 2010. The Impact of Maternal Age on the Effects of Prenatal Alcohol Exposure on Attention. Alcoholism: Clinical and Experimental Research, 34: 1813–1821. doi: 10.1111/j.1530-0277.2010.01269.x

[67] Molina BSG, Donovan JE, Belendiuk KA. 2010. Familial Loading for Alcoholism and Offspring Behavior: Mediating and Moderating Influences. Alcoholism: Clinical and Experimental Research, no. doi: 10.1111/j.1530-0277.2010.01287.x

[68] Kapp ME, O'Malley K. 2001. Watch for the Rainbows; True Stories for Educators and Other Caregivers of Children With Fetal Alcohol Spectrum Disorders. Calgary, Alberta: Frances Kapp Education.

[69] Olson HC, Oti R, Gelo J, Beck S. 2009. "Family Matters:" Fetal Alcohol Spectrum Disorder and the Family. Developmental Disabilities Research Reviews 15 (3): 235-249

[70] Meaney M. 2010. Maternal Care and Gene-environment Interactions Defining Development. Third biennial UBC conference on: Brain Development and Learning: Making Sense of the Science. Vancouver, BC. July 16-20, 2010.

[71] Densmore RJ. 2010. Restoring hope: an adapted attachment parenting DVD series empowers caregivers of children who have FASD. Poster presentation at: 2010 Fetal Alcohol Canadian Expertise (FACE) Research Roundtable. Abstract published: Journal of Population Therapeutics and Clinical Pharmacology 17(2): e284-e301; August 12, 2010. Also viewable at: http://www.cjcp.ca/pubmed.php?articleId=273 p e291.

[72] Singer GHS, Glang A, Williams JM. 1996. Children with Acquired Brain Injury: Educating and Supporting Families. Baltimore: Paul H. Brookes Publishing. p 239.

[73] Robinson B. 1983. Caregiver Strain Index. Journal of Gerontology 38: 344-348

[74] Chudley AE. 2010. Genetic Factors Contributing to FASD. In: Fetal Alcohol Spectrum Disorder: Management and Policy Perspectives of FASD, First Edition. Riley EP, Clarren S, Weinberg J, Jonsson E, editors. Weinheim, Germany: Wiley-VCH Verlag GmbH & Co. KGaA. doi: 10.1002/9783527632510.ch6. pp 109-126.

[75] Lombard Z, Tiffin N, Hofmann O, et al. 2007. Computational selection and prioritization of candidate genes for Fetal Alcohol Syndrome. BMC Genomics 8, 389, http://www.biomedcentral.com/1471-2164/8/389.

[76] Norman AL, Crocker N, Mattson SN, et al. 2009. Neuroimaging and Fetal Alcohol Spectrum Disorders. Developmental Disabilities Research Reviews 15: 209-217

[77] Kamanda T, Lakshmana MK, Komoro H. 2006. Reversal of neuronal migration in a mouse model of fetal alcohol syndrome by controlling second-messenger signalings. Journal of Neuroscience 26: 742-756

[78] Goldsmith HH, Van Hulle CH, Arnesa CL, et al. 2006. A population-based twin study of parentally reported tactile and auditory defensiveness in young children. Journal of Abnormal Child Psychology 34(3): 378-392

[79] Gelernter J. 2009. Symposium 70: Genetic Vulnerabilities for Drug Use and Co-morbid Mental Health Disorders: Approaching Co-morbidity in Addiction Genetics (conference presentation) American Psychiatric Association Annual Meeting, San Francisco. May 16-21, 2009.

[80] Gelernter J, Kranzler HR. 2009. Genetics of alcohol dependence. Human Genetics 126: 91-99

[81] LeStrat Y, Ramoz N, Schuman G, et al. 2008. Molecular Genetics of Alcohol Dependence and Related Endotypes. Current Genomics(9): 444-457

[82] Schuckit MA. 2009. Adolf Meyer Award Lecture. How Alcoholism Develops: Identification of Genetic and Environmental Influences in a 25-year Longitudinal Study. American Psychiatric Association Meeting. San Francisco. May 16-21, 2009.

[83] Kraemer GW, Moore CF, Newman TK, et al. 2008. Moderate level fetal alcohol exposure and serotonin transporter gene promoter polymorphism affect neonatal temperament and limbic-hypothalamic-pituitary-adrenal axis regulation in monkeys. Biological Psychiatry 63: 317-324

[84] Gelernter J, Kanzler HR. 2008. Genetics of Addiction. In: Textbook of Substance Abuse Treatment, 4th edition. Galanter M, Kleber HD, editors. Washington (USA): American Psychiatric Publishing Inc. pp 17-27.

[85] ZERO TO THREE. 2005. Diagnostic Classification of Mental Health and Developmental disorders of Infancy and Early childhood: Revised Edition (DC:0-3R). Washington, DC: ZERO TO THREE Press.

[86] O'Malley KD. 2007. Fetal Alcohol Spectrum Disorders: An Overview. In: O'Malley KD, editor. ADHD and Fetal Alcohol Spectrum Disorders (FASD). New York: Nova Science Publishing Inc. pp 1-24.

[87] Barr RG , Trent RB, Cross J. 2006. Age-related incidence curve of hospitalized Shaken Baby Syndrome cases: convergent evidence for crying as a trigger to shaking. Child Abuse and Neglect 30(1): 7-16 see also: http://www.PURPLECrying.info/

[88] Haycock PC. 2009. Fetal Alcohol Spectrum Disorders: The Epigenetic Perspective. Biology of Reproduction published 27 May 2009; 10.1095/biolreprod.108.074690

[89] Ouko LA, Shantikumar K, Knezovich J, et al. 2009. Effect of alcohol consumption on CpG Methylation in the differentially methylated regions of H19 and IG-DMR in male gametes- implications for Fetal Alcohol Spectrum Disorders. Alcoholism: Clinical and Experimental Research 33(9): 1-13

Appendix: Helpful Websites

This book's website: http://www.fasdrelationships.ca

Dr. Bruce Perry's ChildTrauma Academy website: http://www.childtrauma.org/

Dr. Lucy Miller and Dr. Sarah Schoen's Sensory Processing Disorder website: www.spdfoundation.net/

Dr. Jane Koomar's Sensory Processing Disorder websites: http://www.thespiralfoundation.org/, http://www.otawatertown.com/

Dr. Norman Doige's website for his book: The Brain That Changes Itself (a review of recent studies on neuroplasticity): http://www.normandoidge.com

The (Psychiatric) Diagnostic and Statistical Manual (5th edition) webpage for conditions not yet in the DSM that are proposed for the upcoming (2013) edition: http://www.dsm5.org/ProposedRevisions/Pages/ConditionsProposedbyOutsideSources.aspx

An excellent support programme for high-risk parents (in Vancouver) is Sheway—their website: http://www.vch.ca/media/sheway_brochure.pdf

A similar programme in Seattle is the parent child assistance program (P-CAP): http://depts.washington.edu/chdd/ucedd/ctu_5/parentchildprog_5.html

Family study, NIAAA: This public website discusses ongoing genetic research by National Institute on Alcohol Abuse and Alcoholism: http://pubs.niaaa.nih.gov/publications/arh26-3/214-218.htm

Dr. Daniel Amen's (neuroimaging psychiatric diagnostic clinic) website: http://www.amenclinics.com/

An inspiring theatre company wherein disabled actors work alongside professional actors and directors as equals to produce live theatre: www.chickenshed.org.uk

Developmental optometry websites: http://www.childrensvision.com/OD.htm or http://www.insightlearning.ca/ or http://www.covd.org/

Drs. Fernette and Brock Eide's website regarding learning disabilities: http://www.dyslexicadvantage.com/

Dr. Gordon Neufeld's website on attachment-centered parenting (includes links for purchase of his DVD courses and on line courses: http://www.gordonneufeld.com/

The Canadian ADHD Resource Alliance (CADDRA) sponsors a comprehensive, up to date website on ADHD: http://www.caddra.ca/cms4/

The abstract for poster 6 (Restoring hope: an adapted attachment parenting DVD series empowers caregivers of children who have FASD) can be viewed on page e291 of the Journal of Therapeutics and Clinical Pharmacology (on on line journal incorporating Fetal Alcohol Spectrum Disorder Research). This journal's website: http://www.cjcp.ca/pubmed.php?articleId=273

Diane Malbin's Fetal Alcohol Syndrome Consultation, Education and Training Services, Inc. (FASCETS) website is: www.fascets.org.

A conversation with Mark Ylvisaker, Ph.D., on cognitive rehabilitation for children with brain injuries can be viewed at the International Brain Injury Association website: www.internationalbrain.org/?q=node/71

Tanya Helton's Forest Cottage Centre Inc. offers counseling and support and resources for parents and professionals dealing with attachment problems affecting children in their care; her website is: www.forestcottagecentre.com/

Harvard's Benson-Henry Institute for Mind Body Medicine is a research and resource centre for preventative strategies regarding stress; their website: http://www.mgh.harvard.edu/bhi/

The National Center on Shaken Baby Syndrome maintains a very informative website of user-friendly parent support strategies: www.dontshake.com

West Coast Alternative School (a Vancouver school offering adapted programmes for students with FASD) website:

http://www.vsb.bc.ca/programs/west-coast-alternate-program

FASD Connections is a comprehensive FASD research and resources website run by Jan Lutke, Tina Anterobus and colleaugues: http://www.fasdconnections.ca/

The Washington State FASD clinic website features extensive resources for parents and professionals: Fetal Alcohol Syndrome Diagnostic and Prevention Network (FAS DPN): http://depts.washington.edu/fasdpn/

Toronto Sick Children's Hospital sponsors Motherisk which offers telephone advice to mothers about risks and avoidance of potential harmful substances in pregnancy. Motherisk also maintains an extensive library of resources for professionals and patients on FASD and related topics; the FASD section of their website is: http://www.motherisk.org/FAR/index.jsp

Motherisk's home page is: http://www.motherisk.org/women/index.jsp

Dr. Lisa Najavits is a posttraumatic stress disorder (PTSD) expert and her manualized treatment called Seeking Safety has excellent evidence of effectiveness: www.seekingsafety.org

Interapy is a Netherlands-based online treatment strategy for mental health issues including PTSD: www.interapy.nl

Dr. Alfred Lange's specific PTSD Interapy is discussed at this link: http://alfredlange.interapy.nl/publications/pdf/CBT2003.pdf

Bruce Ritchie, in partnership with St. Michael's Hospital in Toronto runs a comprehensive online database and discussion forum called FASlink; the website: http://www.faslink.org/index.htm

NOFAS is an international organization linking policy makers, parents and professionals. In the USA, their spokeperson is Kathleen Mitchell and their website is: http://www.nofas.org/default.aspx

In the UK, NOFAS's coordinator is Susan Fleisher and their website links to extensive resources for parents and professionals including Fetal Alcohol Forum, an online journal of FASD research. NOFAS-UK's website: http://www.nofas-uk.org/index.htm

Iceberg is an online newsletter about FASD prepared by a parent/professional partnership in Washington State. I do not know of a better source of reliable practical information for parents. Unfortunately, due to funding cuts, the newsletter will not be publishing new editions but their archive is available at: http://www.fasiceberg.org/newsletter.htm

Acknowledgements

I acknowledge, with great appreciation, the incredible kindness of busy clinicians, care providers and researchers who took time to respond generously to my requests and queries. This book is much deeper and more meaningful because of their advice and encouragement. Special thanks go to:

Mark Ylvisaker for his advice about similarities between FASD and Traumatic Brain Injuries

Mary Schneider for her guidance about serotonin receptors and FASD

Kieran O'Malley for his numerous clinical management insights and his emphasis on working within areas of strength

David Pauls for his advice on how to approach research for the Genetics and FASD chapter

Gilles Julien for his encouragement and sharing his family's visionary work called Social Pediatrics about how to optimally support vulnerable children

Michael Meaney for critiquing my proposals for the book

Heather Charmichael Olson for ongoing encouragement of my work with families and suggested refinements of this book

Christine Loock for compassionate care of my family and heartening encouragement of my FASD work

Lucy Miller, Sarah Schoen, Meryle Lehn, Kim Barthell, Diana Henry, and my wife, Shannon, for their training and guidance about sensory problems

Gordon Neufeld for creating training opportunities and for his passion about preserving attachments and empowering caregivers

Martin Bohus from Mannheim, Germany for his insights into brainstem regulation of the amygdala in extreme stress—and the use of his slides

Bruce Perry for his insights about the sequence of neural development and how we can help positively influence development even when kids have had early trauma, neglect, and/or prenatal exposure to alcohol or other teratogens

Myles Himmelreich for his interview—it was a pleasure to work with this young man who has FASD. He inspired me.

Darren Sass for introducing me to the world of developmental optometry

C. Robert Cloninger for introducing me to his concepts of transcendence of mental illness and explaining how patients with developmental disabilities can rise above adversity

Audrey McFarlane and her diagnostic clinic group at Lakeland FASD Center, Cold Lake, Alberta for insisting kids must emerge from their FASD assessment more positive about themselves than before they began, and parents must have less to do after the assessment than before. These attitudes promote patient engagement, caregiver resiliency and clinic staff empathy with the families

Val and Don Massey for their encouragement, wise clinical pearls and delightful sense of humour

Catherine Lebel and her neuroimaging group from the University of Alberta for granting me permission to use their diffusion tensor MRI image of impaired visual processing

Johathan Down for his excellent clinical ideas and indomitable inquisitive energy

Henry Sundquist for his wise counsel in how to plan support and housing strategies

Mark Waage and Donna DeBolt for guidance on how teens with legal troubles can be dealt with effectively

James Jan and Osman Ipsiroglu for their insights on sleep problems in FASD

Nathan Ory for his vivid metaphors and lucid explanations on how to effectively support struggling caregivers and their kids

Linda Fountain from the Social Work and Disabilities Studies Dept. at Mount Royal University, Calgary for her ongoing commitment to acquainting her social work students to FASD

Dan Dubovsky for advice about how to talk to psychiatrists regarding FASD, for his inspiring heart for his son, and for coining the NURMU acronym

Lori Vitale Cox for the DVD of her inspiring community development work in the Maritimes

Renata Johnson, Krystal Oleson, Dawn Grunert, Alison Gaul, Henry Sundquist, Kassie, Leesa and John, Grace Gerry, Ron Jorgenson, Larry Keats, Mary Culshaw and Jonathan Down or their valuable contributions to: Chapter Six: Insights from FASD Stakeholders

My work colleagues at the Kamloops Downtown Health Center, Urban Native Health Clinic, and Armstrong Vision Center for their support as I researched this book, referrals and encouragement of my clinical work

In British Columbia, I serve on a provincial committee overseeing FASD projects. The passion of this group inspires me. I have learned so much from them. I'd like to thank Jan Lutke, Ron Jorgenson, Bobby Boyd, Pat Richardson, Anne Guarasci and past committee members for their ideas, encouragement and support of our family's journey with FASD.

Personal friends have also been incredibly supportive of this project. Sincere thanks go to:

Greg Sczebel for permission to use his song, This is Worth Fighting For, as the musical introduction to the video called: Interview with Myles Himmelreich contained in this book

Patricia Vickers for sharing her First Nations' perspectives on healing from trauma

Several families caring for children that have FASD (that I won't name here to protect their confidentiality) for incredible generosity in sharing poignant personal stories

Brian, Kathy and Paul Robinson for welcoming me during lengthy training sessions

Hanna and Steve Philbert for posing for the book cover

Les Ellenor for great ideas about book set up and proofreading

Steve Goyeche and Ann Seymour for great ideas and helping me get to a number of courses in Toronto

Kitty Bottemiller for inspiring me to write

Susan Fleischer for introducing me to her wonderful parents' group and for publishing some of my materials in NOFAS-UK newsletters

Wally and Liz Cowlard for inspiring me to write and for wise counsel regarding how to approach delays, setbacks and roadblocks encountered over four years of book development

Uncle Roger for putting me up once a week thus supporting my out of town work that has financed this project

Dan and Melody Helm for wise ideas and moral support

I appreciate those who have helped with production /distribution issues including:

Lewis Levin, at L. and L. Production Group, Calgary for his superb video editing—and taking me to the coolest bagel bakery in Calgary

Friesens Corporation for friendly, knowledgeable, and high quality printing

Mareike Klem at The Urban Think Tank for formatting

Natalie Ingram, Fiona Vandergucht and Iris Shewchuk and for proofreading

Suzanne Anderson at Self Publishing in Canada for her encouragement and suggestions on formatting

Ron Marchand the Video Man for video production

Polar Bear Production Ltd. for manufacturing the DVD

Pat Anderson from the "Minga Marketplace" resource centre for FASD at The Asante' Centre for Fetal Alcohol Syndrome for representing my book on a consignment basis

Barb McFadyen-Smuin from the "Mustard Seed Bookstore" for representing my book on a consignment basis

And, as anyone who has written a book knows –it's a family affair! Without the patience, forbearance and support of my family I'd still be researching Chapter One. My daughter Julia, a graduate of Kootenay School of the Arts, has designed the book cover and website. She has also provided some delightful illustrations and single-handedly talked me out of resigning each time Microsoft Word auto-formatting decided to auto-destruct my documents.

Index

A

B

C

D

G

H

I

L

M

N

O

P

Q

R

S

T

V

Y

How to obtain extra copies

This book is available from:

The "Mustard Seed Bookstore"

Contact: Barb McFadyen-Smuin at:

Naramata Centre, Box 68
3375 - 3rd St
Naramata, BC Canada V0H 1N0

Toll Free: 1-877-996-5751 ext. 212
(Alberta & BC)

Phone: 250-496-5751 ext. 212
Fax: 250-496-5800
Email: mustardseed@naramatacentre.net
Web Store: www.naramatacentre.net

The "Minga Marketplace" Resource Centre for FASD at The Asante' Centre for Fetal Alcohol Syndrome (on a consignment basis)

Contact: Pat Anderson at:

The Asante Centre for Fetal
Alcohol Syndrome
#103-22356 McIntosh Avenue
Maple Ridge, BC V2X 3C1
Phone: 604-467-7101
Fax: 604-467-7102
Email: pandersen@asantecentre.org
Website: www.asantecentre.org

Your Notes: